# Current Clinical Oncology

Maurie Markman, MD
Series Editor

More information about this series at http://www.springer.com/series/7631

Antonio Giordano • Marcella Macaluso
Editors

# Gynecological Cancers

## Genetic and Epigenetic Targets and Drug Development

Springer

*Editors*
Antonio Giordano, MD, PhD
Department of Biology
Temple University
Philadelphia, PA, USA

Marcella Macaluso, PhD
Department of Biology
Temple University
Philadelphia, PA, USA

Current Clinical Oncology
ISBN 978-3-319-32905-5 ISBN 978-3-319-32907-9 (eBook)
DOI 10.1007/978-3-319-32907-9

Library of Congress Control Number: 2016943122



Printed on acid-free paper

This Springer imprint is published by Springer Nature
The registered company is Springer International Publishing AG Switzerland

*The Editors, on behalf of all the contributors to this book, dedicate this work to all the women who are fighting with gynecologic cancers and to those involved in the research, prevention, treatment, and care of these diseases.*

# Preface

Over the years, the prevention and treatment of gynecologic cancers has improved as the result of strong multidisciplinary efforts, which allows for early detection of the disease and improved intervention strategies. In this book we have gathered all the molecular and cellular aspects of gynecological cancers together within one volume and provided a comprehensive resource of information on drug discovery and drug development for the treatment of these diseases.

The reader will find an overview of the genetic and epigenetic mechanisms underlying the formation and progression of gynecological cancers as well as detailed, up-to-date information on the etiology, diagnosis, and treatment of these diseases, which include ovarian cancer, uterine cancer, cervical cancer, vaginal cancer, and vulvar cancer. Fertility preservation and available options were also included in the book. In addition, emphasis was placed in providing the public with information on the racial/ethnic disparities in the treatment of gynecological cancers.

Philadelphia, PA, USA

Antonio Giordano
Marcella Macaluso

# Contents

# Contributors

**Robert E. Bristow, MD, MBA** Department of Obstetrics and Gynecology, Division of Gynecologic Oncology, University of California at Irvine, Orange, CA, USA

**Jennifer L. Brown, MD** Division of Gynecologic Oncology, Fox Chase Cancer Center, Philadelphia, PA, USA

**Cristina di Cesare, MD** Division Of Gynecologic Oncology, Agostino Gemelli Hospital, Catholic University of Sacred Heart, Largo Agostino Gemelli, Rome, Italy

**Christina S. Chu, MD** Division of Gynecologic Oncology, Fox Chase Cancer Center, Philadelphia, PA, USA

**Giuseppina D'Andrilli, PhD** Department of Biology, College of Science and Technology, Temple University, Philadelphia, PA, USA

**Selina Davis, MD** Department of Obstetrics and Gynecology, Albert Einstein Medical Center, Philadelphia, PA, USA

**Gavino Faa, MD** Dipartimento di Scienze Chirurgiche, Faculty of Medicine, Istituto di Anatomia Patologica, University Hospital San Giovanni di Dio, University of Cagliari, Cagliari, Italy

**Daniela Fanni, MD, PhD** Dipartimento di Scienze Chirurgiche, Faculty of Medicine, Istituto di Anatomia Patologica, University Hospital San Giovanni di Dio, University of Cagliari, Cagliari, Italy

**Clara Gerosa, MD** Dipartimento di Scienze Chirurgiche, Faculty of Medicine, Istituto di Anatomia Patologica, University Hospital San Giovanni di Dio, University of Cagliari, Cagliari, Italy

**Fong W. Liu, MD, MPH** Division of Gyncologic Oncology, Department of Obstetrics and Gynecology, Beth Israel Deaconess Medical Center, Harvard Medical School, Boston, MA, USA

**Valeria Masciullo, MD, PhD** Division of Gynecologic Oncology, Agostino Gemelli Hospital, Catholic University of Sacred Heart, Rome, Italy

**Ida Paris, MD** Division of Gynecologic Oncology, Agostino Gemelli Hospital, Catholic University of Sacred Heart, Largo Agostino Gemelli, Rome, Italy

**Roberto Piccoli, MD** Department of Gynecology, Outpatient Clinic Center "Piccoli", Naples, Italy

**Giuseppina Pichiri, BSc** Dipartimento di Scienze Chirurgiche, Faculty of Medicine, Istituto di Anatomia Patologica, University Hospital San Giovanni di Dio, University of Cagliari, Cagliari, Italy

**Nicoletta De Rosa, MD** Department of Gynecology, Outpatient Clinic Center "Piccoli", Naples, Italy

**Ang Sun, PhD** Fels Institute of Cancer Research and Molecular Biology, School of Medicine, Temple University, Philadelphia, PA, USA

**Janos L. Tanyi, MD, PhD** Division of Gynecologic Oncology, Department of Obstetrics and Gynecology, University of Pennsylvania Health System, Philadelphia, PA, USA

**Ana I. Tergas, MD, MPH** Division of Gynecologic Oncology, Department of Obstetrics and Gynecology, Columbia University Medical Center, New York, NY, USA

# Part I

# Epigenetic Mechanisms in Gynecological Cancers

# Epigenetic Mechanisms in Gynecological Cancer

1

Gavino Faa, Daniela Fanni, Giuseppina Pichiri, and Clara Gerosa

**Abstract**

The disruption of epigenetic regulatory mechanisms has been demonstrated to represent the prevalent carcinogenetic actor in cancer, aberrant epigenetic silencing of tumor suppressor genes, mainly due to DNA methylation, representing a relevant mechanism able of modifying the expression of key genes during carcinogenesis. In addition, epigenetic regulation has included microRNAs that regulate gene expression leading to inhibition and/or degradation of RNA target. In recent years, epigenetic silencing has been indicated as one of the major causes of gynecological cancer, being able to inactivate multiple pathways including cell cycle control, DNA repair, and apoptosis. In this chapter, the most important environmental factors interfering with the DNA methylation status in mammalian cells, leading to the insurgence of gynecological tumors will be discussed, including the dietary habits that have been indicated as main actors of DNA methylation. The role of epigenetics in the insurgence of ovarian cancer, endometrial cancer, cervical cancer, and endocervical cancer will be discussed. Finally, the role of microbioma in gynecological cancer insurgence and progression will be discussed. Here, a modern view of the relationship between genetics and epigenetics in gynecological cancer is presented. According to this view, genetics might be seen as a piano, a long one with a keyboard of 25,000 keys each one representing one human gene, whereas epigenetics could be represented by the piano tuner and by the pianist. The epigenetic approach is based on changing the pianist, i.e. the hyper- or hypomethylation status of target genes appears much more promising for the therapy of gynecological cancer than the previous ones based on modifying the piano, i.e. the genetic changes accumulating in tumor cells.

G. Faa, MD (✉) • D. Fanni • G. Pichiri • C. Gerosa
Dipartimento di Scienze Chirurgiche, Faculty of Medicine, Istituto di Anatomia Patologica, University Hospital San Giovanni di Dio, University of Cagliari, Via Ospedale N. 56, Cagliari 09124, Italy
e-mail: gavinofaa@gmail.com





A. Giordano, M. Macaluso (eds.), *Gynecological Cancers*, Current Clinical Oncology,
DOI 10.1007/978-3-319-32907-9_1

**Keywords**
Epigenetics • Ovarian cancer • Endometrial cancer • Cervical cancer • Gynecological cancer • Microbioma • DNA methylation • DNA demethylation • Histone methylation/demethylation • Histone acethylation/deacethylation • Histone phosphorelation/dephosphorelation

## Introduction

The term "epigenetics" originates from the acquisition that classical genetics cannot completely explain the diversity of phenotypes within a population, and includes the heritable changes in gene expression that are not due to any alteration in the DNA sequence [1]. Epigenetic factors, and in particular DNA methylation, regulate gene expression, starting from the early phases of human development, the individual methylation pattern being established at the time of implantation. The disruption of epigenetic regulatory mechanisms has been demonstrated to represent the prevalent carcinogenetic actor in cancer [2] (Fig. 1.1). During development, methylation of selected areas of gene promoters might act in a specific pattern, inhibiting differentiation and favoring the maintenance of stemness [3]. The hypothesis that epigenetic alterations might play a significant role in tumor insurgence and progression goes back to the early years of this century, when aberrant epigenetic silencing of tumor suppressor genes, mainly due to DNA methylation, was proposed as a relevant mechanism able of modifying the expression of key genes during carcinogenesis [4]. Further studies evidenced the complexity of the molecular mechanisms through which environment and lifestyle may interfere and regulate gene expression [5]. Nowadays, the most important epigenetic changes may be classified as the following: (a) DNA

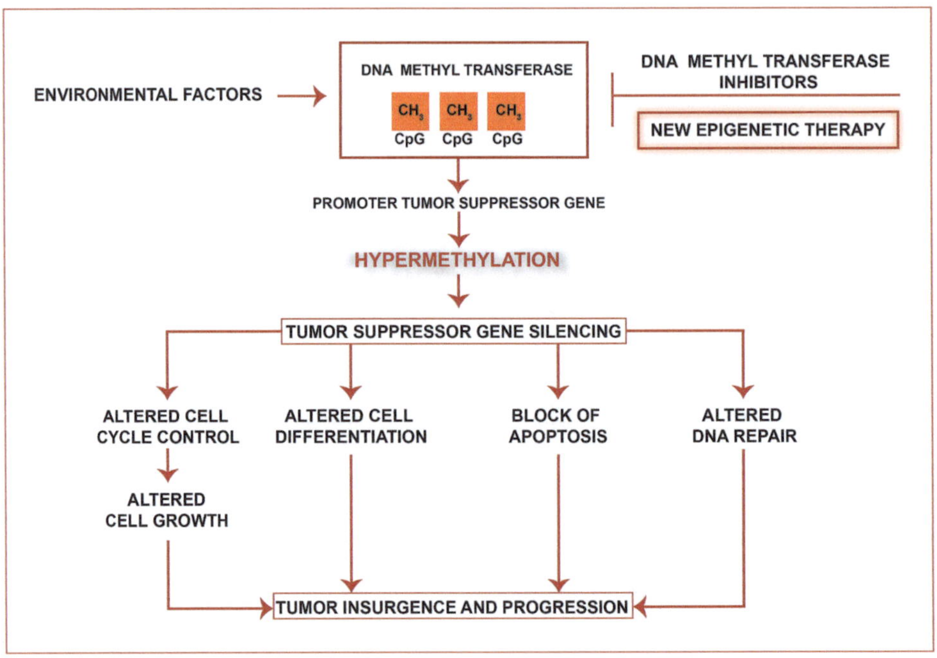


**Fig. 1.1** Epigenetic silencing of tumor suppressor genes

**Fig. 1.2** The most important epigenetic changes in human carcinogenesis

**THE MOST IMPORTANT EPIGENETIC CHANGES IN HUMAN CARCINOGENESIS:**

- DNA HYDROXYMETHYLATION
- DNA METHYLATION
- POLYCOMBS GROUP PROTEINS
- HISTONE ACETHYLATION
- DNA DEMETHYLATION
- LONG NON-CODING RNA METHYLATION
- HISTONE DEACETHYLATION
- HISTONE METHYLATION
- MICRO RNA METHYLATION
- HISTONE DEMETHYLATION

methylation/demethylation [6]; (b) histone methylation/demethylation [7]; (c) histone acethylation/deacethylation [8]; (d) histone phosphorelation/dephosphorelation (Fig. 1.2).

Recently, DNA hydroxymethylation and post-translational modifications (PTMs) of histone proteins affecting nucleosome remodeling have been added to the list of epigenetic mechanisms able to cause aberrant DNA methylation patterns involved in human carcinogenesis [9]. Other epigenetic modifications, including deamination in DNA, ADP ribosylation, and ubiquitylation/sumoylation in histones have been reported in several tumors, including endometrial cancer [10]. In addition, epigenetic regulation has included microRNAs that regulate gene expression leading to inhibition and/or degradation of RNA target [10]. The growing evidence on a major role played by epigenetic dysregulation of microRNAs in cancer insurgence and progression is at the basis of many studies aimed at targeting microRNAs for cancer therapy [11]. Moreover, growing evidence indicates a major role in cancer insurgence for long non-coding ribonucleic acids (LncRNAs), and in particular to their different promoter methylation patterns, aberrant methylation of LncRNAs being involved in cancer development and progression [12]. LncRNAs are involved in multiple biological and pathological processes, including regulations of epigenetics, and their expression patterns in gynecological tumors differ from those of normal tissues and benign tumors, indicating their possible utilization as early diagnostic biomarkers and ideal therapeutic targets in gynecological cancers [13].

In mammalian cells, DNA methylation/demethylation represents the best-known and one of the most popular epigenetic modifications. The development in recent years of new methods for the detection of DNA methylation, including the methylation-specific multiplex ligation-dependent probe amplification (MS-MLPA) [14], the Mass ARRAY mutation method [15], and the MethylCap-Seq analysis [16] facilitated researchers involved in the analysis of the methylation status of tumors originating in several organs, including gynecological cancers [17]. Thanks to these new techniques, the pivotal role of DNA methylation in regulation of gene expression has been highlighted, hypermethylation being able to inactivate and silencing several tumor-suppressor genes and microRNA genes [18, 19]. DNA methylation is catalyzed by DNA methyltransferases (DNMTs), and the regulation of their expression and activity is considered a crucial point in gene expression in mammalian cells [20]. DNMTs consist of three members, DNMT1, DNMT3A, and DNMT3B [21]. DNMT1 catalyzes the methylation of the 5′ cytosine in the CpG islands, whereas DNMT3A and 3B are essential for de novo methylation and for mammalian development [22]. DNA hypermethylation mainly occurs in the promoter region and, in particular, in cytosines preceding guanines (CpGs) [17, 23] (Fig. 1.1). CpGs are frequently found in the 5′ end of the regulatory region of many genes, and are normally not methylated in normal human cells, their methylation representing one of the most important mechanism for the regulation of gene expression in the human genome [24]. DNA methylation occurs in a complex chromatin network and is influenced by peculiar changes in the histone structure, histone modifications representing a risk factor for recurrence in human cancer [25]. The hypothesis that epigenetic changes might play a fundamental role in gene expression, leading to modifications of the checkpoint machinery and to cancer insurgence, is at the basis of the project aimed at defining the human epigenome [26, 27]. The collection of a large series of DNA methylation patterns in human cancers has lead to the definition of MethHC, a database of DNA methylation and gene expression in human cancer. The vast majority of epigenetic events described in gynecological cancers may be found in MethHC (http://MethHC.mbc.notu.edu.tw), including a systematic large collection of DNA methylation data and mRNA/microRNA expression profiles in human cancer [28].

Another epigenetic mechanism able to induce gene silencing has been identified in polycomb group proteins, which are responsible for reversibly repress genes required for differentiation [29]. According to the hypothesis of stem cell origin of cancer, hypermethylation of cancer specific porters in stem cells might transform reversible gene repression into permanent silencing, inducing stem cells in a perpetual state of self-renewal, thereby favoring clonal expansion and malignant transformation [30].

Epigenetic silencing has been indicated by several authors as one of the major causes of gynecological cancer, being able to inactivate multiple pathways including cell cycle control, DNA repair, and apoptosis. Moreover, differential methylation profiles have been revealed in endometrial, cervical, and ovarian cancers, suggesting the existence of different epigenetics-driven molecular pathways among these neoplasms [31]. According to a modern view on pathogenesis of human carcinogenesis, cancer genetics and epigenetics should not be considered as two separate mechanisms, but as two sides of the same coin [32]. Recently, different epigenetic modifiers have been hypothesized to act on the transcription factor NKX6.1 that functions in physiology as a suppressor of epithelial–mesenchymal transition. Hypermethylation and downregulation of the NKH6.1 gene have been detected in several cancers, being associated with the metastatic potential of tumor cells, making this epigenetic change the target for novel therapeutic options in oncology [33].

Regarding the environmental factors interfering with the DNA methylation status in mammalian cells, in health and disease, dietary habits have been indicated in recent years as main actors of DNA methylation (Fig. 1.3). Dietary factors might influence DNA methylation in several ways: (a) modulating the supply of methyl groups for the formation of S-adenosylmethionine; (b) modifying the activity of methyltransferases; (c) regulating the demethylation activity [34]. Multiple food components have been shown to interfere on DNA methylation, including vitamin B6, B12, methionine, folate, and choline [35]. Recently, other dietary components have been indicated as putative conditioners of the DNA methylation status, including alcohol, phytoestrogen, plophenols, and flavonoids in green tea, lycopene [36]. Stress and smoking have also been proposed among the epigenetic factors able to interfere with DNA methylation [37]. Other epigenetic factors have been identified in pollutants altering the endocrine

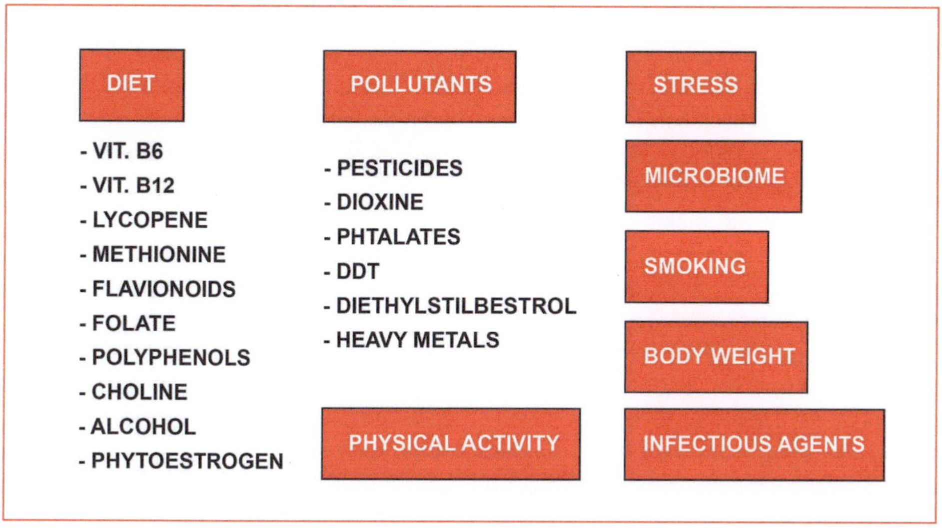


**Fig. 1.3** Environmental factors interfering with DNA methylation

system, also known as endocrine disruptors, which have been hypothesized to have epigenetic adverse effects on the health of future generations. The endocrine disruptors indicated to have a role in human carcinogenesis, and in particular in gynecological cancer insurgence and progression, are pesticides, dioxin, phthalates, DDT, diethylstilbestrol, and heavy metals [38]. In recent years, a new hypothesis has been proposed regarding the influence of a wrong feeding pattern and a modified lifestyle on cancer risk. According to this hypothesis, diet and lifestyle might induce epigenetic changes in human gene expression by inducing changes in the composition of the gut microbiome [39]. A modified microbial community in our gastrointestinal tract has been shown to affect cancer susceptibility, not restricted to gastrointestinal carcinogenesis, but with consequences even in distant organs [40].

## Epigenetic Mechanisms in Endometrial Cancer

The first studies on the epigenetic gene silencing profile of endometrial cancer evidenced the occurrence of hypermethylated alleles in tumor cells, suggesting the existence of aberrant methylation in the vast majority of endometrial tumors. In the first studies aimed at discovering the epigenetically masked tumor suppressor genes in endometrial carcinoma, a hypermethylation status was reported in the progesterone receptor (PR) and estrogen receptor (ER) genes [41]. A specific methylation profile was evidenced in the vast majority of endometrial cancers, characterized by hypermethylation of APC and p16, occasionally associated with aberrant methylation of CASP8, p73, hMLH1, and CDH13 [31]. These preliminary data lead to hypothesize the use of epigenetic markers for a better classification of endometrial cancer, allowing a new sartorial approach to cancer management based on the epigenetic profile of each endometrial tumor. Conflicting results on the target genes of hypermethylation in endometrial cancer were reported by further studies aimed at identifying epigenetic abnormalities specific of endometrial carcinogenesis. Three genes showed significant percentages of hypermethylation, including hMLH1 (40 %), E-cadherin (34 %), and APC (34 %), whereas no aberrant methylation was found in p16 [42]. hMLH1 promoter hypermethylation and silencing was confirmed as a typical epigenetic marker of primary endometrial cancer, in association with histone modifications [43] or with DNA hypermethylation of the CDKN2A/p16 gene [44]. The application of the epigenetic reactivation screening strategy, that combines treatment in vitro of cancer cells with DNA methyltransferase inhibitors and microarray analyses, allowed the identification of new tumor suppressor genes repressed in endometrial cancer, reinforcing the hypothesis of a major role of epigenetic silencing in endometrial carcinogenesis [45]. A further step in the knowledge of the relevance of epigenetic hypermethylation in endometrial cancer is represented by the attempts to introduce methylation inhibitors as anticancer agents. The demonstration that aberrant hypermethylation of the CHFR gene in endometrial carcinoma is correlated with sensitivity of tumor cells to microtubule inhibitors allowed to hypothesize a new therapeutic approach based on the identification of hypermethylated tumor suppressor genes, which could guide a tailored anticancer therapy based on control of methylation [46]. Among the multiple epigenetic factors contributing to abnormal DNA methylation in the setting of endometrial cancer insurgence, recent studies underlined the role of dietary/lifestyle and environmental factors, which might play a relevant role in modifying dynamically gene expression in many cancer types, including endometrial cancer [47]. A study aimed at verifying the presence inside endometrial malignant tumors of tumor cells expressing CD133, a stem cell marker for tumor initiating cells in solid tumors, revealed hypomethylation of the CD133 promoter in malignant endometrial cells relative to benign control [48]. These findings supported the hypothesis that CD133 expression might be epigenetically regulated in endometrial carcinoma, hypomethylation of the CD133 promoter being associated with tumor enrichment of CD133+ tumor cells, influencing tumor aggressivity, recurrences, and prognosis. Downregulation of the Wnt antagonist through epigenetic silencing has been proposed as one of the most relevant mechanisms responsible for deregulation of the Wnt/Beta-catenin signaling pathway in endometrial carcinogenesis [49]. Aberrant DNA hypermethylation in endometrial cancer cells has been indicated as a principal epigenetic mechanism involved in breakdown of the mismatch repair mechanism frequently observed in the development of endometrial cancer, with changes in the expression of the hMLH1 gene playing a particularly relevant role [50]. Moreover, hypermethylation has been proposed as the main responsible mechanism for dysregulation of gene expression by microRNA in tumor cells that frequently underlies the carcinogenetic mechanisms of endometrial cancer [51]. Given that, in endometrial carcinogenesis, tumor-suppressor microRNAs and oncogenic microRNAs are associated with epigenetic dysfunction, they have been hypothesized to have a key role in the therapy of endometrial cancer [52]. Epigenetic inactivation of the epidermal growth factor-containing fibulin-like extracellular matrix protein 1 (EFEMP1) tumor suppressor gene has been identified as a key factor in endometrial carcinogenesis (Fig. 1.4). The altered methylation status, i.e. hypermethylation of the EFEMP1 promoter, was found to be the responsible for downregulation of the EFEMP1 protein with loss of its tumor suppressive function and of its ability to block decreased secretion of metalloproteinases, ending with endometrial cancer insurgence and progression [53]. A possible relevant role for epigenetics in the therapy of endometrial adenocarcinoma was demonstrated in the same study: treatment of tumor xenografts with 5-aza-2′-deoxycytidine and with trichostatin A, two drugs able to restore the physiological methylation status, restored EFEMP1 protein expression in tumor cells, followed by inhibition of tumor cell proliferation, inhibition of tumor growth, decrease in metalloproteinase secretion, and inhibition of invasion. These data clearly indicate EFEMP1 as a candidate tumor suppressor gene in endometrial adenocarcinoma, promoter hypermethylation as the main mechanism responsible for the gene silencing, and suggest target therapy by demethylating agents as the future therapy in endometrial cancer. In further studies on the methylation status of tumor cells in endometrial carcinoma, aberrant CpG methylation was detected in the promoter region of two tumor suppressor genes, GSTP1 and RASSF1A, this epigenetic event being correlated with higher tumor grade, deeper myometrial invasion, and metastasis of pelvic lymph nodes [54]. In the same study, higher percentages

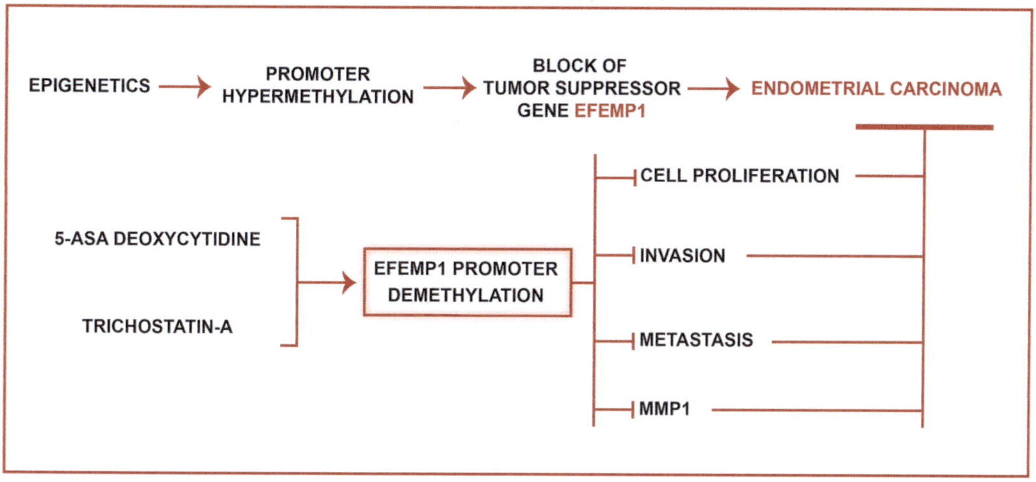


**Fig. 1.4** Epigenetic inactivation of EFEMP1 is associated with tumor suppressive function in endometrial carcinoma

of abnormal methylation were also found in endometrial complex hyperplasia when compared to the healthy endometrium, suggesting a major role for epigenetics also in the early phases of endometrial carcinogenesis, in the progression from complex or atypical endometrial hyperplasia to endometrial carcinoma.

A study based on a novel integrative epigenome–transcriptome–interactome analysis revealed that HAND2, a typical tumor suppressor gene, represents the hub of the most highly ranked differential methylation hotspots in endometrial cancer, HAND2 hypermethylation being paralleled by a decrease in RNA and protein levels [17]. Moreover, increased HAND2 methylation was detected as a typical feature of complex atypical endometrial hyperplasia, suggesting the hypothesis that HAND2 methylation analysis of endometrial secretions from women with postmenopausal bleeding might be utilized as a biomarker for early detection of endometrial cancer. Among women with endometrial hyperplasia, high levels of HAND2 methylation were associated with a low response to progesterone treatment, indicating this epigenetic marker as a predictor of treatment response in endometrial precancerous lesions. All these data taken together, the potential clinical usefulness of HAND2 methylation analysis emerges: it might be applied to triage women with postmenopausal bleeding as an epigenetic test to early diagnosis of endometrial cancer and to predict response to treatment. A methylation analysis in endometrioid carcinoma evidenced significantly higher methylation of the promoter CpG islands of CDH13, WT1, and GATA5 genes. Hypermethylation of the GATA5 gene was also shown to be associated with a poor prognosis, its epigenetic silencing characterizing the poorly differentiated endometrioid carcinomas [55]. A hypermethylation status has been detected in the gene encoding for a microRNA, miR-196b, its epigenetic silencing causing the absence of its regulatory function on c-myc and Bcl-2 expression [56]. PTEN, a critical tumor suppressor gene regulating the PI3K-AKT pathway, has been found to be repressed in endometrial carcinogenesis not only for mutations and deletion, but even through epigenetically silencing by promoter hypermethylation [57]. The hypothesis of a relevant role of epigenetics on PTEN silencing in endometrial cancer has been confirmed by a recent study, showing that Piwil7, a member of the Piwi family, could promote the loss of function of the tumor suppressor gene PTEN by increasing hypermethylation of its promoter through upregulation of DNA methyltransferase 1 (DMT1) [58].

Promoter hypermethylation patterns have been reported, in recent years, in other tumor

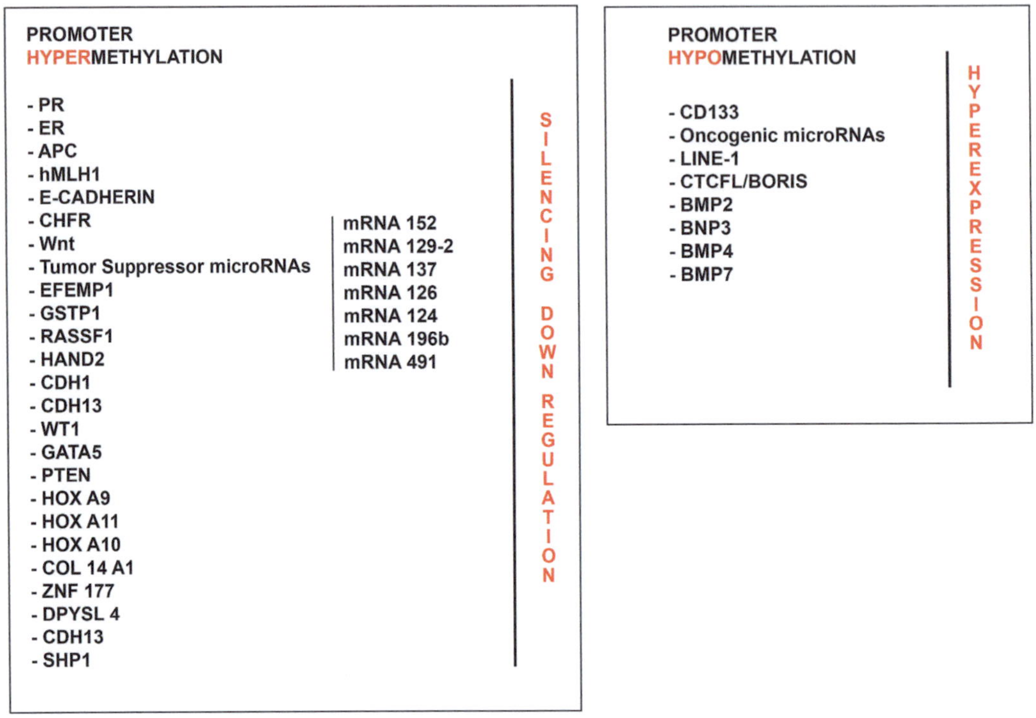


**Fig. 1.5** Epigenetic factors involved in endometrial carcinogenesis

suppressor genes involved in endometrial carcinogenesis, including the E-cadherin gene [59], the cadherin13 (CDH13) gene [60], the cadherin 1 (CDH1), and the Ras-associated domain gene family 1 (RASSF1) [54] (Fig. 1.5). Epigenetic dysregulation has been reported in some members of the homeobox (HOX) family, acting as tumor suppressors in endometrial carcinogenesis. Promoter hypermethylation was found in HOXA11 [61] and HOXA10, the latter involved in epithelial–mesenchymal transition, the mechanism facilitating tumor cell invasion and metastasis [62]. The hypothesis that the carcinogenic mechanisms of endometrial cancer may involve both genetic and epigenetic changes has been reinforced by a recent study by Banno and coworkers [63]. In that article, hypermethylation of genes of the mismatch repair (MMR) system and of suppressor microRNAs including mir124, mir126, mir 137, mir129-2, mir152, and mir491 have been proposed as the mechanism responsible for development of new treatment strategies in endometrial carcinoma, based on targeting epigenetically hypermethylated genes. Further genes have been shown to be hypermethylated in their promoter region in endometrial carcinoma by using the real-time methylation-specific polymerase chain reaction amplification method [58]. Promoter hypermethylation of collagen type XIV alpha-1 (COL14A1), zinc finger protein 177 (ZNF177), dihydropyrimidinase-like 4 (DPYSL4), homeobox A9 (HOXA9), and transmembrane protein with epidermal growth factor-like and two follistatin-like domains 2 (TMEFF2) was found to represent a frequent epigenetic event in endometrial carcinogenesis. The combined testing of ZNF177 and COL14A1 methylation had the highest specificity (100 %) for the diagnosis of endometrial cancer. The hypothesis that epigenetic changes in endometrial cancer and in precancerous lesions might be utilized as markers for the early diagnosis of endometrial cancer has been reinforced by a recent study aimed at exploring the epigenetic regulation of endometrial carcinogenesis [33]. In that study, promoter methylation of the CDH13 gene was detected in complex endometrial hyperplasia and in atypical endometrial hyperplasia as well as in well differentiated endometrial carcinoma, indicating a role for CDH13 epigenetic changes in the early phases of endometrial carcinogenesis. Hypermethylation of another suppressor gene, SHP1, was restricted to endometrial carcinoma cells, being absent in endometrial hyperplasia. As a consequence, SHP1 epigenetic hypermethylation changes have been proposed as a useful biomarker for diagnosis of endometrial cancer. A systematic analysis of the multiple mechanisms underlying downregulation of progesterone receptors (PRs) in endometrial cancer allowed the identification of different epigenetic mechanisms responsible for the decrease of PRs in the more advanced and less differentiated forms of endometrial cancer. Recruitment of the polycomb repressor complex 2 to the PR promoter probably represents the initial mechanism of PR gene silencing, followed by hypermethylation that suppresses completely PR transcription, inactivating progesterone, the natural inhibitor of endometrial carcinogenesis [64].

Targeting epigenetic changes in endometrial cancer has been suggested by several authors as a promising field in the therapy of endometrial cancer, with the aim of developing new drugs able to reactivate tumor suppressor gene function silenced by epigenetic changes [65]. A new epigenetic pathway dysregulation has been reported in endometrial cancer by a recent immunohistochemical study focused on the role of G9a, a histone methyltransferase [66]. Increased G9a immunoreactivity in endometrial cancer cells was associated with deep myometrial invasion, suggesting a major role for G9a in endometrial carcinoma progression. Moreover, a significant negative correlation between G9a and E-cadherin expression was observed in endometrial cancer cells, suggesting that E-cadherin loss probably mediates the effects of G9a on cancer invasion. On the basis of these data, targeting the G9a-mediated epigenetic dysregulation has been suggested as a new therapeutic strategy for endometrial cancer.

Another epigenetic mechanism involved in gynecological carcinogenesis is represented by hypomethylation, also known as demethylation, of the promoter region of oncogenes, a mechanism that plays an important role in human carcinogenesis and in particular in endometrial cancer [10]. A hypomethylation status has been detected in numerous familial and sporadic cancer types, including endometrial cancer. Demethylation of the promoter of the long interspersed element-1 (LINE-1) has been indicated as a putative marker for the early diagnosis of endometrial carcinoma [67]. Hypomethylation of the promoter of the CTCFL/BORIS gene has been described in the early phases of endometrial carcinogenesis, leading to overexpression of the protein product, associated with poor prognosis of endometrial adenocarcinomas [68]. Hypomethylation has been indicated also as a prognostic marker of recurrence in endometrial carcinoma: hypomethylation of bone morphogenic protein (BMP) members, including BMP2, 3, 4, and 7 was associated with recurrence and poor survival in women affected by endometrial cancer [69]. Hypermethylation and demethylation often work as two sides of the same coin in ovarian cancer: an overall global decrease of heterochromatin, and in particular a demethylation status of the promoter region of several oncogenes, is associated with hypermethylation of specific CpG islands in the promoter of several tumor suppressor genes [70].

## Epigenetic Factors in Ovarian Cancer

The knowledge that epigenetic factors might play a relevant role in ovarian carcinogenesis, in particular in the precursor lesions and early events of ovarian cancer insurgence, goes back to the beginning of this century [71] (Fig. 1.6). DNA hypomethylation of SAT2 in chromosome 1 was one of the first epigenetic change reported in ovarian cancer, being associated with advanced stage or high grade of the neoplasm [72]. Further studies on the epigenetic gene-silencing methylation-related profile of ovarian cancer revealed hypermethylation of APC and p16 genes in the majority of cases, occasionally associated

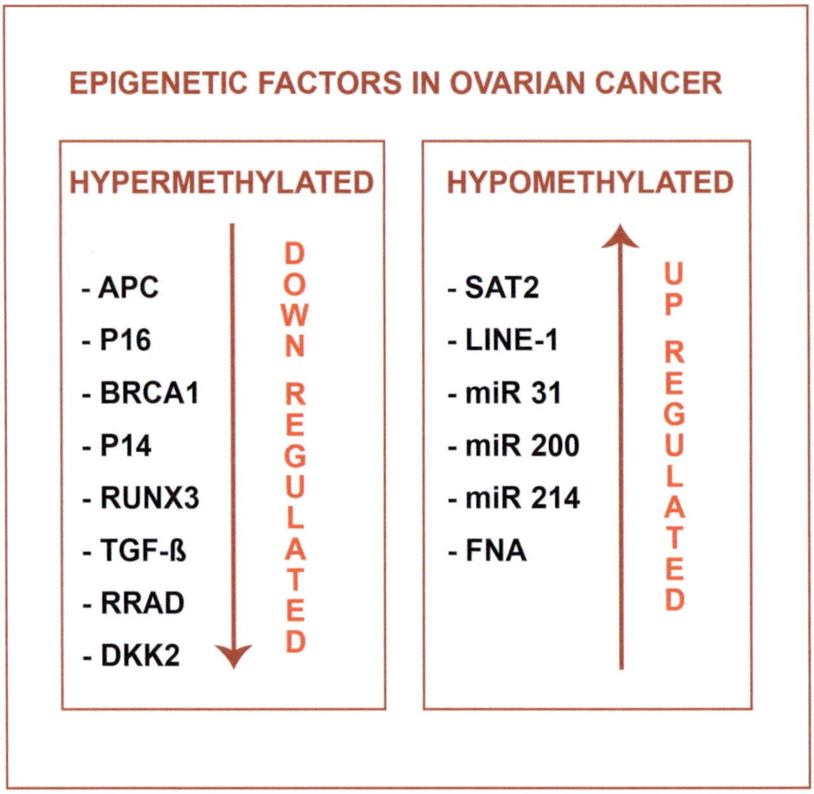


**Fig. 1.6** Epigenetic factors in ovarian cancer

with BRCA1 and p14, and only rarely with PTEN hypermethylation [31]. Studies carried out on genome methylation status in epithelial ovarian cancer evidenced a progressive decrease in the level of methylation in the promoter of the long interspersed element 1 (LINE-1) gene, lower levels correlating with advanced tumor grade and a poorer mean overall survival. On this basis, LINE-1 hypomethylation has been proposed as a useful marker to be included among the clinic-pathological parameters in the prognosis, and a potential marker for a target therapy of ovarian cancer [73]. The epigenetic origin of the inactivation of the RUNX3 gene has been demonstrated by a methylation-specific PCR analysis that demonstrated hypermethylation of the promoter region of RUNX3 in 86 % of the analyzed endometrial cancers. In the same study, immunohistochemistry confirmed the loss of the RUNX3 protein in the majority of endometrial carcinomas, the increase in the percentage of negative cases paralleling the increase of the tumor grade, thus indicating epigenetic RUNX silencing as an important factor in carcinogenesis of the endometrium [74]. All these data taken together, DNA methylation was proposed as a relevant tool for early diagnosis, prognosis, and treatment of ovarian cancer [75].

Epigenetic regulation has been associated also with ovarian cancer stem cells. The finding of ovarian cancer cells immunoreactive for CD133, a typical marker of stem/progenitor cells, induced Baba and coworkers to analyze the methylation state of these progenitors. This study evidenced a hypomethylated state in CD133-positive cancer stem cells, reinforcing the hypothesis that the activity of ovarian cancer stem cells may be epigenetically regulated [76]. The application of the high-throughput profiling method for the identification of the DNA hypermethylation profile in different subtypes of ovarian cancer allowed to reveal the existence of a unique hypermethylation pattern in different subtypes, suggesting the existence of different epigenetic mechanisms involved in different histotypes of ovarian cancer [77].

Epigenetic factors related to age have been shown to may play a relevant role in ovarian carcinogenesis. A study carried out utilizing the expression microarray analysis on ovarian cancer revealed the age-related progressive epigenetic silencing of the TGF-beta pathway activity, associated with hypermethylation of the TGF-beta gene, leading to suppression of the TGF-beta signaling contributing to ovarian carcinogenesis [78]. A study aimed at shedding light on the role of epigenetic gene silencing in ovarian carcinogenesis revealed the enrichment of methylation in multiple genes related to cell differentiation and proliferation inhibition, their silencing promoting tumor cell proliferation [3]. These data reinforced the hypothesis on a major role of epigenetic gene silencing in ovarian cancer insurgence and progression, and suggests that the study of the methylation pattern in ovarian cancer might represent an additional tool for prognostic and therapeutic purposes. The potential reversibility of epigenetic mechanisms made them particularly attractive candidates for development of new therapies of ovarian carcinoma, the definition of a specific epigenetic signature facilitating the development of a personalized and tailored cancer treatment [70]. The Ras-related associated with diabetes (RRAD) gene, encoding for a Ras-related GTPase, has been found to be hypermethylated in the promoter region in ovarian cancer, hypermethylation being associated with concomitant loss of expression [79]. In the same study, treatment of ovarian cancer cells with DNA methyltransferase inhibitors resulted in demethylation of the RRAD promoter and restored RRAD expression, followed by inhibition of tumor growth. These data clearly evidence the relevant role played by RRAD epigenetic silencing in ovarian carcinogenesis and reinforce the hypothesis on a major role that targeted epigenetic therapies might play in ovarian cancer.

Targeting the epigenome has become one of the most important challenges for researchers involved in gynecological cancer and, in particular in ovarian carcinogenesis. Two main reasons are at the basis of this assumption: (a) the small number of distinct genetic mutations contributing to ovarian carcinogenesis; (b) the always more numerous evidences of the prominent role played by epigenetic deregulation in silencing tumor suppressor genes and activating proto-oncogenes. On this basis, epigenetic therapies represent the new challenge in ovarian oncology, with the potential of the new epigenetic drugs to modify the epigenetic programming in ovarian cancer cells, reactivating tumor suppressors and repressing proto-oncogenes [80]. DKK2, a member of the Dickkopf family, is a Wnt antagonist that has been found to be highly downregulated in ovarian cancer cells, due to its promoter hypermethylation. Epigenetic silencing of the DKK2 gene has been proposed as a major molecular mechanism responsible for ovarian carcinogenesis. Downregulation of the DKK2 protein expression causes overexpression of the downstream genes of the Wnt signaling pathway, including beta-catenin, c-Myc, and cyclin D1, supporting a major role for DKK2 dysregulation in human ovarian carcinogenesis. Moreover, DKK2 silencing has been associated with overexpression of matrix metalloproteinase 2, indicating a role for DKK2 dysregulation in ovarian cancer cell migration and invasion. These findings suggest that DKK2 probably represents a hypermethylated target gene in ovarian cancer, its epigenetic silencing playing a fundamental role in human ovarian cancer insurgence and progression [81]. As a consequence, development of new epigenetic drugs aimed at demethylating and reactivating the DKK2 gene expression might represent one of the most important challenges in human ovarian oncology [82].

Targeting epigenetic mechanisms associated with miRNAs upregulation may represent another promising field in the treatment of ovarian cancer. Many microRNAs have been found to be characterized by altered expression in ovarian cancer tumor cells, including miR31, miR200, and miR214, and inhibition of their upregulation might be effective for development of new strategies in the target therapy of ovarian carcinomas [63]. In the search of agents for a targeted therapy of ovarian cancer, sorafenib, a multiple kinase inhibitor able to block tumor growth and epithelial–mesenchymal transition, has been shown to also act at epigenetic level, altering the histone acethylation pattern [83].

DNA hypomethylation has been indicated as the epigenetic mechanism responsible for glycosilation changes in the cell membrane of epithelial ovarian cancer cells, leading to altered cell signaling [84]. In particular, FNA hypomethylation has been indicated as the main mechanism at the basis of a decreased expression of MGAT3, one of the enzymes involved in the synthesis of cell membrane glycans, leading to the synthesis of the unique "bisecting GlcNAc" type N glycans on the cell membrane of ovarian cancer cells that might potentially be useful for the development of new anti-glycan anticancer drugs.

A peculiar problem in gynecological carcinogenesis is represented by ovarian endometriosis and, in particular, by factors involved in malignant transformation of the ectopic endometrium. A recent study on the methylation status of the SPOCK2 gene in ovarian endometriosis, combined with the analysis of the SPOCK2 protein expression pattern, revealed the hypermethylation state of SPOCK2 in endometriosis-related ovarian endometrioid carcinoma. These data suggest a major role of epigenetics in malignant transformation of ovarian endometriosis, abnormal methylation of the SPOCK2 gene leading to loss of expression of the SPOCK2 protein, ending with insurgence of ovarian endometrioid cancer [85]. The role of epigenetics in the insurgence of endometrioid carcinoma in ovarian endometriosis has been confirmed by the finding that epigenetic inactivation of the hMLH1 gene represents an early event in the malignant transformation of ectopic endometrium [86]. According to these findings, the methylation status of the hMLH1 gene has been proposed as a useful molecular marker for the early diagnosis of cancer progression in ovarian endometriosis. A recent study focused on the role of genetic and epigenetic mechanisms involved in the development of endometriosis-related ovarian carcinoma, evidenced a major role for epigenetics in the development of endometrioid ovarian carcinoma. Three main phases were identified in this process: (a) the uterine initial phase, represented by the inheritance of a genetic background characterized by endometriosis susceptible genes; (b) the second phase with epigenetic disruption of tumor suppressor genes' expression, due to hypermethylation of their promoter; (c) the third phase consisting in retrograde menstruation causing iron storage, leading to Fenton reaction-mediated oxidative stress and accumulation of somatic mutations [87]. A recent study aimed at investigating the role of the epigenetic inactivation of the runt-related transcription factor 3 (RUNX3) gene in the malignant transformation of ovarian endometriosis evidenced that RUNX3 inactivation by promoter hypermethylation plays a significant role in the progression of endometriosis toward endometrioid carcinoma [88]. The methylation status was inversely correlated with the expression of the RUNX protein, indicating immunohistochemistry for the RUNX protein as an early diagnostic marker in patients with ovarian endometriosis at increased risk for developing adenocarcinoma.

## Epigenetic Mechanisms in Cervical Carcinoma

Human papilloma virus has been identified as the unique, or better as the major etiological factor responsible for the insurgence of carcinoma of the uterine cervix. The long interval between HPV infection and the diagnosis of cervical cancer clearly indicates the existence of multiple factors, including epigenetic events, that should be responsible for the multiple steps of development and progression of cervical carcinoma. According to this hypothesis, viral proteins have been shown to interact with cell cycle proteins of infected cervical cells, including cyclin D, cyclin E, p16, p21, and p27, leading to alterations of the cell cycle checkpoint machinery, playing a fundamental role in cervical carcinogenesis [89]. First studies aimed at defining the differential methylation profiles of gynecological cancers evidenced hypermethylation of the APC, p16, and DAPK genes as typical markers of cervical cancer cells. These preliminary data suggested the existence of a specific methylation gene silencing profile in cervical cancer cells, able to differentiate it from endometrial and ovarian cancer cells [31]. The search for other epigenetic cofactors contributing to cervical neoplasm insurgence and progression evidenced the aberrant methylation status of two suppressor genes, namely BLU and RASSF1A. The highest levels of hypermethylation were detected in the promoter of the BLU gene, with percentages ranging from 23 % in low-squamous intraepithelial lesion (SIL), to 57 % in high-SIL, up to 77 % in squamous cell carcinoma (SCC). Lower percentages of methylation were found in the RASSF1A suppressor gene, ranging from 0 % in L-SIL, to 15% in SCC, and 18 % in H-SIL [90]. These data clearly indicate the association between hypermethylation of the BLU gene and the insurgence and progression of cervical cancer, assigning a minor role to hypermethylation of the RASSF1 gene.

Further studies on the molecular mechanisms involved in cervical carcinogenesis clearly evidenced that infection and integration of high-risk human papilloma viruses in the host genome of basal cell of the human cervix is insufficient for cervical carcinogenesis, suggesting the existence of environmental factors responsible for the epigenetic inactivation of tumor suppressor genes [91]. Epigenetic alterations have been indicated as the major factor involved in the multistep process starting from HPV infection and ending with the insurgence and progression of cervical cancer. According to this hypothesis, cervical carcinogenesis should be characterized by the accumulation of epigenetic and genetic changes in regulatory genes, ending with the inactivation of key tumor suppressor genes by promoter hypermethylation [91]. The study of the methylation level in a pool of DNA from in situ cervical cancers (CIN3 lesions) using a methylation bead array revealed significant hypermethylation in fourteen genes: AJAP1, ADRA1D, COL6A2, EDN3, EPO, MAG12, POU4F3, PTGDR, SOX8, SOX17, ST6GAL2, SYT9, ZNF614, and HS3ST2. Since five of these hypermethylated genes are implicated in beta-cathenin signaling, these findings suggested the epigenetic dysregulation in this signaling pathway during cervical carcinogenesis [92]. Moreover, the concurrent hypermethylation of several genes in cervical cancer, including in situ lesions, induced the authors to hypothesize the existence of a specific driver of methylation phenotype in cervical carcinogenesis. Epigenetic mutations have been indicated as responsible for aberrant expression of the human riboflavin transporter 2 (hRFT2) in cervical squamous cell carcinoma, hypermethylation of two CpG sites in its promoter region being associated with translocation of the hRFT2 protein from the cytoplasm and cell membrane into the nucleus of tumor cells [93]. Epigenetic silencing of the CXCR4 gene, due to hypermethylation of its promoter, has been shown to promote loss of cell adhesion in cervical cancer, a key event in favoring invasion and metastasis [94]. Interestingly, in the same study, treatment of cervical cancer cell lines with a DNA hypomethylating drug (5-aza-2′-deoxycytidine) and a histone deacethylase inhibitor (Trichestatin) was able to reactivate CXCR4 transcription and protein expression, promoting tumor cell adhesion.

A recent study focused on new candidate biomarkers associated with poor prognosis and able to predict sensitivity to treatment of cervical cancer evidenced a major role for epigenetic biomarkers in this neoplasm. In particular, hypermethylation of the checkpoint with forkhead and ring finger gene was indicated as a useful marker for predicting sensitivity of tumor cells to paclitaxel, whereas the hypermethylation status of the Werner DNA helicase gene was suggested as a marker indicating sensitivity of cervical cancer cells to another anticancer agent, CPT-11 [95]. Epigenetic changes, and in particular hypermethylation of the Keap1 gene promoter, have been found to be at the basis of the nuclear overexpression of NRF2 in cervical cancer cells, NRF2 immunoreactivity and Keap1 negativity being associated with more advanced cervical cancer. Overexpression of NRF2 was associated with increased proliferation, inhibition of apoptosis, and enhanced cell migration and metastasis, suggesting a major role for epigenetics in cervical cancer progression [96].

The role of epigenetics in cervical carcinogenesis has been recently reinforced by the report of an epigenetic role of HPV on the retinoblastoma 1 (RB1) gene. HPV has been shown to inactivate RB1 by inducing its promoter hypermethylation. In a recent study on the association between HPV infection and the methylation status in cervical lesions, only cervical cancer cases presented RB1 promoter hypermethylation, the dysregulation of the methylation status increasing with cancer progression [97]. All these data taken together indicate that RB1 promoter hypermethylation is a tumor-associated epigenetic event in HPV-related cervical cancer.

## Epigenetic Mechanisms in Endocervical Carcinogenesis

More than 30 years ago, the hypothesis that epigenetic mechanisms might contribute to the insurgence of adenocarcinoma of the endocervix was introduced in the literature, based on the evidence of the downregulation of lactoferrin expression during the neoplastic transformation of the endocervix [98]. A further study on the aberrant methylation status in adenocarcinoma of the endocervix revealed the occurrence of hypermethylation of two suppressor genes, BLU (44 %) and RASSF1A (26 %) [90].

## Microbioma and Cancer Insurgence and Progression

The role of the intestinal microbioma in human health and disease is becoming always more important, starting from the perinatal period and extending into adulthood [99]. In physiology, the indigenous intestinal commensal bacteria are able to modulate the expression of host genes, and play an important role in maintaining human homeostasis and health [100]. In recent years, changes in the human gut microbiome have been implicated in cancer insurgence [101]. The linkage between the intestinal microbiome and cancer insurgence has been found in the modification of dietary compounds that might influence cancer risk, in patients affected by pathological changes in the composition of colonic bacteria. The modification of the microbial metabolism of macronutrients by activating diverse metabolic pathways has been shown to induce the production of new microbial metabolites that may function as epigenetic activators/inhibitors of human gene expression, influencing cancer risk. The epigenetic influence of microbial metabolites may be exerted through inhibition of enzymes involved in epigenetic pathways, including methyltransferases. The action of microbial metabolites produced by a pathological microbiome may be exerted on colon enterocytes, being the colonic mucosa directly exposed to the toxic microbial metabolites, but their production may also affect risk of cancer in tissues outside the gastrointestinal tract, including gynecological cancer [102]. A complex and dynamic interplay between the composition of the gut microbiome, dietary exposure to xenobiotics, including drugs and carcinogens, and the host immune system is emerging as a new fascinating field of research in oncology. Recently, some strains of microorganisms harbored in the human gut that might affect the metabolic pathways responsible for carcinogenesis, increasing susceptibility to develop cancer, have been identified [103].

The human cervicovaginal microbiome plays a fundamental role in female reproductive health, affecting susceptibility to many sexually transmitted infections, including human paillomavirus (HPV) [104]. Recently, a major role for vaginal microbiome has been suggested in the persistence of HPV infection and in cervical carcinogenesis [105]. In particular, increasing vaginal microbiome diversity associated with low levels of Lactobacillus ssp. were associated with viral persistence and progression of cervical intraepithelial neoplasia (CIN) [106]. According to these data, changes in vaginal microbiota might represent a fundamental epigenetic event in cervical carcinogenesis, explaining why the vast majority (about 90 %) of HPV infections are transient and clear within 2 years, and only a small proportion of infected women develop CIN and invasive cervical cancer [107, 108]. These data taken together, studying how microbiota may amplify cervical carcinogenesis, assigning causal roles to specific components of the vaginal microbiome, represents an area of intensive interest for exploiting a better knowledge for cervical cancer prevention, diagnosis, and therapy [109].

## Conclusions

The concept that epigenetic events can modify gene expression is spreading, in recent years, through the scientific community. In a modern view of the relationship between genetics and epigenetics, genetics might be seen as a piano, a long one with a keyboard of 25,000 keys each one representing one human gene, whereas epigenetics could be represented by the piano tuner and by the pianist. In this example, the roles of the pianist and of the piano tuner appear predominant on the quality of the piano and of the keyboard for obtaining a good performance. Everybody might prefer an excellent pianist playing a low-quality piano than a fantastic keyboard played by an incompetent pianist. According to a modern view of health and disease, genetics (our keyboard) should be considered as a good or bad predisposition to health or to a disease status, whereas epigenetics (the environment, our life style, our microbiome) should be seen as the most important factors responsible for the realization of the health status or for our susceptibility to develop a disease.

In the balance between genetics and epigenetics in oncology, accumulating evidences suggest that much of the risk of cancer insurgence and progression is highly influenced by the environment and lifestyle, the epigenome serving as the interface between the genome and the environment [110]. All data here reported lay stress on a major role played by environmental (including changes in microbioma) epigenetic mechanisms of gene regulation not only in normal cellular function, but even in disease and in particular in human carcinogenesis.

The better comprehension of epigenetic factors involved in gynecological carcinogenesis reached in recent years is shedding light on the several aspects of the mechanisms of gynecological cancer insurgence and progression that remained unclear for many years, given that genetic variations and mutations of cancer-related genes did not provide a complete explanation of the several steps of tumor insurgence and progression in the vast majority of patients [111]. Hypermethylation of the promoter region of tumor suppressor genes and hypomethylation of oncogenes appear, at the best of our actual knowledge, as the most important epigenetic molecular mechanism involved in gynecological carcinogenesis. A better definition of the potential role of DNA methylation/demethylation in different types of gynecological cancer might represent the basis for utilizing the epigenetic profile of a single tumor entity for developing a tailored therapeutic approach in oncology [31].

One of the most intriguing findings emerging from the analysis of the epigenetic events reported in gynecological tumors is that epigenetic changes are different in different organs and the epigenetic profile differs from one tumor type to the next, hypermethylation of specific tumor suppressor genes representing a hallmark of many gynecological cancers. These findings lead to some considerations regarding both the pathogenesis and the future therapy of gynecological tumors. The finding of peculiar epigenetic profiles clearly indicates different pathogenetic mechanisms acting in endometrial, cervical, and ovarian tumors. Moreover, recent data show that even among neoplasms originating from the same tissue, the definition of the epigenetic profile may be able to differentiate multiple tumor subtypes. These data lead to hypothesize the use of epigenetic markers for a better new classification of endometrial, cervical, and ovarian cancers, allowing a new sartorial approach to cancer management based on the epigenetic profile of each single gynecological tumor [31].

The second consideration regards the use of the epigenetic profile for the development of a new sartorial and individualized cancer therapy, mainly based on targeting the aberrant hyper- or hypomethylation of target genes. This approach appears promising, in our opinion, since epigenetic changes are reversible. According to the example of the piano and the pianist, the epigenetic approach is based on changing the pianist, i.e. the hyper- or hypomethylation status of target genes appears much more promising than the previous ones based on modifying the piano, i.e. the genetic changes accumulating in tumor cells. Further attempts to use methylation inhibitors as anticancer agents and epigenetic abnormalities may be useful as biomarkers of anticancer drug sensitivity and to identify biological characteristics of tumor cells for determination of treatment options based on the restoration of physiological levels of methylation in tumor cells [46]. With the goal of improved diagnosis and treatment based on control of the epigenetic changes of cancer cells and, in particular of the abnormal methylation status of oncogenes and of tumor suppressor genes.

## References


1. Holliday R. The inheritance of epigenetic defects. Science (New York, NY). 1987;238(4824):163–70.
2. Sandoval J, Esteller M. Cancer epigenomics: beyond genomics. Curr Opin Genet Dev. 2012;22(1):50–5. Epub 2012/03/10. eng.
3. Michaelson-Cohen R, Keshet I, Straussman R, Hecht M, Cedar H, Beller U. Genome-wide de novo methylation in epithelial ovarian cancer. Int J Gynecol Cancer. 2011;21(2):269–79. Epub 2011/01/29. eng.
4. Berger J, Daxenbichler G. DNA methylation of nuclear receptor genes—possible role in malignancy. J Steroid Biochem Mol Biol. 2002;80(1):1–11. Epub 2002/02/28. eng.
5. Barrow TM, Michels KB. Epigenetic epidemiology of cancer. Biochem Biophys Res Commun. 2014;455(1-2):70–83. Epub 2014/08/16. eng.
6. Ooi SK, Bestor TH. The colorful history of active DNA demethylation. Cell. 2008;133(7):1145–8. Epub 2008/07/01. eng.
7. Rotili D, Mai A. Targeting histone demethylases: a new avenue for the fight against cancer. Genes Cancer. 2011;2(6):663–79. Pubmed Central PMCID: Pmc3174264, Epub 2011/09/24. eng.
8. Ropero S, Esteller M. The role of histone deacetylases (HDACs) in human cancer. Mol Oncol. 2007;1(1):19–25. Epub 2007/06/01. eng.
9. Paska AV, Hudler P. Aberrant methylation patterns in cancer: a clinical view. Biochem Med. 2015;25(2):161–76. Pubmed Central PMCID: Pmc4470106, Epub 2015/06/26. eng.
10. Ma X, Gao X. Epigenetic modifications and carcinogenesis of human endometrial cancer. Austin J Clin Pathol. 2014;1(3):1014.
11. Kasinski AL, Slack FJ. Epigenetics and genetics. MicroRNAs en route to the clinic: progress in validating and targeting microRNAs for cancer therapy. Nat Rev Cancer. 2011;11(12):849–64. Pubmed Central PMCID: Pmc4314215, Epub 2011/11/25. eng.
12. Zhi H, Ning S, Li X, Li Y, Wu W, Li X. A novel reannotation strategy for dissecting DNA methylation patterns of human long intergenic non-coding RNAs in cancers. Nucleic Acids Res. 2014;42(13):8258–70. Pubmed Central PMCID: Pmc4117791, Epub 2014/07/12. eng.
13. Zhao M, Qiu Y, Yang B, Sun L, Hei K, Du X, et al. Long non-coding RNAs involved in gynecological cancer. Int J Gynecol Cancer. 2014;24(7):1140–5. Epub 2014/08/01. eng.
14. Nygren AO, Ameziane N, Duarte HM, Vijzelaar RN, Waisfisz Q, Hess CJ, et al. Methylation-specific MLPA (MS-MLPA): simultaneous detection of CpG methylation and copy number changes of up to 40 sequences. Nucleic Acids Res. 2005;33(14), e128. Pubmed Central PMCID: Pmc1187824, Epub 2005/08/18. eng.
15. Jurinke C, Denissenko MF, Oeth P, Ehrich M, van den Boom D, Cantor CR. A single nucleotide polymorphism based approach for the identification and characterization of gene expression modulation using MassARRAY. Mutat Res. 2005;573(1-2):83–95. Epub 2005/04/15. eng.
16. Bock C, Tomazou EM, Brinkman AB, Muller F, Simmer F, Gu H, et al. Quantitative comparison of genome-wide DNA methylation mapping technologies. Nat Biotechnol. 2010;28(10):1106–14. Pubmed Central PMCID: Pmc3066564, Epub 2010/09/21. eng.
17. Jones PA. Functions of DNA methylation: islands, start sites, gene bodies and beyond. Nat Rev Genet. 2012;13(7):484–92. Epub 2012/05/30. eng.
18. Merlo A, Herman JG, Mao L, Lee DJ, Gabrielson E, Burger PC, et al. 5′ CpG island methylation is associated with transcriptional silencing of the tumour suppressor p16/CDKN2/MTS1 in human cancers. Nat Med. 1995;1(7):686–92. Epub 1995/07/01. eng.
19. Saito Y, Liang G, Egger G, Friedman JM, Chuang JC, Coetzee GA, et al. Specific activation of microRNA-127 with downregulation of the proto-oncogene BCL6 by chromatin-modifying drugs in human cancer cells. Cancer Cell. 2006;9(6):435–43.
20. Kinney SR, Pradhan S. Regulation of expression and activity of DNA (cytosine-5) methyltransferases in mammalian cells. Prog Mol Biol Transl Sci. 2011;101:311–33. Epub 2011/04/22. eng.
21. Szyf M, Bozovic V, Tanigawa G. Growth regulation of mouse DNA methyltransferase gene expression. J Biol Chem. 1991;266(16):10027–30. Epub 1991/06/05. eng.
22. Okano M, Bell DW, Haber DA, Li E. DNA methyltransferases Dnmt3a and Dnmt3b are essential for de novo methylation and mammalian development. Cell. 1999;99(3):247–57. Epub 1999/11/11. eng.
23. Herman JG, Baylin SB. Gene silencing in cancer in association with promoter hypermethylation. N Engl J Med. 2003;349(21):2042–54. Epub 2003/11/25. eng.
24. Weber M, Hellmann I, Stadler MB, Ramos L, Paabo S, Rebhan M, et al. Distribution, silencing potential and evolutionary impact of promoter DNA methylation

in the human genome. Nat Genet. 2007;39(4):457–66. Epub 2007/03/06. eng.
25. Seligson DB, Horvath S, Shi T, Yu H, Tze S, Grunstein M, et al. Global histone modification patterns predict risk of prostate cancer recurrence. Nature. 2005;435(7046):1262–6. Epub 2005/07/01. eng.
26. Jones PA, Martienssen R. A blueprint for a Human Epigenome Project: the AACR Human Epigenome Workshop. Cancer Res. 2005;65(24):11241–6. Epub 2005/12/17. eng.
27. Bernstein BE, Meissner A, Lander ES. The mammalian epigenome. Cell. 2007;128(4):669–81. Epub 2007/02/27. eng.
28. Huang WY, Hsu SD, Huang HY, Sun YM, Chou CH, Weng SL, et al. MethHC: a database of DNA methylation and gene expression in human cancer. Nucleic Acids Res. 2015;43(Database issue):D856–61. Pubmed Central PMCID: Pmc4383953, Epub 2014/11/16. eng.
29. Mills AA. Throwing the cancer switch: reciprocal roles of polycomb and trithorax proteins. Nat Rev Cancer. 2010;10(10):669–82. Pubmed Central PMCID: Pmc4068012, Epub 2010/09/25. eng.
30. Widschwendter M, Fiegl H, Egle D, Mueller-Holzner E, Spizzo G, Marth C, et al. Epigenetic stem cell signature in cancer. Nat Genet. 2007;39(2):157–8. Epub 2007/01/04. eng.
31. Yang HJ, Liu VW, Wang Y, Tsang PC, Ngan HY. Differential DNA methylation profiles in gynecological cancers and correlation with clinicopathological data. BMC Cancer. 2006;6:212. Pubmed Central PMCID: Pmc1560388, Epub 2006/08/25. eng.
32. You JS, Jones PA. Cancer genetics and epigenetics: two sides of the same coin? Cancer Cell. 2012;22(1):9–20. Pubmed Central PMCID: Pmc3396881, Epub 2012/07/14. eng.
33. Li HJ, Yu PN, Huang KY, Su HY, Hsiao TH, Chang CP, et al. NKX6.1 functions as a metastatic suppressor through epigenetic regulation of the epithelial-mesenchymal transition. Oncogene. 2015. Epub 2015/08/11.Eng.
34. Ross SA. Diet and DNA methylation interactions in cancer prevention. Ann N Y Acad Sci. 2003;983:197–207. Epub 2003/05/02. eng.
35. Brunaud L, Alberto JM, Ayav A, Gerard P, Namour F, Antunes L, et al. Effects of vitamin B12 and folate deficiencies on DNA methylation and carcinogenesis in rat liver. Clin Chem Lab Med. 2003;41(8):1012–9. Epub 2003/09/11. eng.
36. Lim U, Song MA. Dietary and lifestyle factors of DNA methylation. Methods Mol Biol (Clifton, NJ). 2012;863:359–76.
37. Mathers JC, Strathdee G, Relton CL. Induction of epigenetic alterations by dietary and other environmental factors. Adv Genet. 2010;71:3–39. Epub 2010/10/12. eng.
38. Del Pup L, Mantovani A, Luce A, Cavaliere C, Facchini G, Di Francia R, et al. Endocrine disruptors and female cancer: Informing the patients (Review). Oncol Rep. 2015;34(1):3–11. Epub 2015/05/23. eng.
39. Zarrinpar A, Chaix A, Yooseph S, Panda S. Diet and feeding pattern affect the diurnal dynamics of the gut microbiome. Cell Metab. 2014;20(6):1006–17. Pubmed Central PMCID: Pmc4255146, Epub 2014/12/04. eng.
40. Hullar MA, Burnett-Hartman AN, Lampe JW. Gut microbes, diet, and cancer. Cancer Treat Res. 2014;159:377–99. Pubmed Central PMCID: Pmc4121395, Epub 2013/10/12. eng.
41. Ghabreau L, Roux JP, Niveleau A, Fontaniere B, Mahe C, Mokni M, et al. Correlation between the DNA global methylation status and progesterone receptor expression in normal endometrium, endometrioid adenocarcinoma and precursors. Virchows Arch. 2004;445(2):129–34. Epub 2004/06/29. eng.
42. Banno K, Yanokura M, Susumu N, Kawaguchi M, Hirao N, Hirasawa A, et al. Relationship of the aberrant DNA hypermethylation of cancer-related genes with carcinogenesis of endometrial cancer. Oncol Rep. 2006;16(6):1189–96. Epub 2006/11/08. eng.
43. Xiong Y, Dowdy SC, Eberhardt NL, Podratz KC, Jiang SW. hMLH1 promoter methylation and silencing in primary endometrial cancers are associated with specific alterations in MBDs occupancy and histone modifications. Gynecol Oncol. 2006;103(1):321–8. Pubmed Central PMCID: Pmc3273419, Epub 2006/05/17. eng.
44. Guida M, Sanguedolce F, Bufo P, Di Spiezio Sardo A, Bifulco G, Nappi C, et al. Aberrant DNA hypermethylation of hMLH-1 and CDKN2A/p16 genes in benign, premalignant and malignant endometrial lesions. Eur J Gynaecol Oncol. 2009;30(3):267–70. Epub 2009/08/25. eng.
45. Takai N, Narahara H. Array-based approaches for the identification of epigenetic silenced tumor suppressor genes. Curr Genomics. 2008;9(1):22–4. Pubmed Central PMCID: Pmc2674306, Epub 2008/03/01. eng.
46. Muraki Y, Banno K, Yanokura M, Kobayashi Y, Kawaguchi M, Nomura H, et al. Epigenetic DNA hypermethylation: clinical applications in endometrial cancer (Review). Oncol Rep. 2009;22(5):967–72. Epub 2009/09/30. eng.
47. Tao MH, Freudenheim JL. DNA methylation in endometrial cancer. Epigenetics. 2010;5(6):491–8. Pubmed Central PMCID: Pmc2954259, Epub 2010/06/15. eng.
48. Friel AM, Zhang L, Curley MD, Therrien VA, Sergent PA, Belden SE, et al. Epigenetic regulation of CD133 and tumorigenicity of CD133 positive and negative endometrial cancer cells. Reprod Biol Endocrinol. 2010;8:147. Pubmed Central PMCID: Pmc3027593, Epub 2010/12/03. eng.
49. Dellinger TH, Planutis K, Tewari KS, Holcombe RF. Role of canonical Wnt signaling in endometrial carcinogenesis. Expert Rev Anticancer Ther. 2012;12(1):51–62. Epub 2011/12/14. eng.
50. Banno K, Kisu I, Yanokura M, Masuda K, Ueki A, Kobayashi Y, et al. Epigenetics and genetics in endometrial cancer: new carcinogenic mechanisms and relationship with clinical practice. Epigenomics. 2012;4(2):147–62. Epub 2012/03/28. eng.

51. Banno K, Kisu I, Yanokura M, Masuda K, Kobayashi Y, Ueki A, et al. Endometrial cancer and hypermethylation: regulation of DNA and microRNA by epigenetics. Biochem Res Int. 2012;2012:Article ID 738274.
52. Banno K, Yanokura M, Kisu I, Yamagami W, Susumu N, Aoki D. MicroRNAs in endometrial cancer. Int J Clin Oncol. 2013;18(2):186–92. Epub 2013/02/06. eng.
53. Yang T, Qiu H, Bao W, Li B, Lu C, Du G, et al. Epigenetic inactivation of EFEMP1 is associated with tumor suppressive function in endometrial carcinoma. PLoS One. 2013;8(6), e67458. Pubmed Central PMCID: Pmc3696089, Epub 2013/07/11. eng.
54. Fiolka R, Zubor P, Janusicova V, Visnovsky J, Mendelova A, Kajo K, et al. Promoter hypermethylation of the tumor-suppressor genes RASSF1A, GSTP1 and CDH1 in endometrial cancer. Oncol Rep. 2013;30(6):2878–86. Epub 2013/09/27. eng.
55. Dvorakova E, Chmelarova M, Laco J, Palicka V, Spacek J. Methylation analysis of tumor suppressor genes in endometroid carcinoma of endometrium using MS-MLPA. Biomedical Papers of the Medical Faculty of the University Palacky, Olomouc, Czechoslovakia. 2013;157(4):298–303. Epub 2013/06/06. eng.
56. Abe W, Nasu K, Nakada C, Kawano Y, Moriyama M, Narahara H. MiR-196b targets c-myc and Bcl-2 expression, inhibits proliferation and induces apoptosis in endometriotic stromal cells. Hum Reprod (Oxford). 2013;28(3):750–61.
57. Dellas A, Jundt G, Sartorius G, Schneider M, Moch H. Combined PTEN and p27kip1 protein expression patterns are associated with obesity and prognosis in endometrial carcinomas. Clin Cancer Res. 2009;15(7):2456–62. Epub 2009/03/19. eng.
58. Chen Z, Che Q, Jiang FZ, Wang HH, Wang FY, Liao Y, et al. Piwil1 causes epigenetic alteration of PTEN gene via upregulation of DNA methyltransferase in type I endometrial cancer. Biochem Biophys Res Commun. 2015;463(4):876–80. Epub 2015/06/10. eng.
59. Leal Rojas P, Anabalon Rodriguez L, Garcia Munoz P, Tapia Escalona O, Guzman Gonzalez P, Araya Orostica JC, et al. [Promoter hypermethylation gene patterns in gynecological tumors]. Med Clin. 2009;132(10):371–6.
60. Seeber LM, Zweemer RP, Marchionni L, Massuger LF, Smit VT, van Baal WM, et al. Methylation profiles of endometrioid and serous endometrial cancers. Endocr Relat Cancer. 2010;17(3):663–73. Epub 2010/05/22. eng.
61. Whitcomb BP, Mutch DG, Herzog TJ, Rader JS, Gibb RK, Goodfellow PJ. Frequent HOXA11 and THBS2 promoter methylation, and a methylator phenotype in endometrial adenocarcinoma. Clin Cancer Res. 2003;9(6):2277–87. Epub 2003/06/11. eng.
62. Yoshida H, Broaddus R, Cheng W, Xie S, Naora H. Deregulation of the HOXA10 homeobox gene in endometrial carcinoma: role in epithelial-mesenchymal transition. Cancer Res. 2006;66(2):889–97. Epub 2006/01/21. eng.
63. Banno K, Yanokura M, Iida M, Masuda K, Aoki D. Carcinogenic mechanisms of endometrial cancer: involvement of genetics and epigenetics. J Obstet Gynaecol Res. 2014;40(8):1957–67. Epub 2014/08/19. eng.
64. Yang S, Jia Y, Liu X, Winters C, Wang X, Zhang Y, et al. Systematic dissection of the mechanisms underlying progesterone receptor downregulation in endometrial cancer. Oncotarget. 2014;5(20):9783–97. Pubmed Central PMCID: Pmc4259437, Epub 2014/09/18. eng.
65. Amadio G, Masciullo V, Ferrandina MG, Scambia G. Emerging drugs for endometrial cancer. Expert Opin Emerg Drugs. 2014;19(4):497–509. Epub 2014/10/22. eng.
66. Hsiao SM, Chen MW, Chen CA, Chien MH, Hua KT, Hsiao M, et al. The H3K9 methyltransferase G9a represses E-cadherin and is associated with myometrial invasion in endometrial cancer. Ann Surg Oncol. 2015;22 Suppl 3:1556–65. Epub 2015/01/24. eng.
67. Pavicic W, Joensuu EI, Nieminen T, Peltomaki P. LINE-1 hypomethylation in familial and sporadic cancer. J Mol Med (Berlin). 2012;90(7):827–35.
68. Hoivik EA, Kusonmano K, Halle MK, Berg A, Wik E, Werner HM, et al. Hypomethylation of the CTCFL/BORIS promoter and aberrant expression during endometrial cancer progression suggests a role as an Epi-driver gene. Oncotarget. 2014;5(4):1052–61. Pubmed Central PMCID: Pmc4011582, Epub 2014/03/25. eng.
69. Hsu Y-T, Gu F, Huang Y-W, Liu J, Ruan J, Huang R-L, et al. Promoter hypomethylation of EpCAM-regulated bone morphogenetic protein gene family in recurrent endometrial cancer. Clin Cancer Res. 2013;19(22):6272–85.
70. Koukoura O, Spandidos DA, Daponte A, Sifakis S. DNA methylation profiles in ovarian cancer: implication in diagnosis and therapy (Review). Mol Med Rep. 2014;10(1):3–9.
71. Cvetkovic D. Early events in ovarian oncogenesis. Reprod Biol Endocrinol. 2003;1:68. Pubmed Central PMCID: Pmc239895, Epub 2003/10/28. eng.
72. Widschwendter M, Jiang G, Woods C, Muller HM, Fiegl H, Goebel G, et al. DNA hypomethylation and ovarian cancer biology. Cancer Res. 2004;64(13):4472–80. Epub 2004/07/03. eng.
73. Pattamadilok J, Huapai N, Rattanatanyong P, Vasurattana A, Triratanachat S, Tresukosol D, et al. LINE-1 hypomethylation level as a potential prognostic factor for epithelial ovarian cancer. Int J Gynecol Cancer. 2008;18(4):711–7. Epub 2007/10/20. eng.
74. Yoshizaki T, Enomoto T, Fujita M, Ueda Y, Miyatake T, Fujiwara K, et al. Frequent inactivation of RUNX3 in endometrial carcinoma. Gynecol Oncol. 2008;110(3):439–44. Epub 2008/06/24. eng.

75. Barton CA, Hacker NF, Clark SJ, O'Brien PM. DNA methylation changes in ovarian cancer: implications for early diagnosis, prognosis and treatment. Gynecol Oncol. 2008;109(1):129–39. Epub 2008/02/01. eng.
76. Baba T, Convery PA, Matsumura N, Whitaker RS, Kondoh E, Perry T, et al. Epigenetic regulation of CD133 and tumorigenicity of CD133+ ovarian cancer cells. Oncogene. 2009;28(2):209–18. Epub 2008/10/07. eng.
77. Yoon MS, Suh DS, Choi KU, Sol MY, Shin DH, Park WY, et al. High-throughput DNA hypermethylation profiling in different ovarian epithelial cancer subtypes using universal bead array. Oncol Rep. 2010;24(4):917–25. Epub 2010/09/03. eng.
78. Matsumura N, Huang Z, Mori S, Baba T, Fujii S, Konishi I, et al. Epigenetic suppression of the TGF-beta pathway revealed by transcriptome profiling in ovarian cancer. Genome Res. 2011;21(1):74–82. Pubmed Central PMCID: Pmc3012928, Epub 2010/12/16. eng.
79. Wang Y, Li G, Mao F, Li X, Liu Q, Chen L, et al. Ras-induced epigenetic inactivation of the RRAD (Ras-related associated with diabetes) gene promotes glucose uptake in a human ovarian cancer model. J Biol Chem. 2014;289(20):14225–38. Pubmed Central PMCID: Pmc4022888, Epub 2014/03/22. eng.
80. Murphy SK. Targeting the epigenome in ovarian cancer. Future Oncol (London). 2012;8(2):151–64.
81. Zhu J, Zhang S, Gu L, Di W. Epigenetic silencing of DKK2 and Wnt signal pathway components in human ovarian carcinoma. Carcinogenesis. 2012;33(12):2334–43. Epub 2012/09/12. eng.
82. Matei DE, Nephew KP. Epigenetic therapies for chemoresensitization of epithelial ovarian cancer. Gynecol Oncol. 2010;116(2):195–201. Pubmed Central PMCID: Pmc2813995, Epub 2009/10/27. eng.
83. Smolle E, Taucher V, Petru E, Haybaeck J. Targeted treatment of ovarian cancer—the multiple – kinase – inhibitor sorafenib as a potential option. Anticancer Res. 2014;34(4):1519–30. Epub 2014/04/03. eng.
84. Anugraham M, Jacob F, Nixdorf S, Everest-Dass AV, Heinzelmann-Schwarz V, Packer NH. Specific glycosylation of membrane proteins in epithelial ovarian cancer cell lines: glycan structures reflect gene expression and DNA methylation status. Mol Cell Proteomics. 2014;13(9):2213–32. Pubmed Central PMCID: Pmc4159645, Epub 2014/05/24. eng.
85. Ren F, Wang DB, Li T. [Epigenetic inactivation of SPOCK2 in the malignant transformation of ovarian endometriosis]. Zhonghua fu chan ke za zhi. 2011;46(11):822–5.
86. Ren F, Wang D, Jiang Y, Ren F. Epigenetic inactivation of hMLH1 in the malignant transformation of ovarian endometriosis. Arch Gynecol Obstet. 2012;285(1):215–21. Epub 2011/05/11. eng.
87. Kobayashi H, Imanaka S, Nakamura H, Tsuji A. Understanding the role of epigenomic, genomic and genetic alterations in the development of endometriosis (review). Mol Med Rep. 2014;9(5):1483–505. Epub 2014/03/19. eng.
88. Guo C, Ren F, Wang D, Li Y, Liu K, Liu S, et al. RUNX3 is inactivated by promoter hypermethylation in malignant transformation of ovarian endometriosis. Oncol Rep. 2014;32(6):2580–8. Epub 2014/10/22. eng.
89. Kim YT, Zhao M. Aberrant cell cycle regulation in cervical carcinoma. Yonsei Med J. 2005;46(5):597–613. Pubmed Central PMCID: Pmc2810564, Epub 2005/11/01. eng.
90. Lai HC, Lin YW, Chang CC, Wang HC, Chu TW, Yu MH, et al. Hypermethylation of two consecutive tumor suppressor genes, BLU and RASSF1A, located at 3p21.3 in cervical neoplasias. Gynecol Oncol. 2007;104(3):629–35. Epub 2006/11/14. eng.
91. Minaguchi T, Yoshikawa H. [Molecular mechanism of cervical carcinogenesis]. Gan to kagaku ryoho Cancer Chemother. 2010;37(1):18–22.
92. Chen YC, Huang RL, Huang YK, Liao YP, Su PH, Wang HC, et al. Methylomics analysis identifies epigenetically silenced genes and implies an activation of beta-catenin signaling in cervical cancer. Int J Cancer. 2014;135(1):117–27. Epub 2013/12/07. eng.
93. Ma JQ, Kurban S, Zhao JD, Li QZ, Hasimu A. Epigenetic regulation of human riboflavin transporter 2(hRFT2) in cervical cancers from Uighur women. Asian Pac J Cancer Prev. 2014;15(6):2485–9. Epub 2014/04/26. eng.
94. Yadav SS, Prasad SB, Das M, Kumari S, Pandey LK, Singh S, et al. Epigenetic silencing of CXCR4 promotes loss of cell adhesion in cervical cancer. BioMed Res Int. 2014;2014:Article ID 581403.
95. Iida M, Banno K, Yanokura M, Nakamura K, Adachi M, Nogami Y, et al. Candidate biomarkers for cervical cancer treatment: potential for clinical practice (Review). Mol Clin Oncol. 2014;2(5):647–55. Pubmed Central PMCID: Pmc4106747, Epub 2014/07/24. Eng.
96. Ma JQ, Tuersun H, Jiao SJ, Zheng JH, Xiao JB, Hasim A. Functional role of NRF2 in cervical carcinogenesis. PLoS One. 2015;10(8), e0133876. Pubmed Central PMCID: Pmc4527737, Epub 2015/08/08. eng.
97. McCormick TM, Canedo NH, Furtado YL, Silveira FA, de Lima RJ, Rosman AD, et al. Association between human papillomavirus and Epstein–Barr virus DNA and gene promoter methylation of RB1 and CDH1 in the cervical lesions: a transversal study. Diagn Pathol. 2015;10:59. Pubmed Central PMCID: Pmc4450846, Epub 2015/06/03. eng.
98. Farley J, Loup D, Nelson M, Mitchell A, Esplund G, Macri C, et al. Neoplastic transformation of the endocervix associated with downregulation of lactoferrin expression. Mol Carcinog. 1997;20(2):240–50. Epub 1997/11/19. eng.
99. Faa G, Gerosa C, Fanni D, Nemolato S, van Eyken P, Fanos V. Factors influencing the development of a personal tailored microbiota in the neonate, with particular emphasis on antibiotic therapy. J Matern

Fetal Neonatal Med. 2013;26 Suppl 2:35–43. Epub 2013/09/27. eng.
100. Maukonen J, Saarela M. Human gut microbiota: does diet matter? Proc Nutr Soc. 2015;74(1):23–36. Epub 2014/08/27. eng.
101. Hullar MA, Fu BC. Diet, the gut microbiome, and epigenetics. Cancer J (Sudbury, MA). 2014;20(3):170.
102. Hullar MA, Burnett-Hartman AN, Lampe JW. Gut microbes, diet, and cancer. Advances in nutrition and cancer. New York, NY: Springer; 2014. p. 377–99.
103. Hagland HR, Søreide K. Cellular metabolism in colorectal carcinogenesis: influence of lifestyle, gut microbiome and metabolic pathways. Cancer Lett. 2015;356(2):273–80.
104. Smith BC, McAndrew T, Chen Z, Harari A, Barris DM, Viswanathan S, et al. The cervical microbiome over 7 years and a comparison of methodologies for its characterization. PLoS One. 2012;7(7), e40425.
105. Martin DH. The microbiota of the vagina and its influence on women's health and disease. Am J Med Sci. 2012;343(1):2.
106. Mitra A, MacIntyre D, Lee Y, Smith A, Marchesi J, Lehne B, et al. Cervical intraepithelial neoplasia disease progression is associated with increased vaginal microbiome diversity. Sci Rep. 2015;5.
107. Richardson H, Kelsall G, Tellier P, Voyer H, Abrahamowicz M, Ferenczy A, et al. The natural history of type-specific human papillomavirus infections in female university students. Cancer Epidemiol Biomarkers Prev. 2003;12(6):485–90.
108. Gravitt PE. The known unknowns of HPV natural history. J Clin Invest. 2011;121(12):4593.
109. Garrett WS. Cancer and the microbiota. Science (New York, NY). 2015;348(6230):80–6.
110. Jones A, Teschendorff AE, Li Q, Hayward JD, Kannan A, Mould T, et al. Role of DNA methylation and epigenetic silencing of HAND2 in endometrial cancer development. PLoS Med. 2013;10(11), e1001551. Pubmed Central PMCID: Pmc3825654, Epub 2013/11/23. eng.
111. Banno K, Kisu I, Yanokura M, Masuda K, Kobayashi Y, Ueki A, et al. Endometrial cancer and hypermethylation: regulation of DNA and microRNA by epigenetics. Biochem Res Int. 2012;2012:738274. Pubmed Central PMCID: Pmc3324134, Epub 2012/05/02. eng.

# Pharmacoepigenomics and Pharmacovigilance in Gynecological Cancers

2

Ang Sun

**Abstract**

Aberrant epigenetic changes have been reported in gynecological cancers and contribute to the tumorigenesis. Patients with the same type of cancer may carry different epigenetic defects. In fact, each tumor harbors a different set of epigenetic changes, demonstrating a heteroepigeneity among the tumors. The patients may respond differently to the same treatment due to the differences in epigenetic alterations they're harboring. Epigenetic changes are associated with loss of drug sensitivity and contribute to drug-resistance development. Pharmacoepigenomics include two aspects. One that has been emphasized previously is the interindividual differences at epigenome level that lead to different responses to the same drug. Another aspect that should not be overlooked is the effect of a treatment on the epigenome of patients. The emerging epigenetic therapies alone or in combination with chemotherapy or radiotherapy change the epigenome of patients, which in turn change the response of the patients to the drugs. Although currently most of the studies use loci-specific biomarkers to reflect epigenome changes, the advancement of next-generation sequencing will make more and more studies directly demonstrate the changes at the epigenome level. It is worth to notice that epigenetic therapy is still at its infancy. Lacking of specific targeting to reverse the epigenetic changes raise concerns of pharmacovigilance or drug safety. In this chapter, I focus on ovarian cancer, cervical cancer, and uterine cancer to discuss the pharmacoepigenomics and pharmacovigilance. For ovarian cancer, I emphasize that epigenetic alterations in patients cause chemoresistance acquisition and cancer recurrence, however, epigenetic therapies change the epigenome of cancer cells to resensitize them to chemotherapy. As for cervical cancer, the combination epigenetic therapies using both DNA

A. Sun, PhD (✉)
Fels Institute for Cancer Research and Molecular Biology, School of Medicine, Temple University, 3307 N Broad Street, Philadelphia, PA 19140, USA
e-mail: angsun@temple.edu; angsunbio@gmail.com


A. Giordano, M. Macaluso (eds.), *Gynecological Cancers*, Current Clinical Oncology,
DOI 10.1007/978-3-319-32907-9_2

methyltransferase (DNMT) inhibitors (DNMTIs) and histone deacetylase (HDAC) inhibitors (HDACIs) are emphasized. Regarding uterine cancer, application of epigenetic therapy to revive the hormonal therapy is discussed.

**Keywords**
Ovarian Cancer • Cervical Cancer • Gynecological Cancers • Endometrial cancer • Epigenetics • DNA Methylation • Histone Acetylation • Histone Deacetylase • Drug resistance • Pharmacoepigenomics • Pharmacovigilance • Combination Thearpy

## I. Gynecological Cancers, Pharmacoepigenomics, and Pharmacovigilance

Gynecological cancers are cancers that arise in a woman's reproductive system. Besides the rare fallopian tube cancer, there are primarily five types of gynecological cancers, including ovarian cancer, cervical cancer, uterine cancer, vaginal cancer, and vulvar cancer.

Even patients with the same type of gynecological cancer may respond to drug treatments differently. It is defined previously that the influence of interindividual epigenomic polymorphisms on drug response is pharmacoepigenomics [1]. In fact, pharmacoepigenomics should be defined to involve the studies of two aspects: one is drug treatments induce different epigenetic changes genome-wide in the patients, and the other is patients with various epigenomic backgrounds response to the drugs differently. Although the latter has attracted more efforts, more and more studies of the first aspect would emerge along the booming of the next generation sequencing. These two aspects of pharmacoepigenomics are actually intertwined. On the one hand, the effects of a drug on a patient's epigenome also depends on the existing epigenetic modifications in the patient; on the other hand, the epigenome contributing to the different responses to drugs can be affected by drug treatments, in particular the epigenetic therapeutics.

The epigenomic changes, besides the expression changes regulated by microRNA, mainly refer to the global changes of DNA methylation, or histone modifications primarily including histone phosphorylation, methylation, and acetylation. Different epigenomic backgrounds, such as different DNA methylation at genome-wide level (methylome) and at specific loci in the genome, have been shown to be associated with or even responsible for drug resistance in gynecological cancer cells as discussed in detail later.

When talking about treating gynecological cancers, we cannot get around pharmacovigilance, which refers to drug safety and is a major concern for drug development. In the process of drug development, preclinical trials using rodents and non-rodent animals, clinical trials I and II, and even post-market clinical trials all involve pharmacovigilance studies. It is one of the two most important aspects affect the decision of the regulatory agencies when the approval of a new drug is in concern.

## II. Pharmacoepigenomics and Pharmacovigilance in Ovarian Cancer

### Ovarian Cancer and Its Key Statistics

Ovarian cancer is the uncontrolled growth of malignant cells that originally arises in the ovaries. There are a few different types of ovarian cancer, including epithelial ovarian cancer (EOC), germ cell carcinoma, stromal carcinoma, and small cell carcinoma of the ovary (SCCO). EOC accounts about 90 % of all the ovarian cancer cases. According to American Cancer Society, in the USA in 2015, it estimates there are 21,290 newly diagnosed cases of ovarian cancer, and 14,180 women die from it. It accounts for 1.3% of new cancer cases, but 2.4% of all cancer deaths. It causes more deaths than any other gynecological cancers [2, 3]. It is the fifth most leading cause of cancer death in women, although it is only the eighth most common cancer among women. In the past two decades, the diagnosed rate of ovarian cancer has been slowly falling; however, during a woman's lifetime, her risk of getting ovarian cancer is still about 1 in 75, and risk of dying from ovarian cancer is one in 100 [4–6]. Based on the data in the SEER (Surveillance, Epigemiology, and End Results) Cancer Statistics Factsheets, the 5-year survival rate is 45.6% for ovarian cancer patients [7].

More than 90% of EOC are clonal progenies of a single cell. There are about 10% of ovarian cancer patients are familial and predisposed with germ-line mutations in BRCA1 (breast cancer susceptibility gene 1), BRCA2 (breast cancer susceptibility gene 2), mismatch repair genes, or p53. In sporadic ovarian cancers, somatic mutations have been found activating oncogenes or resulting in loss of tumor suppressor gene function [8].

## Pharmacoepigenomics in Ovarian Cancer

### Different Epigenetic Changes Contribute to Tumorigenesis of Ovarian Cancer

As many other cancers, ovarian cancer is also heterogeneous. Tumors from different patients or even from the same patient harbor different genetic mutations. In fact, tumors are also hetero-epigeneous, meaning they are different in terms of their epigenome. Many different epigenetic changes, including aberrant DNA methylation of gene promoters, histone modifications, and miRNA activities, contribute to the transformation of the ovarian epithelium and tumorigenesis of ovarian cancer [8, 9].

### Tumor Suppressors can be Silenced by Promoter DNA Methylation, Histone Modification, and miRNA Activity

In ovarian cancer, it has been observed that there are specific CpG islands hypermethylation within the promoter regions of some tumor suppressor genes to inactivate their expression [10, 11]. High frequency of de novo promoter methylation in hMLH1 (human MutL homologue-1), CDKN2A (cyclin-dependent kinase inhibitor 2A), and MGMT (O-6-methylguanine-DNA methyltransferase) was detected by methylation-specific polymerase chain reaction (MSP) assay on bisulfite-converted DNA from 18 primary ovarian carcinomas [12]. PTEN haploinsufficiency caused by epigenetic events may possibly contribute to development of some histological types of ovarian cancer and may be an adverse prognostic factor [13]. Secreted protein acidic and rich in cysteine (SPARC) promoter is methylated in 68% of primary ovarian tumors, which downregulates the level of SPARC protein and promotes the progress of cancer [14]. Argininosuccinate synthetase 1 (ASS1) gene expression may be lost due to epigenetic silencing of its promoter and has been associated with relapse of ovarian cancer [15, 16]. ZAC is an imprinted gene that only paternally expressed. Epigenetic silencing of this gene by DNA methylation has been reported as an early event in the progression of human ovarian cancer [17]. Another tumor suppressor has been observed being epigenetically silenced via DNA hypermethylation in ovarian cancer is retinoic acid receptor-beta2 (RAR-β2) [18]. In addition, the promoter of XPG gene, which is a nucleotide excision repair (NER) gene, has been reported being methylated in a significant proportion of ovarian tumors [19].

As aforementioned, there are about 10% of EOC are familiar. These hereditary ovarian cancer cases are primarily due to germ line mutations in the BRCA1 tumor suppressor gene. Mutations in BRCA1 predispose women to EOC [20, 21]. Besides genetic mutations, BRCA1 can also lose function due to epigenetic inactivation, which has been reported in sporadic ovarian cancer [21, 22].

The gene coding for mitochondrial Hinge protein, the ubiquinol-cytochrome C reductase hinge gene (UQCRH) was reported epigenetically inactivated in two ovarian cell lines. Demethylating agent 5-azacytidine (AZA) was able to restore UQCRH expression in OAW42 ovarian cancer cells [23].

Moreover, methylation of four tumor suppressor genes (MINT31, HIC1, RASSF1, and CABIN1) has been reported in ovarian cancer. The silencing of these genes is significantly associated with ovarian cancer development. Aberrant methylation of three genes (MINT31, RASSF1, and CDH13) upregulated Her-2/neu expression [24].

However, promoter methylation analysis showed silencing of the transforming growth factor-beta (TGFβ) signaling component km23 through promoter hypermethylation is rare in ovarian cancer [25].

Table 2.1 lists genes that can be silenced by promoter DNA hypermethylation in ovarian cancer. It includes some genes conveying chemoresistance by epigenetically silencing and will be discussed in details later.

**Table 2.1** List of genes that can be silenced in ovarian cancer by promoter DNA methylation

| Gene name | Reference |
|---|---|
| hMLH1 | [12] |
| CDKN2A | [12] |
| MGMT | [12] |
| PTEN | [13] |
| SPARC | [14] |
| ASS1 | [15, 16] |
| BRCA1 | [21, 22] |
| UQCRH | [23] |
| ZAC | [17] |
| RAR-β2 | [18] |
| MINT31 | [24] |
| HIC1 | [24] |
| RASSF1 | [24, 41] |
| CABIN1 | [24] |
| XPG | [19] |
| ARHI | [38, 42] |
| ZIC1 | [49] |
| ZIC4 | [49] |
| HSulf-1 | [68, 69] |
| annexin A11 | [70] |
| Plk2 | [74] |
| GREB1 | [77] |
| TGIF | [77] |
| TOB1 | [77] |
| BLU (ZMYND10) | [51] |
| TIMP3 | [53] |
| CDH1 | [53] |

In addition to DNA methylation, histone methylation can also play critical roles in many neoplastic processes, including silencing of tumor suppressor genes. For instance, histone methylation of H3K9 and H3K27 has been linked to aberrant gene silencing in cancer cells. In ovarian cancer cells, RASSF1 (Ras-associated domain family 1) was shown to be a direct target of H3K27 methylation-mediated silencing. Loss of methylation at H3K27 increased expression of tumor suppressor genes and resensitized drug-resistant ovarian cancer cells to the chemotherapeutic agent cisplatin [26].

The microRNAs (miRNAs) are a class of non-coding RNAs that posttranscriptionally, and thus epigenetically, inhibit gene expression. The miRNAs themselves can be epigenetically regulated as well [27–29]. One example is the miR-193a can target c-KIT mRNA for degradation and thus may play a crucial role in ovarian cancer development [30].

### Aberrant Promoter DNA Hypomethylation and Histone Acetylation Activate Oncogenes and Contribute to Ovarian Cancer Tumorigenesis

Although most of the efforts have focused on the epigenetic inactivation of tumor suppressor genes during tumorigenesis [11], there are reports about the epigenetic activation of cancer-associated genes by DNA hypomethylation and through the loss of repressive histone modifications [31].

Similar to many other cancers, ovarian cancer has an overall global decrease in DNA methylation of heterochromatin leading to demethylation of some oncogenes [11]. Comparing with the wild-type SK-OV-3 cells, aberrant hypomethylation of interferon-induced transmembrane protein 1 (IFITM1) promoter was observed in metastatic implants of human ovarian carcinoma xenografts in mice. Demethylating agent 5-aza-2′-deoxycytidine (DAC), an inhibitor of DNMTs, enhanced IFITM1 expression in a dose-dependent manner. IFITM1 overexpression caused increased migration and invasiveness in SK-OV-3 cells [3]. Another example is, TMPRSS3 gene variants A and D (TMPRSS3-A/D) were significantly hypomethylated in high-grade serous EOC tumors, compared with low-grade tumors and normal tissue, suggesting the frequently observed upregulation of different members of the type II serine proteases gene family in advanced cancer could be due to aberrant DNA hypomethylation [32].

Besides being affected by DNA hypomethylation alone, the expression of some putative oncogenes is regulated by both DNA hypomethylation and histone modifications. CLDN4, a gene encoding claudin-4, which is a member of a large family of tight junction proteins, is overexpressed in ovarian cancer. Ovarian cancer cells overexpressing CLDN4 exhibit low DNA methylation and high histone H3 acetylation of the critical CLDN4 promoter region. The CLDN4-negative cells can be induced to express CLDN4 by demethylating and/or acetylating agents [33]. In addition, in ovarian cancer, the expression of the cell surface marker CD133, which identifies cancer-initiating cells in EOC and attributes to cancer recurrence, is also directly regulated by both histone modifications and promoter DNA methylation. Sorted CD133–negative cancer cells treated with DNMT and HDAC inhibitors show a synergistic increase in cell surface CD133 expression [34].

### Different Aberrant Signaling Pathways and Cellular Processes in Ovarian Cancer Can Be Disrupted by Epigenetic Changes

Different ovarian cancers exhibit aberrant autocrine and/or paracrine growth regulation with alteration in the expression of growth factors and their receptors [8]. Human epidermal growth factor receptor (EGFR) family, poly(ADP-ribose) polymerase (PARP), and mammalian target of rapamycin (mTOR) signaling pathway, are aberrant in ovarian cancer tissues [35].

EGFR pathway can be abnormally activated in ovarian cancer [36, 37]. Ras signaling downstream EGFR regulates DNA methylation [37, 38]. EGFR inhibitor PD153035 has been shown be able to stimulate expression of RAR-β, which was epigenetically silenced via DNA hypermethylation in OVCAR-3 ovarian carcinoma cells [18]. Another EGFR inhibitor, erlotinib, has been used together with a DNMT inhibitor in a phase I clinical trial [39].

Members of Ras signaling may also be disrupted by epigenetic changes, for example, RASSF1A (Ras-associated domain family 1A) [24, 26, 40, 41]. Another member in the Ras superfamily, ARHI (Ras homologue member I) is one of the first reported tumor suppressors. It is expressed consistently in normal ovarian epithelial cells, but dramatically downregulated in more than 70 % of ovarian cancers. ARHI is maternally imprinted in the maternal allele of normal cells [38, 42]. Loss of ARHI expression can occur through epigenetic mechanisms. It has been reported that acetylation and methylation of chromatin associated with the ARHI promoter leads to loss of both ARHI expression and the ability to suppress tumor growth. Reactivation of both the silenced paternal and imprinted maternal alleles can be achieved by demethylation and inhibition of histone deacetylation [42]. Epigenetic therapy targeting imprinted ARHI has been reported in ovarian cancer [38].

PARP (poly(ADP-ribose) polymerase) inhibitors are mainly used in ovarian cancer susceptibility gene-mutated patients [35]. Epigenetic losses of BRCA1/2 and PTEN in ovarian cancer have been reported being used to predict sensitivity to PARP inhibitors [36].

For ovarian cancer, epigenetic alterations could affect the activation of PI3K/AKT/mTOR pathway [43]. mTOR inhibitors are also attractive treatments, either alone or in combination with chemotherapy [35].

Epigenetic mechanisms play a key role in epithelial-to-mesenchymal transition (EMT), a key step in the process of metastasis. In ovarian cancer, disruption of TGF-β/SMAD signaling may lead to epigenetic silencing of its target genes through histone modifications or promoter hypermethylation [44]. TGF-β induces expression of DNMT-1, -3A, and -3B, and global changes in DNA methylation during the EMT in ovarian cancer cells. Treatment with the DNMT inhibitor SGI-110 prevented TGF-β-induced EMT [45]. Epigenetic drugs also regulate EMT to potentiate the efficacy of low-dose cisplatin [46].

Reactive oxygen species (ROS) induced by live-attenuated measles virus (MV) vaccine in ovarian cancer may upregulate DNMT3a and thus epigenetically silence E-cadherin [47].

Ubiquitination and protein degradation can also be affected by epigenetic changes. PDLIM2 is critical to promote ubiquitination of nuclear p65. It has been reported that PDLIM2 is epigenetically repressed in ovarian cancer. Epigenetic repression of PDLIM2 promoted ovarian cancer growth both in vivo and in vitro via NOS2-derived nitric oxide signaling [48].

In addition, members of sonic hedgehog pathway, ZIC1 and ZIC4, which are putative tumor suppressors, may be herpermethylated and silenced in ovarian tumors and ovarian cancer cell lines [49].

Moreover, epigenetic dysregulations of genes have been reported interfered p53 signaling in ovarian cancer and contributed to the failure of phase II/III trial of p53 gene-therapy [50].

Many other pathways or cellular processes can be regulated by epigenetic changes as well. For example, CLDN4 involved in tight junction [33], ubiquinol-cytochrome C reductase hinge gene (UQCRH) that encodes a mitochondrial Hinge protein [23], cancer stem cell/initiating cell surface marker CD133 [34], and recruitment of CD8+ T-cell in early stage ovarian cancer [34].

The epigenetic regulation of apoptosis [51, 52] and angiogenesis [53] will be discussed later in the section for chemoresistance.

In summary, as discussed above, a variety of epigenetic changes both at genome-wide level and at specific loci have been reported. These DNA hypermethylation and hypomethylation, histone acetylation and deacetylation, histone methylation, and miRNA activity, either activating oncogenes or inactivating tumor suppressor genes, contribute to the tumorigenesis and development of ovarian cancer. Not all of these epigenetic changes affect expression of tumor suppressor genes or oncogenes in all the ovarian tumors. Each tumor has its own set of aberrant epigenetic modifications and is epigenomically different from other tumors, showcasing an interindividual difference and a populational heteroepigeneity. These aberrant epigenetic changes disrupt the function of different genes and pathways in different patients, make a patient would respond to some drugs or treatments, but not others. This lays the logic foundation to further explore the pharmacoepigenomics, which in turn would be important for treating patients with ovarian cancer with personalized medicine.

As it has been discussed before, ovarian cancer is the most lethal gynecological cancer. The high mortality rate is resulted from lacking of early diagnosis, as well as the eventual development of chemoresistance and the unfortunate recurrence of the cancer. Many epigenetic changes are not only involved in the tumorigenesis and development of the ovarian cancer, thus establishing the interindividual epigenomic variances, an important part of the pharmacoepigenomics, but also contribute to the chemoresistance development. As different ovarian cancer patients may have different epigenetic modifications attributing to chemoresistance, interindividual epigenomic variances certainly play roles in the chemoresistance.

## The Aberrant Epigenetic Changes Contribute to Chemoresistance of Ovarian Cancer

Currently, surgical tumor debulking, followed by taxane (paclitaxel or docetaxel) and platinum (cisplatin or carboplatin) chemotherapy is the standard treatment used in the treatment of ovarian cancer [21]. As aforementioned, the mortality rate of ovarian cancer patients is high. The low 5-year survival rate is partially due to the eventual development of drug resistance and recurrence, despite the initial response to therapy is high [4, 21, 35, 54–56].

## Epigenetic Markers Are Important for Early Detection and Predict Therapy-Response

The 5-year survival rate is strongly related to the diagnosed stage of the ovarian cancer. Patients diagnosed at early stage has a 90 % 5-year survival rate comparing with the 30 % 5-year survival rate for patients diagnosed with cancer metastasized into the peritoneal cavity [5]. Unfortunately, most ovarian cancer patients are diagnosed at the advanced-stage of the disease, because of few early symptoms and a lack of early detection strategies [3, 56, 57]. There are only a small number of distinct genetic mutations, such as mutations in BRAC1 and BRAC2, are known to contribute to ovarian carcinogenesis [20–22, 58–60]. Cancer-specific DNA methylation changes, may be exploreded to identify epigenetic-(in)activation-associated downregulated or upregulated genes as biomarkers or even signatures for ovarian cancer to improve early-stage diagnosis and better predict prognosis [5, 57, 61].

Besides DNA hypermethylation, DNA hypomethylation of promoter of oncogenes can be used as biomarkers as well. For example, DNA hypomethylation within the IFITM1 promoter region could be a biomarker indicating metastatic progression in ovarian cancer [3].

Additionally, MSI (microsatellite instability). which may be resulted from epigenetic inactivation of DNA mismatch repair genes, could be a biomarker for good prognosis after some chemotherapeutic treatments. For example, it has been reported that the majority of MSI-positive ovarian cell lines are hypersensitive to bleomycin, a DNA double-strand-break (DSB) producing chemotherapeutic drug [62].

In addition to examining the DNA methylation of specific genes, people have also performed genome-wide methylation detection arrays and high-throughput sequencing, which have provided profound information regarding ovarian cancer-specific methylation that may serve as biomarkers for diagnosis or prognosis [63].

Potential biomarkers, including miRNAs, which may predict prognosis, are listed in Table 2.2.

**Table 2.2** Potential epigenetic markers in ovarian cancer for therapy response

| Biomarker | Epigenetic change | Prognosis | Reference |
|---|---|---|---|
| IFITM1 promoter | DNA hypomethylation | Poor | [3] |
| BRAC1 promoter | DNA hypermethylation | Good | [21, 59, 60, 67] |
| XPG promoter | DNA hypermethylation | Poor | [19] |
| HSulf-1 promoter | DNA hypermethylation | Poor | [68, 69] |
| annexin A11 promoter | DNA hypermethylation | Poor | [70] |
| CABIN1 promoter | DNA hypermethylation | Poor | [24] |
| RASSF1 promoter | DNA hypermethylation | Poor | [24, 41] |
| ASS1 promoter | DNA hypermethylation | Poor | [15, 16] |
| LINE1 | DNA hypomethylation | Poor | [73] |
| Plk2 promoter | DNA hypermethylation | Poor | [74] |
| 6p21.3 in the R class | DNA hypomethylation | Good | [80] |
| GREB1 | DNA hypomethylation | Good | [77] |
| TGIF | DNA hypomethylation | Good | [77] |
| TOB1 | DNA hypomethylation | Good | [77] |
| TMCO5 | DNA hypermethylation | Good | [77] |
| PTPRN | DNA hypermethylation | Good | [77] |
| GUCY2C | DNA hypermethylation | Good | [77] |
| hMLH1 promoter | DNA hypermethylation | Poor | [12, 78] |
| BLU promoter | DNA hypermethylation | Poor | [51] |
| TIMP3 promoter | DNA hypermethylation and repressive histone methylation | Poor | [53] |
| CDH1 promoter | DNA hypermethylation and repressive histone methylation | Poor | [53] |
| Low level of miR-130b | Possible DNA hypermethylation | Poor | [27] |
| High level of miR-152 | | Good | [83] |
| High level of miR-185 | | Good | [83] |
| Low level of miR-199b-5p | DNA hypermethylation | Poor | [28] |
| High level of miR-370 | | Good | [85] |
| MSI or mismatch mutator phenotype | | Good | [62] |

## The Drug Resistance May Be Due to Epigenetic Modifications

Drug resistance may result from genetic changes. For example, it has been reported that ovarian tumor cell lines that retain RASSF1A expression commonly harbor polymorphisms in the region of Ser131, while the S131F polymorphism conveys resistance to DNA-damaging agents [40, 64].

Besides genetic mutations, drug resistance is contributed to by the epigenetic changes, including aberrant DNA methylation, atypical histone modifications and dysregulated expression of distinct microRNAs [4, 54, 65, 66]. Pharmacoepigenomic modulators of genes and pathways, such as promoter methylation (MLH1 and BRCA1 genes) and miRNA regulation (PTEN/AKT and NF-kappaB pathways) have been associated with ovarian cancer chemoresponse [1].

It has been reported the downregulated expression of XPG due to the promoter hypermethylation contributes to the drug resistance to nemorubicin, a doxorubicin derivative, and could affect the response to therapy using platinum [19].

BRCA1 deficiency predicts enhanced response to platinum [21, 59, 67]. It also has been reported that in both cancer cell lines and xenografted tumors, hypermethylation of BRCA1 CpG island promoter silences BRCA1 and enhances sensitivity to platinum-derived drugs to the same extent as BRCA1 mutations. Epigenetic inactivation of BRCA1 proves to be a predictor of longer time to relapse and improved overall survival in ovarian cancer patients undergoing chemotherapy with cisplatin [59, 60]. More interestingly, in both human and murine models of BRCA1-associated ovarian carcinoma, BRCA1-deficient ovarian carcinoma cells exhibit hypermethylation within a p73 regulatory region, which abrogates the binding of a p73 transcriptional repressor, ZEB1, and thus increases the expression of transactivating p73 isoforms (TAp73). This helps to explain the mechanism why BRCA1-deficient ovarian carcinoma cells are sensitive to platinum therapy [67].

It has been observed that HSulf-1 expression is downregulated in ovarian cancer, which is partly mediated by epigenetic silencing and can be reversed by DAC treatment. The downregulation of HSulf-1 expression in OV167 and OV202 ovarian cancer cells leads to decreased response to cisplatin [68, 69]. Epigenetic silencing of annexin A11, CABIN1, and RASSF1 in ovarian cancer has been linked to chemoresistance [24, 70]. Platinum sensitive primary ovarian cancer is characterized by ASS1 overexpression. Downregulation of ASS1 by epigenetic silencing has been associated with the development of platinum-based chemoresistance in ovarian cancer [15, 16]. Overexpression of Enhancer of Zeste Homologue 2 (EZH2), a specific histone 3 lysine 27 (H3K27) methyltransferase has been associated with other cancer [71]. In ovarian cancer cells both in vitro and in tumor xenograft implants, it contributes to acquired cisplatin resistance [72].

LINE1 DNA hypomethylation has been reported as a prognostic factor for both overall and progression-free survival in mucinous ovarian cancers [73]. Polo-like kinase (Plk2) promoter methylation was associated with drug-resistant human EOC cell lines and a higher risk of relapse in patients treated postoperatively with carboplatin and paclitaxel [74].

There is evidence showing that intercellular adhesion molecule (ICAM)-1, which is epigenetically silenced in ovarian cancer, is associated with cisplatin sensitivity [75]. It also has been proposed that epigenetic changes may precede the increased expression and amplification of mdr1 (the multidrug resistance locus) sequences found in multidrug-resistant ovarian carcinoma cells [76].

Besides the study at specific loci, a genome-wide study performed on twenty advanced ovarian cancer samples by using Illumina HumanMethylation27 BeadChip revealed longer survival was associated with hypomethylation in some genes (e.g., GREB1, TGIF, and TOB1) and hypermethylation in some other genes (e.g., TMCO5, PTPRN, and GUCY2C) [77].

A very interesting example of pharmacoepigenomics in ovarian cancer, which shows the two aspects of pharmacoepigenomics study, is the methylation of the DNA mismatch repair (MMR) gene hMLH1. As aforementioned, high frequency of de novo promoter methylation in hMLH1 was detected by MSP in primary ovarian carcinoma

[12]. A study revealed that hMLH1 has a direct role in conferring cisplatin sensitivity when reintroduced into cells *in vitro* [78]. While this can be interpreted as how the interindividual epigenetic difference causes different responses to the same drug, another study is on the other hand demonstrating how the same drug treatment causes different epigenetic changes in patients: after chemotherapy, plasma DNA from patients with ovarian cancer showed acquisition of methylation of hMLH1. This acquisition of methylation of hMLH1 associated with poor prognosis [79].

Patients with different epigenomic modifications respond to the same treatment differently. Different sensitivities to the same chemotherapy may be resulted from specific epigenetic modifications affecting certain signaling pathways, for instance, the apoptosis cascade, which is critical to cancer cell survival. An example is BLU (ZMYND10) could upregulate the expression of BAX and enhance the effect of paclitaxel-induced apoptosis in ovarian cancer cells. Methylation of BLU disrupted the apoptosis and confers chemoresistance to ovarian cancer cells resulted in significantly shorter progression-free survival in patients [51]. The study of the docking protein 2 (DOK2), an adapter protein downstream of tyrosine kinase, is another example for how epigenetic deregulation of genes target chemotherapeutics-induced apoptosis and resulte in chemoresistance in ovarian cancer. DOK2 was identified by analyzing epigenomes of 45 ovarian samples. Loss of DOK2 decreased the level of apoptosis in response to carboplatin [52].

Besides genes affecting apoptosis, the ones related to angiogenesis can be epigenetically regulated and thus affect the recurrence of ovarian cancer as well. For example, it has been shown in both cultured ovarian cells and xenografts, the expression of the antiangiogenic genes TIMP3 and CDH1 (cadherin 1) can be regulated by promoter DNA methylation and histone methylation [53].

Genes in immune-related pathways can also be regulated epigenetically and therefore affect the prognosis. An example is hypomethylation of CpGs located in 6p21.3 in the R class is associated with cis upregulation of genes (TAP1, PSMB8, PSMB9, HLA-DQB1, HLA-DQB2, HLA-DMA, and HLA-DOA) enriched in immune response processes and with longer time to recurrence of high-grade serous epithelial ovarian cancer [80].

Developing a method using epigenetic features of ovarian cancer to predict platinum-free survival has been attempted [81]. By employing microarray, people have evaluated the predisposition of drug response by aberrant methylation in ovarian cancer. Consistent with many other studies have been discussed in this chapter earlier, the result from this microarray study indicates that the hypermethylation-induced loss of gene activity confers a predisposition in certain cancer types and is an early event in disease progression. Methylation profiles of ovarian cancer might be useful for early cancer detection and prediction of chemotherapy outcome in a clinical context [82].

In addition to DNA methylation and histone modification, the miRNAs have been reported associated with acquired chemoresistance in ovarian cancer [27, 28, 83–85]. Partially by targeting the 3′-UTR of CSF-1, downregulation of miR-130b, possibly through DNA methylation, promotes the development of multidrug resistant ovarian cancer [27]. The miR-152 and miR-185 have been reported to be able to target DNMT1 directly and thus co-contribute to ovarian cancer cells cisplatin sensitivity [83]. Another study shows that epigenetic silencing of miR-199b-5p is associated with acquired chemoresistance via activation of JAG1-Notch1 signaling in ovarian cancer [28]. By directly and negatively regulating Endoglin (ENG), miR-370 suppresses proliferation and promotes endometrioid ovarian cancer chemosensitivity to cDDP [85]. The miRNAs could be further explored as biomarkers of response and survival to therapy in ovarian cancer [84].

Of course, further studies are needed to clarify some controversies. For example, as it has been discussed earlier that, after chemotherapy, acquisition of methylation of hMLH1 was found in plasma DNA in patients with ovarian cancer [79]; however, in another study chemotherapy did not change promoter DNA methylation of MLH1, or another two genes: BRAC1 and FANCF. The researchers conducted the later study suggested that recurrent ovarian carcinomas commonly with increased BRCA1 and/or BRCA2 protein expression post chemotherapy exposure, which in turn could mediate resistance to platinum based therapies; however, alterations in expression of these proteins after chemotherapy are not commonly mediated by promoter methylation, and other regulatory mechanisms are likely to contribute to these alterations [86].

## Epigenetic Therapy Is a Promising Therapeutic Strategy for Treating Ovarian Cancers, in Particular, for Resensitizing Chemoresistant Ovarian Cancers

The preponderance evidence discussed above, supports aberrant epigenetic changes contribute to chemoresistance and recurrence of ovarian cancer. In contrast to genetic alterations, aberrant gene-repressive epigenetic modifications are more "plastic" and thus are potentially reversible by epigenetic therapies [11, 56, 87]. Therefore, using epigenetic therapies to reverse the aberrant epigenetic changes and resensitize chemoresistant ovarian cancers is emerging as a promising therapeutic strategy [58, 88].

Small interfering RNA (siRNA) has been explored as a tool to reactivate silenced tumor suppressor genes by using DNMTs targeting siRNAs to induce DNA hypomethylation [10]. A high level of YIN YANG 1 (YY1) enhanced taxane sensitivity in ovarian cancer [89].

### Histone Deacetylase (HDAC) Inhibitor Treatment

It has been reported that, in a variety of ovarian cancer cell lines, HDAC inhibitors (HDACIs) were able to inhibit cell growth, arrest cell cycle progression, induce apoptosis, and inhibit the expression of genes related to the malignancy [90]. In human ovarian carcinoma cells, treatments of HDACIs were able to induce the acetylation of the p21(WAF1) gene chromatin and increased the p21 in a dose-dependent manner in 2008/C13 cells [90, 91]. In xenograft models, some of HDACIs have demonstrated antitumor activity with few side effects. Some clinical trials indicate that HDACI are new mechanism-based therapeutics for ovarian cancer [90].

Class I HDAC-biased HDACIs have shown potent antitumor effects in preclinical models and therapeutic potential for ovarian cancer cells [2]. Preclinical studies show that class I biased HDAC inhibitor, romidepsin (FK228) and its two analogues, thailandepsin A (TDP-A) and thailandepsin B (TDP-B), induce DNA damage response, suppress cell viability, and induce apoptosis at nanomolar drug concentrations in four out of the five ovarian cancer cell lines [92].

Sorafenib, a multiple kinase inhibitor, has also been shown be able to alter the histone acetylation pattern. Clinical I, II, III trials using this drug have been conducted in ovarian cancer either alone or in combination with other chemotherapeutics. Although complete response was rarely observed, it has been proposed that due to clear cell ovarian cancer has different molecular characteristics from other ovarian cancers and is less sensitive to standard chemotherapy, sorafenib might work particularly well in treating clear cell ovarian cancer [6].

### DNA Demethylating Treatments

DNA methylation within CpG islands of the promoters of tumor suppressor genes plays a crucial role in drug-resistance development in ovarian cancers.

Demethylating agent zebularine [1-(beta-D-ribofuranosyl)-1,2-dihydropyrimidin-2-one] and DAC were used to treat ovarian cancer cell lines Hey, A2780, and the cisplatin-resistant A2780/CP. Zebularine significantly induced demethylation of the tumor suppressors RASSF1A and hMLH1. Both Zebularine and DAC demethylated DNA globally in a similar way with differences at specific loci [40].

EGFR inhibitor PD153035 has been shown be able to stimulate expression of RAR-β, which was epigenetically silenced via DNA hypermethylation in OVCAR-3 ovarian carcinoma cells. Reactivation of RAR-β by PD153035 was associated with demethylation of the RAR-β2 gene promoter P2 as demonstrated by MSP [18].

### Combination Therapy Using Epigenetic Therapeutics and Chemotherapeutics

Although using epigenetic therapies alone has rarely shown activity against solid tumors, including ovarian cancer, preclinical studies suggest that when epigenetic therapies are used in combination with one another or with conventional chemotherapeutics, improved antitumor activity may be achieved. Thus, combinatorial epigenetic therapy regiments are being examined in cancer clinical trials [87].

The rationale of using combination therapy of DNMT inhibitors and HDAC inhibitors in ovarian cancer was supported by a study using quantitative real-time reverse transcription polymerase chain reaction (qRT-PCR) and immunohistochemical staining to examine the mRNA and protein expression in 22 cases of ovarian cancer and 8 normal ovaries. This study revealed that: (1) DNMT1, DNMT3b and class I HDACs were increased in ovarian cancers, while the expression of DNMT3a was not different between cancer tissues and normal ovaries; (2) Comparing with stage I/II ovarian carcinomas, DNMT1, DNMT3b, HDAC1, and HDAC2 were significantly higher in advanced tumors (stage III/IV); (3) Expression of HDAC2 was positively correlated with HDCA1, HDAC3, and HDAC8, DNMT1 was positively correlated with DNMT3b, and DNMT3b was correlated with HDAC1 and HDAC2 [93].

HDAC inhibitor valproic acid (VPA), in combination with Aurora kinase inhibitors, has shown promising results for a more effective therapy of ovarian cancer. In an investigation, VPA and the Aurora kinase inhibitor VE465 were used to treat four ovarian cancer cell lines (2008/C13, OVCAR3, SKOV3, and A2780VPA). Enhanced cytotoxic effects were observed in three (2008/C13, A2780, and OVCAR3) of the four cell lines. Co-treatment with VPA (2 mM) and VE465 (1 μM) induced more apoptosis in 2008/C13 cells than monotreatment [91].

Combination therapy using epidermal growth factor receptor (EGFR) inhibitor, erlotinib, and AZA has been used to treat advanced ovarian cancer in a phase I clinical trial, in the hope the epigenetic therapeutic would enhance the antiproliferative effect of erlotinib. Partial response was observed [39].

Combination treatments using trichostatin A (TSA) and DAC was conducted on human ovarian cancer cell lines. Combination treatment had greater efficacy than single drugs [46].

Different ovarian cancer cell lines (SKOV3 and HEY) have different status of estrogen receptor (ER) beta promoter methylation. DAC and the histone deacetylase (HDAC) inhibitor, trichostatin (TSA) were found be able to inhibit ovarian cancer cell growth [94].

In the same kind of cell lines, another study using DAC in combination with another HDAC inhibitor (suberoylanilide hydroxamic acid [SAHA]) synergistically inhibit Hey and SKOv3 cell growth by apoptosis and cell cycle arrest, and reactivate expression of imprinted tumor suppressor genes ARHI and PEG3 (paternally expressed 3) in both cultured cells and in xenografts, correlating with growth inhibition. DAC treatment induced autophagy in Hey cells that was enhanced by SAHA [38].

### Combination Therapy to Overcome Drug Resistance

As it has been discussed, epigenetic modifications contribute to the development of drug resistance in the ovarian cancer. Thus, it is logic to think epigenetic therapy may reverse the "plastic" epigenetic modifications and resensitize ovarian tumors to conventional chemotherapeutics [95, 96].

Zebularine could resensitize the drug-resistant cell line A2780/CP to cisplatin, with a 16-fold reduction in the $IC_{50}$ of that conventional agent [40].

Combination treatments using trichostatin A (TSA) and DAC with low-dose cisplatin was conducted on human ovarian cancer cell lines. The epigenetic drugs potentiate the anticancer efficacy of low-dose cisplatin through regulation of EMT and pluripotency [46].

A study enrolled 17 patients with platinum resistant ovarian cancer showed that combination therapy with DAC and carboplatin resensitized chemoresistant ovarian cancer to platinum [97].

In ovarian cancer cell lines and animal models, epigenetic therapeutic agents have been shown to enhance gene expression and drug sensitivity.

Phase I trial of DAC has completed in ovarian cancer [96]. A phase II clinical trial showed that low-dose DAC altered DNA methylation of genes and cancer pathways, which restored sensitivity to carboplatin in patients with heavily pretreated ovarian cancer and resulted in higher response rate (RR) and longer progression-free survival (PFS) [98].

The results of a phase II study reported in 2007 and involved seven patients with refractory ovarian cancer support the claim that the epigenetic therapy with hydralazine and magnesium valproate overcomes chemotherapy resistance [99].

After combination treatment of AZA, VPA, and carboplatin, minor responses or stable disease lasting ≥4 months were achieved by three patients with platinum-resistant or platinum-refractory ovarian cancer. The combination treatment also induced death receptor 4 (DR4) methylation decrease in a subset of patients, but which was not related to tumor response or number of cycles received [100].

Loss of RASSF1A expression has been observed strongly correlated with the development of Taxol resistance in primary ovarian cancer samples. It has been reported after using a combination of small molecule inhibitors of DNMTs, RASSF1A expression and Taxol sensitivity were restored [41].

In OVCAR-3 and MDAH-2774 ovarian cancer cells, combination treatment using AT-101 and cisplatin, inhibited both DNMT and HDAC activities, overcame chemoresistance by inducing apoptosis [101].

Beside siRNA can be used to target DNMTs and reactivates silenced tumor suppressor genes [10], lentivirus-mediated RNAi silencing targeting excision repair cross-complementing gene 1 (ERCC1) reversed cisplatin resistance in cisplatin-resistant ovarian carcinoma cell line [102].

## Pharmacovigilance in Ovarian Cancer

There are reports indicating epigenetic therapies may have little side effects. One report is for the study in xenograft models, some of HDACIs have demonstrated antitumor activity with only few side effects [90]. Also, a phase I clinical trial showed that combination treatment of erlotinib and AZA was well tolerated in ovarian cancer patients [39].

However, the clinical trials investigating Sorafenib (a multiple kinase inhibitor with histone acetylation altering ability) in ovarian cancer revealed that adverse effects occurred frequently, including rash, diarrhea, edema, and weight gain [6].

People have to realize that when applying epigenetic therapies, under certain situations, it may be complex. For instance, although DNA demethylating reagent, such as DAC, is able to activate the expression of promoter-DNA-methylation-silenced tumor suppressor genes, it may also activate some oncogenes, such as IFITM1 [3].

Besides, promoter DNA hypomethylation, histone acetylation may activate putative oncogenes [33, 34]. Expression of ABCG2, a member of ATP binding cassette (ABC) transporters, has been linked to multidrug resistance (MDR) in ovarian cancer cell line (IGROV-1). Interestingly, ABCG2 can be upregulated by histone hyperacetylation. Thus, HDAC inhibitors may lead to MDR development in some ovarian cancer cell lines [103].

So, epigenetic therapeutics used to treat ovarian cancers may also cause side effects due to unwanted oncogene activations. This should be taken as a precaution when carrying on preclinical studies and clinical trials. However, as discussed thoroughly earlier and being supported by many studies, particularly in ovarian cancer, using epigenetic therapies in combination with chemotherapies is a very promising strategy to overcome chemoresistance and improve antitumor efficacy of conventional drugs. More efforts on looking for epigenetic therapies more specifically targeting tumor suppressors for DNA demethylation and histone acetylation are needed.

## Pharmacoepigenomics and Pharmacovigilance in Cervical Cancer

Every year, there are about 500,000 cervical cancer cases are diagnosed worldwide [104]. According to SEER cancer statistics fact sheets, in 2015, it is estimated that there will be 12,900 new cases diagnosed in the USA [105]. The standard treatment of advanced cervical cancers (International Federation of Gynecology and Obstetrics staging system (IFGO) starting from stage IIB) is combined radiotherapy with concomitant chemotherapy [104].

Human papilloma virus (HPV) infection is the major cause of cervical cancer development [105]. It can cause genomic instability, affect immune system and also induce DNA methylation changes in host cells. In fact, it may cause many epigenetic changes in the cervical precancerous lesions, which strongly indicate it is the causative agent for cervical cancer.

## Pharmacoepigenomics in Cervical Cancer

Epigenetic changes in cervical cancer and precancerous lesions have been reported during all stages of cervical carcinogenesis in both human papillomavirus and host cellular genomes [106–108]. These epigenetic changes, including global DNA hypomethylation, hypermethylation of key tumor suppressor genes, and histone modifications, are clinical relevant. For example, tumor suppressor genes: retinoic acid receptor-β (RARβ), cadherin 1 (CDH1), death-associated protein kinase-1 (DAPK1), and GSTP1 have been reported can be silenced by promoter DNA hypermethylation in cervical cancers [109–112]. Furthermore, a study identified a high frequency of promoter hypermethylation in the Slit-Robo pathway genes (SLIT1, SLIT2, SLIT3, ROBO1, and ROBO3 genes). The Slit family of secreted proteins modulates chemokine-induced cell migration of distinct somatic cell types. Slit genes mediate their effect by binding to its receptor Roundabout (Robo). The promoter hypermethylation of these genes occurs early in tumor progression and results in gene expression downregulation in invasive cervical cancer [113]. In addition, there are reports that aberrant HDAC activity and the resulted histone hypoacetylation, are associated with cervical cancer development [114, 115]. Additionally, a few epigenetic modifications of IFN-γ gene, increasing IFN-γ expression in Th1 lymphocytes and reducing IFN-γ expression in Th2 lymphocytes, have been described and may appear to confer a susceptibility to cervical cancer [116]. These aberrant epigenetic changes can be used in early cervical screening, diagnosis, and management of cervical precancerous lesions and cancers [106–108]. For instance, as has been reported, epigenetic changes were able to distinguish early from advanced transforming cervical intraepithelial neoplasia (CIN) lesions [108]. And the aforementioned promoter methylation of Slit-Robo genes could be an epigenetic signature to identify precancerous lesions at risk to progress to cervical cancer [113]. Interestingly, a potential chemotherapeutic agent in cervical cancer, plant alkaloid berberine, was thought to be able to bind to DNA and may contribute to epigenetic modifications [117].

### Tumor Suppressor Epigenetically Silenced in Cervical Cancer

Silencing by DNA methylation of tumor suppressor gene GADD45G, adenomatous polyposis coli (APC), and tumor suppressor in lung cancer 1 (TSLC1), has been detected in some cervical cancer cell lines, which could be reversed by either DAC treatment, genetic double knockout of DNMT1 and DNMT3B, or other DNMT1 inhibitors [118, 119].

Recently, it has been reported that the cell adhesion molecule 1 (CADM1), a tumor suppressor, is downregulated in human papillomavirus (HPV)-infected cervical cancer cell lines via its hypermethylation. Demethylation using DAC reactivated the expression of CADM1 protein [120].

Besides the epigenetic silencing by DNA methylation, it has been reported that the tumor suppressor genes, RARβ2, E-cadherin, p21 (CIP1), and p53, could be epigenetically silenced through histone deacetylation, which is important for cervical carcinogenesis [109, 110, 121].

### Epigenetic Change Predicts the Prognosis After Chemoradiotherapy

A study using methylation-specific multiplex ligation-dependent probe amplification (MS-MLPA) showed promoter hypermethylation in the XRCC2 gene was significantly associated with occurrence of late grade III–IV toxicity in cervical cancer patients treated by chemoradiotherapy [104].

Unmethylated MYOD1, unmethylated ESR1, methylated hTERT promoter, and lower ESR1 transcript levels could predict chemoradiation resistance in locally advanced invasive cervical carcinoma (IFGO IIB/III) patients treated with standard chemoradiation therapy [122].

Epigenetic inactivation of TRAIL decoy receptors in cervical cancer cell lines effectively activate downstream caspases and extrinsic apoptotic pathway, suggesting decoy receptor gene inactivation may be used as a biomarker of response to Apo2L/TRAIL-combination therapy [123].

In addition, the epigenetic regulation of p73 expression via DNA methylation was investigated in 103 cervical cancers and 124 normal cervices. Hypermethylation of p73 gene was observed in 38.8 % of cervical cancers and significantly associated with reduced or absent p73 expression. Because p73 expresses in samples that are sensitive to radiotherapy and overexpression of p73 predicted a better prognosis in cervical cancer patients [124], hypermethylation of p73 in cervical cancer may be used as a marker for poor prognosis.

## Epigenetic Monotherapy

### Epigenetic Therapy Using DNMT Inhibitors in Treating Cervical Cancer

In human cervical cancer cell lines, HeLa and CaSki, trichosanthin (TSC, a component isolated from a Chinese medicinal herb) decreased expression of DNMT1, reduced DNMT1 enzyme activity, induced demethylation, and reactivated expression of APC and TSLC1, two tumor suppressor genes silenced by methylation [119].

### Epigenetic Therapy Using HDAC Inhibitors to Treat Cervical Cancer

As mentioned previously, aberrant HDAC activity and resulted histone hypoacetylation, have been associated with cervical cancer development [114, 115]. Based on the logic to use HDAC inhibitors (HDACIs) to reverse the aberrant HDAC activity, HDACIs have been used to treat a variety of cervical cancer cell lines, xenograft tumors, and patients enrolled in colonial trials. HDACIs exhibited antitumor abilities, including inhibiting cell growth, arresting cell cycle progression, inducing apoptosis, and may be cervical cancer cell differentiation in these studies. In addition, in the xenograft model and a Phase I study, limited side effects were observed [109, 110, 114, 115, 125].

In a phase I study, HDAC activity was inhibited and histones were hyperacetylated in cervical tumor tissues from patients, who had been newly diagnosed with cervical cancer and taken 20 and 40 mg/kg magnesium valproate orally [114].

It has been widely reported that HDACIs could induce apoptosis in cervical cancer cell lines, such as Hela and Caski [125]. The mechanism of inducing apoptosis in cervical cancer cell lines, but not in normal human keratinocyte line HaCaT, could be TSA, a HDACi, could downregulate DNMT3B in cervical cancer cells but not in the normal cells [125]. This raises an interesting question as whether or not de novo DNA methylation is required by cervical cancer cell survival.

## Combination Therapy

### Combination Therapy Using Both HDACIs and DNMTIs

In addition to using HDACIs alone to treat cervical cancer, combination therapies using other drugs together with HDACIs have been explored [91, 109, 110].

A group of Mexican scientists have conducted a series of studies of using HDACIs and DNMTIs in combination to treat cervical cancers [126–130]. By using microarray analysis, they compared the transcriptional profiles of ten pairs of pre- and post-treatment cervical tumors, and found that combination therapy using both a DNMTI (hydralazine) and a HDACI (magnesium valproate) reactivated genes and enhanced protein acetylation in primary cervical tumors. The 964 genes being upregulated are involved in ribosome protein, the oxidative phosphorylation, MAPK signaling, as well as other pathways. It was thought the pathways are related to energy production and may promote apoptosis [126]. In a double-blind, placebo-controlled, randomized phase III trial for advanced cervical cancer, the same group of researchers investigated the advantage of using hydralazine (DNMTI) and valproate (HDACI) (HV) in combination with chemotherapy (cisplatin topotecan, CT). There were 36 patients (17 CT+HV and 19 CT+placebo) were enrolled. Epigenetic therapy began 1 week before the chemotherapy. The median progression-free survival was statistically different as 6 months for CT+placebo and 10 months for CT+HV. This preliminary study indicates that epigenetic therapy in combination with chemotherapy has significant advantage over one of the current standard chemotherapies in cervical cancer in terms of progression-free survival [129].

Another group of scientists performed a study in Hela cells showed that a green tea catechin, (−)-epigallocatechin-3-gallate (EGCG), was able to inhibit both DNMT and HDAC enzymatic activities, and reduce the expression of DNMT3B. By inducing hypomethylation at the promoter DNA, EGCG activated the expression of tumor suppressor genes: retinoic acid receptor-β (RARβ), cadherin 1 (CDH1) and death-associated protein kinase-1 (DAPK1) [111]. In another study, this group of scientists investigated the epigenetic effects of sulforaphane in Hela cells. They found that sulforaphane was able to inhibit both the enzymatic activity and the expression of DNMT3B and HDAC1. This is slightly different from the effect of EGCG, which only reduced the expression of DNMT3B, but not HDAC1. Furthermore, similarly to what they found in the study of EGCG, they observed the reactivation of tumor suppressor genes: RARβ, CDH1, DAPK1, and GSTP1, after treatment of sulforaphane [112].

#### Combination Therapy Using HDACIs with Inhibitors Other Than DNMTIs

A study using VPA and ATRA (all-trans retinoic acid, a retinoid selective for tumor suppressor RARβ2), could reactivate expression of histone-deacetylation-silenced RARβ2. The expression of RARβ2 was upregulated 50–90 folds in cervical cancer cells by this combination treatment. There is an additive effect both in vitro and in vivo of combining these two drugs together. Significant upregulation of p21(CIP1) and p53 as well as a pronounced decrease in p-Stat3 was observed. More interestingly, instead of inducing apoptosis, this combination therapy mainly induced differentiation in cervical cancer cells through PI3K/Akt pathway [109]. Very similar results have been reported in another study conducted by this group of scientists. This time, instead of using only VPA, SAHA was also used in combination with ATRA. Upregulation of RARβ2 was also observed which might be resulted from acetylation of histones in the RARβ2-RARE promoter region. In a xenograft model, VPA could restore RARβ2 expression via epigenetic modulation, and showed additive antitumor effect when it was used with ATRA. Differentiation of cervical cells, reactivation of RARβ2, E-cadherin, p21 (CIP1), and p53 and reduced the level of p-Stat3 were also observed [110].

It has also been reported that combined treatment using VPA and the aurora kinase inhibitor VE465 enhanced cytotoxic effects in a cervical cell line, ME180 [91].

#### Epigenetic Therapy to Reverse Drug-resistance

In cervical cancer, epigenetic changes, in particular DNA methylation changes have been shown to be responsible for drug resistance. It has been shown by a methylation specific microarray that oxaliplatin-resistant cervical cancer cell S3 has methylation changes both genome-wide and within individual loci compared with its parental cell line SiHa. S3 treated by DNA demethylating agent restored the sensitivity of S3 cells to cisplatin, taxol, and oxaliplatin to the same level as that of SiHa. Methylation of gene Casp8AP2 was shown be sufficient to increase drug resistance [131].

In a gemcitabine-resistant cervical cancer cell line (CaLoGR), downregulation of hENT1 and dCK genes was observed not associated with promoter methylation. Treatment with hydralazine reversed gemcitabine resistance and led to hENT1 and dCK gene reactivation, which is independent of DNA promoter methylation or histone acetylation at these promoters, but through inhibition of G9A histone methyltransferase [128].

Cisplatin resistance caused by overexpression of multi drug resistant proteins MRP1 and Pgp1 in SiHa-derived cervical cancer cell line SiHaR could be overcome by curcumin. Curcumin treatment could inhibit HDACs and HPV expression, and differentially increase acetylation and upregulation of p53, pRb, p21, and p27, in both SiHa and SiHaR, leading to cell cycle arrest at G1/S phase. Using curcumin could also lower the chemotherapeutic dose of cisplatin [132].

Radiosensitization of SiHa cervical cancer cell line could be increased by treatment with hydralazine in combination with valproic acid. This effect can be further increased by adding cisplatin [133].

### Epigenetic Therapy of Cervical Cancer in the Future

In the future, along with further understanding of the epigenetic regulations of many other genes, more epigenetic therapies may be developed. For example, ASXL1, ASXL2, and ASXL3 are epigenetic scaffolds for BAP1, EZH2, NCOA1, nuclear receptors, and WTIP. It has been observed that copy number gains of ASXL1 occur in cervical cancer. The cell context-dependent epigenetic code of ASXLs should be deciphered to develop therapeutics for cervical cancer [134].

In addition to understanding more about the epigenetic regulation of some genes, more tools and technologies will be available for epigenetic therapy. For instance, the RNA-guided nuclease CRISPR-Cas9 (clustered regularly interspaced short palindromic repeats-CRISPR associated nuclease 9) and its variants such as nickase Cas9, dead Cas9, guide RNA scaffolds and RNA-targeting Cas9 are convenient and versatile platforms for site-specific epigenomic modulations. Epigenetic modifications of cancer microenvironment with CRISPR-Cas9 systems for therapeutic purposes represent a promising area in cervical cancer research [135].

## Pharmacovigilance in Cervical Cancer

HPV infection is the major cause of cervical cancer. Due to the availability of anti-HPV vaccine since about a decade ago, the infection rate of HPV is declining. Beside, different from ovarian cancer, which lacks efficient means for early diagnosis, early diagnosis of cervical cancer can be achieved by routine Pap test/smear. The availability of early diagnosis of cervical cancer contributes to a lower mortality rate than ovarian cancer.

Although DNA demethylating agents can reactivate tumor suppressors silenced by DNA methylation, there is a possibility that they may also activate HPV oncoproteins, as comparing HPV genome methylation in pre-invasive and invasive cervical lesions suggesting that neoplastic transformation can be suppressed by gene hypermethylation. Thus, epigenetic therapy may have the risk to promote cancer progression by enhancing HPV oncoprotien expression in cervical cancer [121].

In a study testing hydralazine and valproate either alone or in combination on cervical cancer cell lines. The expression of HPV oncoprotein E6/E7 was upregulated correlating with DNA hypomethylation and histone acetylation at the long control region (LCR). Fortunately, in the majority of patients with cervical cancer, treatment with hydralazine, valproate, or both did not enhance the expression of E6/E7 [121]. Thus, it seems hydralazine and valproate can be safely administered to patients with cervical cancer.

Hydralazine and valproate were also shown being well-tolerated and safe when administered with cisplatin chemoradiation as supported by the results of a clinical trial performed in IFGO Stage IIIB patients [130].

In fact, not only in cervical cancer, but also in other cancers, hydralazine (DNMTI) and valproate (HDACI) have been tested are safe to be used alone or in combination with chemotherapy or chemoradiation [127].

Using MSP, a study investigated the promoter methylation of the mitotic checkpoint gene CHFR (checkpoint with forkhead and ring finger) in both cervical cancer specimens and cell lines. Aberrant methylation of CHFR was detected in 12.3 % (2/14) of adenocarcinoma specimens but not in normal cervical cells or squamous cell carcinoma cells. Out of 6 of human cervical carcinoma cell lines, SKG-IIIb and HeLa cells had aberrant methylation of CHFR and showed high sensitivity to taxanes, but became taxane-resistant upon treatment with DAC. Moreover, suppression of CHFR expression in siRNA-transfected SKG-IIIa cells caused increased sensitivity to taxanes [136]. All of these indicate that promoter DNA methylation caused silencing of CHFR increased sensitivity to treatment of taxanes. Thus, DNA hypomethylating reagent, such as DAC, may make it worse for treating the cervical cancer patients with hypermethylated CHFR.

The Werner (WRN) gene encodes a DNA helicase contributing to genomic stability. Aberrant DNA hypermethylation and decreased expression of WRN were detected in 7/21 cases of primary cervical cancer and in 2/6 cervical cancer cell lines. These two cell lines showed high sensitivity to a topoisomerase I inhibitor, CPT-11, but became resistant to CPT-11 after treatment with DAC. It indicates that aberrant DNA hypermethylation of WRN increased the sensitivity of cervical cancer cells to CPT-11 [137]. So inappropriate using DNA demathylating agent in cervical cancer cells with methylated Werner gene will increase drug resistance to CPT-11 and cause adverse prognosis.

Besides epigenetic therapies may activate unwanted oncogenes, paradoxically, they may also activate some genes, which are traditionally thought as tumor suppressors and silenced epigenetically, but indeed whose activities are harmful in cervical cancer. It has been reported that paradoxically tumor suppressor p16(INK4A) is necessary for survival of cervical carcinoma cell lines, although its activity has been epigenetically silenced in many tumors p16(INK4A) [138].

Another example may further showcase how complex cancer is, and epigenetic inactivation and therapies can be. As it has been discussed earlier, some genes in Slit-Robo pathway are epigenetically silenced in invasive cervical cancer; however, the inhibitors of DNA methylation and HDACs failed to effectively reactivate the downregulated expression of Slit-Robo genes in cervical cancer cell lines [113].

## Pharmacoepigenomics and Pharmacovigilance in Uterine Cancer

Uterine cancers include uterine sarcomas and endometrial carcinomas. Uterine sarcomas only consist about 3–7 % of malignant uterine tumors [139]. According to reports from American Cancer Society, most of the endometrial carcinomas are endometrioid adenocarcinoma (endometrioid-type endometrial cancer). There are uterine carcinosarcomas as well. Endometrial cancer is the seventh most common cancer worldwide among women and is the most common gynecological cancer affecting women [140–142]. Follows ovarian cancer, it is the second-most fatal gynecologic cancer [4]. According to American Cancer Society, in the USA in 2015, it estimated that there would be 54,870 new cases of cancer of uterine body with 10,170 deaths. Type II endometrial carcinoma is often poorly differentiated. Patients diagnosed with Type II disease (~11 %) are disproportionately represented in annual endometrial cancer deaths (48 %) [142]. For most women, surgery is the main method of treatment for endometrial cancer, with radiotherapy and chemotherapy as subsidiary treatments. In addition, hormone (progestin-based) therapy has proven be effective in a subset of patients, particularly in patients with progesterone receptor (PR) expression [143].

## Pharmacoepigenomics in Uterine Cancer

### Epigenetic Changes in Uterine Cancer Contribute to Carcinogenesis and Responses to Treatments

Some cases of endometrial cancer may be hereditary. For instance, patients with Lynch syndrome, which is a hereditary disease, have a higher risk for developing endometrial cancer than the general population [141]. However, epigenetic effects, such as silencing of genes by DNA hypermethylation, hereditary epimutation of DNA mismatch repair genes, and regulation of gene expression by miRNAs, also play roles in carcinogenesis of endometrial cancer [141].

Similar to what have been discussed in ovarian cancer and cervical cancer, there are genes are silenced through hypermethylation in endometrial cancer [144]. BRCA1 expression can also be a biomarker of chemosensitivity response and prognosis in uterine cancer in addition to ovarian cancer [145]; epigenetic inactivation of hMLH1, CDKN2A, and MGMT may be a common and early event in the development of synchronous primary endometrial cancer [12]; and frequent epigenetic silencing of tumor suppressor genes PTEN and progesterone receptor were also reported in uterine cancer [146]. It has also been known that endometrial cancer has overexpression of HDAC and DNMT enzymes [146]. In endometrial cancer, HAND2 DNA methylation has been reported as a common and crucial molecular alteration that could potentially be employed as a biomarker for early detection of endometrial cancer and as a predictor of treatment response [147]. Promoter DNA hypomethylation signatures of candidate bone morphogenetic protein (BMP) genes, which is associated with EpCAM-mediated expression, may be used as biomarkers to predict poor survival in endometrial cancer [148]. There are also efforts for looking for new candidate biomarkers for endometrial cancer include those for molecular epigenetic mutations, such as miRNAs [149]. In endometrial cancer, miRNAs are associated with regulation of epigenetic dysfunction and carcinogenesis and may be explored as biomarkers for endometrial cancer diagnosis and prognosis [150]. PHC3, a polycomb group gene (PcG) member and an epigenetic effector, may be of worth to be explored as a biomarker for predicting poorer prognosis in uterine carcinomas [151].

Recent advances in research have shown that DNA methylation-based assays may be a useful in diagnosing uterine cancer. Epigenetic modification agents, including inhibitors for DNA methyltransferases and histone deacetylases, may be used alone or in combination with conventional chemotherapy to treat endometrial cancer. Epigenetic reactivation of the progesterone receptor provides a novel approach for resensitization of advanced, PR-negative endometrial cancers to progestin-based therapy [152]. New therapies include targeting epigenetic changes using histone deacetylase inhibitors and noncoding microRNA, have been explored [91, 139, 141, 146, 153, 154].

### Epigenetic Monotherapy and Combination Therapy

Although it is rarely reported, epigenetic monotherapy has been explored. For instance, HCI2509, a lysine specific demethylase 1 (LSD1) inhibitor, was used to treat two poorly differentiated Type II endometrial cancer cell lines, AN3CA and KLE, and demonstrated anticancer properties. HCI2509 showed single-agent efficacy in orthotopic xenograft studies as well [142].

Using cell lines representing different stages of endometrioid cancers, effects of DAC and TSA on cell cycle and apoptosis were examined. DAC and TSA exhibited strong cytostatic and apoptotic effects in endometrial cancer cell lines, and a strong synergy has been observed by using the tow inhibitors together [155].

Previously, we discussed that combination treatment using both HDAC inhibitor valproic acid and aurora kinase inhibitor VE465 to enhance the cytotoxicity in ovarian cancer cell lines. In fact, this combination therapy also enhanced cytotoxicity in endometrial cancer cell line HEC-1B [91].

Treated endometrial sarcoma cell lines, ESS-1 and MES-SA, with the tumor necrosis factor-related apoptosis-inducing ligand (TRAIL/Apo-2L) combined with HDAC inhibitor SAHA induced apoptosis by reactivating epigenetic silenced genes that are involved in the intrinsic apoptotic pathway. DAC treatment induced promoter DNA hypomethylation and reactivated expression of caspase-8 and DR 4/TRAIL-R1 in ESS-1 and MES-SA cells, respectively, and increased the sensitivity of both cell lines against TRAIL-induced apoptosis [139].

### Epigenetic Approach to Revive Hormonal Therapy

Because the expression of progesterone receptors has been shown to be upregulated and downregulated by various epigenetic mechanisms [156], the epigenetic therapy may be beneficial and should be considered when choosing hormone therapy for patients.

The progesterone receptor (PR) gene is transcribed from one gene by two alternative promoters and translated into PR-B, a potent transcriptional activator, and PR-A, the shorter isoform, necessary to oppose the effects of PR-B [156]. Because PR-B gene expression is regulated by epigenetic factors including DNA methylation [157, 158], MBD (methyl-CpG-binding domain) binding [157], histone modifications [157, 158], MeCP2 (methyl-CpG-binding protein 2) occupancy [157], as well as miRNAs [158], epigenetic reactivation of PR-B could be a potential strategy to sensitize the PR-B-negative endometrial cancers to progestational therapy [157, 158].

People have described approaches to restore expression of PR at the epigenetic level in endometrial cancer, which is believed to reestablish PR expression and resensitize endometrial tumors to progestin therapy [143, 154, 159]. The PR-B negative endometrioid cancer cell lines KLE and HEC-1B treated by DAC and TSA revealed that epigenetically silenced PR-B gene remains sensitive to changes in DNA demethylation and histone acetylation. Treatment with DAC and/or TSA results in a robust and sustainable PR-B upregulation [159]. In addition, it has been reported that in Type I endometrial cancer cells with low basal PR, LBH589, an HDAC inhibitor, induced a profound upregulation of PR mRNA and restored PR protein expression even in the presence of progesterone. The restored PR in turn upregulated FoxO1, p21, and p27 and downregulated cyclin D1 in a ligand-dependent manner and induced cell cycle arrest in G1 that was further augmented by progesterone [154]. These studies suggest that reestablishing PR expression by epigenetic modulators can resensitize endometrial tumors to progestin therapy and enhance the efficacy of hormonal therapy for endometrial cancer.

The efforts that have been discussed above are focused on targeting PR expression in tumors; however, a very exciting research provided strong support that through epigenetic derepression to reactivate PR expression in the stroma, the tumor environment, is sufficient for resensitize hormone-refractory tumors to progesterone therapy [160].

## Pharmacovigilance in Uterine Cancer

Similar to what have been discussed for ovarian and cervical cancers, application of epigenetic agents may reactivate silenced oncogenes as well. For instance, since promoter DNA hypomethylation of candidate BMP genes is associated with poor survival in endometrial cancer [148], using DNA demethylating agent should be weighted for its benefits and risks first, as it may induce promoter DNA hypomethylation of candidate BMP genes.

Therefore, personalized epigenetic therapy based on a patient's epigenomic background is more ideal and should be recommended.

## Pharmacoepigenomics and Pharmacovigilance in Other Gynecological Cancers

Mainly due to the rareness of the cases of vaginal cancer, vulval cancer, and fallopian tube cancer, the studies of pharmacoepigenomics and pharmacovigilance in these cancers are few and just emerged [161, 162]. Epigenetic alterations affect the carcinogenesis of these cancers as well [161, 162]. For instance, diethylstilboestrol (DES), an endocrine disrupter, may have acted as an obesogen, can cause epigenetic alterations. Vaginal clear cell adenocarcinoma may develop in some of the daughters of the women who have been treated with DES [162]. Similar to what has been discussed in ovarian cancer, cervical cancer, and uterine cancer, different patients may response differently to the same drug treatment due to different epigenetic aberrances present in their tumors. More studies of pharmacoepigenomics and pharmacovigilance are needed in these cancers to make personalized treatments possible, improve therapeutic efficacy, and reduce mortality.

## References

1. Paige AJW, Brown R. Pharmaco(epi)genomics in ovarian cancer. Pharmacogenomics. 2008;9(12):1825–34.
2. Khabele D. The therapeutic potential of class I selective histone deacetylase inhibitors in ovarian cancer. Front Oncol. 2014;4:111.

3. Kim NH, Sung HY, Choi EN, Lyu D, Choi HJ, Ju W, et al. Aberrant DNA methylation in the IFITM1 promoter enhances the metastatic phenotype in an intraperitoneal xenograft model of human ovarian cancer. Oncol Rep. 2014;31(5):2139–46.
4. Balch C, Matei DE, Huang THM, Nephew KP. Role of epigenomics in ovarian and endometrial cancers. Epigenomics. 2010;2(3):419–47.
5. Gloss BS, Samimi G. Epigenetic biomarkers in epithelial ovarian cancer. Cancer Lett. 2014; 342(2):257–63.
6. Smolle E, Taucher V, Petru E, Haybaeck J. Targeted treatment of ovarian cancer – the multiple – kinase – inhibitor sorafenib as a potential option. Anticancer Res. 2014;34(4):1519–30.
7. Institute NC. Ovary Cancer. SEER cancer statistics factsheets 2005–2011.
8. Bast Jr RC, Mills GB. Alterations in oncogenes, tumor suppressor genes, and growth factors associated with epithelial ovarian cancers. Methods Mol Med. 2001;39:37–48.
9. Barton CA, Hacker NF, Clark SJ, O'Brien PA. DNA methylation changes in ovarian cancer: implications for early diagnosis, prognosis and treatment. Gynecol Oncol. 2008;109(1):129–39.
10. Leu Y-W, Rahmatpanah F, Shi H, Wei SH, Liu JC, Yan PS, et al. Double RNA interference of DNMT3b and DNMT1 enhances DNA demethylation and gene reactivation. Cancer Res. 2003;63(19):6110–5.
11. Koukoura O, Spandidos DA, Daponte A, Sifakis S. DNA methylation profiles in ovarian cancer: Implication in diagnosis and therapy (Review). Mol Med Rep. 2014;10(1):3–9.
12. Furlan D, Carnevali I, Marcomini B, Cerutti R, Dainese E, Capella C, et al. The high frequency of de novo promoter methylation in synchronous primary endometrial and ovarian carcinomas. Clin Cancer Res. 2006;12(11):3329–36.
13. Kolasa IK, Rembiszewska A, Janiec-Jankowska A, Dansonka-Mieszkowska A, Lewandowska AM, Konopka B, et al. PTEN mutation, expression and LOH at its locus in ovarian carcinomas. Relation to TP53, K-RAS and BRCA1 mutations. Gynecol Oncol. 2006;103(2):692–7.
14. Socha MJ, Said N, Dai YS, Kwong J, Ramalingan P, Trieu V, et al. Aberrant promoter methylation of SPARC in ovarian cancer. Neoplasia. 2009;11(2): 126-U37.
15. Delage B, Fennell DA, Nicholson L, McNeish I, Lemoine NR, Crook T, et al. Arginine deprivation and argininosuccinate synthetase expression in the treatment of cancer. Int J Cancer. 2010;126(12): 2762–72.
16. Nicholson LJ, Smith PR, Hiller L, Szlosarek PW, Kimberley C, Sehouli J, et al. Epigenetic silencing of argininosuccinate synthetase confers resistance to platinum-induced cell death but collateral sensitivity to arginine auxotrophy in ovarian cancer. Int J Cancer. 2009;125(6):1454–63.
17. Kamikihara T, Arima T, Kato K, Matsuda T, Kato H, Douchi T, et al. Epigenetic silencing of the imprinted gene ZAC by DNA methylation is an early event in the progression of human ovarian cancer. Int J Cancer. 2005;115(5):690–700.
18. Grunt TW, Puckmair K, Tomek K, Kainz B, Gaiger A. An EGF receptor inhibitor induces RAR-beta expression in breast and ovarian cancer cells. Biochem Biophys Res Commun. 2005;329(4):1253–9.
19. Sabatino MA, Marabese M, Ganzinelli M, Caiola E, Geroni C, Broggini M. Down-regulation of the nucleotide excision repair gene XPG as a new mechanism of drug resistance in human and murine cancer cells. Mol Cancer. 2010;9.
20. Wang R-H, Zheng Y, Kim H-S, Xu X, Cao L, Luhasen T, et al. Interplay among BRCA1, SIRT1, and survivin during BRCA1-associated tumorigenesis. Mol Cell. 2008;32(1):11–20.
21. Quinn JE, Carser JE, James CR, Kennedy RD, Harkin DP. BRCA1 and implications for response to chemotherapy in ovarian cancer. Gynecol Oncol. 2009;113(1):134–42.
22. Meisel JL, Hyman DM, Garg K, Zhou Q, Dao F, Bisogna M, et al. The performance of BRCA1 immunohistochemistry for detecting germline, somatic, and epigenetic BRCA1 loss in high-grade serous ovarian cancer. Ann Oncol. 2014;25(12):2372–8.
23. Modena P, Testi MA, Facchinetti F, Mezzanzanica D, Radice MT, Pilotti S, et al. UQCRH gene encoding mitochondrial Hinge protein is interrupted by a translocation in a soft-tissue sarcoma and epigenetically inactivated in some cancer cell lines. Oncogene. 2003;22(29):4586–93.
24. Feng Q, Deftereos G, Hawes SE, Stern JE, Willner JB, Swisher EM, et al. DNA hypermethylation, Her-2/neu overexpression and p53 mutations in ovarian carcinoma. Gynecol Oncol. 2008;111(2):320–9.
25. Campbell IG, Phillips WA, Choong DYH. Genetic and epigenetic analysis of the putative tumor suppressor km23 in primary ovarian, breast, and colorectal cancers. Clin Cancer Res. 2006;12(12):3713–5.
26. Abbosh PH, Montgomery JS, Starkey JA, Novotny M, Zuhowski EG, Egorin MJ, et al. Dominant-negative histone H3 lysine 27 mutant derepresses silenced tumor suppressor genes and reverses the drug-resistant phenotype in cancer cells. Cancer Res. 2006;66(11):5582–91.
27. Yang C, Cai J, Wang Q, Tang H, Cao J, Wu L, et al. Epigenetic silencing of miR-130b in ovarian cancer promotes the development of multidrug resistance by targeting colony-stimulating factor 1. Gynecol Oncol. 2012;124(2):325–34.
28. Liu MX, Siu MK, Liu SS, Yam JW, Ngan HY, Chan DW. Epigenetic silencing of microRNA-199b-5p is associated with acquired chemoresistance via activation of JAG1-Notch1 signaling in ovarian cancer. Oncotarget. 2014;5(4):944–58.
29. Zhang S, Lu Z, Unruh AK, Ivan C, Baggerly KA, Calin GA, et al. Clinically relevant microRNAs in ovarian cancer. Mol Cancer Res. 2015;13(3): 393–401.
30. Cheng FHC, Aguda BD, Tsai J-C, Kochanczyk M, Lin JMJ, Chen GCW, et al. A mathematical model of

bimodal epigenetic control of miR-193a in ovarian cancer stem cells. PLoS One. 2014;9(12):e116050.
31. Kwon MJ, Shin YK. Epigenetic regulation of cancer-associated genes in ovarian cancer. Int J Mol Sci. 2011;12(2):983–1008.
32. Guerrero K, Wang Z, Bachvarova M, Gregoire J, Renaud M-C, Plante M, et al. A novel genome-based approach correlates TMPRSS3 overexpression in ovarian cancer with DNA hypomethylation. Gynecol Oncol. 2012;125(3):720–6.
33. Honda H, Pazin MJ, Ji H, Wernyj RP, Morin PJ. Crucial roles of Sp1 and epigenetic modifications in the regulation of the CLDN4 promoter in ovarian cancer cells. J Biol Chem. 2006;281(30):21433–44.
34. Baba T, Convery PA, Matsumura N, Whitaker RS, Kondoh E, Perry T, et al. Epigenetic regulation of CD133 and tumorigenicity of CD133+ovarian cancer cells. Oncogene. 2009;28(2):209–18.
35. Itamochi H. Targeted therapies in epithelial ovarian cancer: molecular mechanisms of action. World J Biol Chem. 2010;1(7):209–20.
36. Weberpals JI, Koti M, Squire JA. Targeting genetic and epigenetic alterations in the treatment of serous ovarian cancer. Cancer Genet. 2011;204(10):525–35.
37. Samudio-Ruiz SL, Hudson LG. Increased DNA methyltransferase activity and DNA methylation following epidermal growth factor stimulation in ovarian cancer cells. Epigenetics. 2012;7(3):216–24.
38. Chen M-Y, Liao WSL, Lu Z, Bornmann WG, Hennessey V, Washington MN, et al. Decitabine and suberoylanilide hydroxamic acid (SAHA) inhibit growth of ovarian cancer cell lines and xenografts while inducing expression of imprinted tumor suppressor genes, apoptosis, G2/M arrest, and autophagy. Cancer. 2011;117(19):4424–38.
39. Bauman J, Verschraegen C, Belinsky S, Muller C, Rutledge T, Fekrazad M, et al. A phase I study of 5-azacytidine and erlotinib in advanced solid tumor malignancies. Cancer Chemother Pharmacol. 2012;69(2):547–54.
40. Balch C, Yan P, Craft T, Young S, Skalnik DG, Huang THM, et al. Antimitogenic and chemosensitizing effects of the methylation inhibitor zebularine in ovarian cancer. Mol Cancer Ther. 2005;4(10):1505–14.
41. Kassler S, Donninger H, Birrer MJ, Clark GJ. RASSF1A and the taxol response in ovarian cancer. Mol Biol Int. 2012;2012:263267.
42. Yu YH, Fujii S, Yuan J, Luo RZ, Wang L, Bao J, et al. Epigenetic regulation of ARHI in breast and ovarian cancer cells. In: Verma M, Dunn BK, Umar A, editors. Epigenetics in cancer prevention: early detection and risk assessment. Ann N Y Acad Sci. 2003;983:268–77.
43. Mazzoletti M, Broggini M. PI3K/AKT/mTOR inhibitors in ovarian cancer. Curr Med Chem. 2010;17(36):4433–47.
44. Chou J-L, Chen L-Y, Lai H-C, Chan MWY. TGF-beta: friend or foe? The role of TGF-beta/SMAD signaling in epigenetic silencing of ovarian cancer and its implication in epigenetic therapy. Expert Opin Ther Targets. 2010;14(11):1213–23.
45. Cardenas H, Vieth E, Lee J, Segar M, Liu Y, Nephew KP, et al. TGF-beta induces global changes in DNA methylation during the epithelial-to-mesenchymal transition in ovarian cancer cells. Epigenetics. 2014;9(11):1461–72.
46. Meng F, Sun G, Zhong M, Yu Y, Brewer MA. Anticancer efficacy of cisplatin and trichostatin A 5-aza-2′-deoxycytidine on ovarian cancer. Br J Cancer. 2013;108(3):579–86.
47. Zhou S, Li Y, Huang F, Zhang B, Yi T, Li Z, et al. Live-attenuated measles virus vaccine confers cell contact loss and apoptosis of ovarian cancer cells via ROS-induced silencing of E-cadherin by methylation. Cancer Lett. 2012;318(1):14–25.
48. Zhao LYC, Zhou S, Lau WB, Lau B, Luo Z, Lin Q, Yang H, Xuan Y, Yi T, Zhao X, Wei Y. Epigenetic repression of PDZ-LIM domain-containing protein 2 promotes ovarian cancer via NOS2-derived nitric oxide signaling. Oncotarget. 2015.
49. Huang R-L, Gu F, Kirma NB, Ruan J, Chen C-L, Wang H-C, et al. Comprehensive methylome analysis of ovarian tumors reveals hedgehog signaling pathway regulators as prognostic DNA methylation biomarkers. Epigenetics. 2013;8(6):624–34.
50. Zeimet AG, Marth C. Why did p53 gene therapy fail in ovarian cancer? Lancet Oncol. 2003;4(7):415–22.
51. Chiang Y-C, Chang M-C, Chen P-J, Wu M-M, Hsieh C-Y, Cheng W-F, et al. Epigenetic silencing of BLU through interfering apoptosis results in chemoresistance and poor prognosis of ovarian serous carcinoma patients. Endocr Relat Cancer. 2013;20(2):213–27.
52. Lum E, Vigliotti M, Banerjee N, Cutter N, Wrzeszczynski KO, Khan S, et al. Loss of DOK2 induces carboplatin resistance in ovarian cancer via suppression of apoptosis. Gynecol Oncol. 2013;130(2):369–76.
53. Lyu T, Jia N, Wang J, Yan X, Yu Y, Lu Z, et al. Expression and epigenetic regulation of angiogenesis-related factors during dormancy and recurrent growth of ovarian carcinoma. Epigenetics. 2013;8(12):1330–46.
54. Balch C, Nephew KP. The role of chromatin, microRNAs, and tumor stem cells in ovarian cancer. Cancer Biomark. 2010;8(4-5):203–21.
55. Marsh S. Pharmacogenomics of taxane/platinum therapy in ovarian cancer. Int J Gynecol Cancer. 2009;19:S30–4.
56. Seeber LMS, van Diest PJ. Epigenetics in ovarian cancer. Methods Mol Biol. 2012;863:253–69.
57. Wittenberger T, Sleigh S, Reisel D, Zikan M, Wahl B, Alunni-Fabbroni M, et al. DNA methylation markers for early detection of women's cancer: promise and challenges. Epigenomics. 2014;6(3):311–27.
58. Murphy SK. Targeting the epigenome in ovarian cancer. Future Oncol. 2012;8(2):151–64.
59. Stefansson OA, Villanueva A, Vidal A, Marti L, Esteller M. BRCA1 epigenetic inactivation predicts sensitivity to platinum-based chemotherapy in breast and ovarian cancer. Epigenetics. 2012;7(11):1225–9.

60. De Luca P, De Siervi A. Critical role for BRCA1 expression as a marker of chemosensitivity response and prognosis. Front Biosci (Elite Ed). 2016;8:72–83.
61. Kumar G, Breen EJ, Ranganathan S. Identification of ovarian cancer associated genes using an integrated approach in a Boolean framework. BMC Syst Biol. 2013;7.
62. Li HR, Shagisultanova EI, Yamashita K, Piao Z, Perucho M, Malkhosyan SR. Hypersensitivity of tumor cell lines with microsatellite instability to DNA double strand break producing chemotherapeutic agent bleomycin. Cancer Res. 2004;64(14):4760–7.
63. Tang J, Fang F, Miller DF, Pilrose JM, Matei D, Huang TH-M, et al. Global DNA methylation profiling technologies and the ovarian cancer methylome. In: Verma M, editor. Cancer epigenetics: risk assessment, diagnosis, treatment, and prognosis. Methods Mol Biol. 2015;1238:653–75.
64. Hamilton G, Yee KS, Scrace S, O'Neill E. ATM regulates a RASSF1A-dependent DNA damage response. Curr Biol. 2009;19(23):2020–5.
65. Maldonado L, Hoque MO. Epigenomics and ovarian carcinoma. Biomark Med. 2010;4(4):543–70.
66. Maradeo ME, Cairns P. Translational application of epigenetic alterations: ovarian cancer as a model. FEBS Lett. 2011;585(13):2112–20.
67. Ibrahim N, He L, Leong C-O, Xing D, Karlan BY, Swisher EM, et al. BRCA1-associated epigenetic regulation of p73 mediates an effector pathway for chemosensitivity in ovarian carcinoma. Cancer Res. 2010;70(18):7155–65.
68. Staub J, Chien J, Pan Y, Qian X, Narita K, Aletti G, et al. Epigenetic silencing of HSulf-1 in ovarian cancer: implications in chemoresistance. Oncogene. 2007;26(34):4969–78.
69. Liu P, Khurana A, Rattan R, He X, Kalloger S, Dowdy S, et al. Regulation of HSulf-1 expression by variant hepatic nuclear factor 1 in ovarian cancer. Cancer Res. 2009;69(11):4843–50.
70. Song J, Shih I-M, Chan DW, Zhang Z. Suppression of annexin A11 in ovarian cancer: implications in chemoresistance. Neoplasia. 2009;11(6):605-U121.
71. Mattioli E, Vogiatzi P, Sun A, Abbadessa G, Angeloni G, Ugo DD, et al. Immunohistochemical analysis of pRb2/p130, VEGF, EZH2, p53, p16(INK4A), p27(KIP1), p21(WAF1), Ki-67 expression patterns in gastric cancer. J Cell Physiol. 2007;210(1):183–91.
72. Hu S, Yu L, Li Z, Shen Y, Wang J, Cai J, et al. Overexpression of EZH2 contributes to acquired cisplatin resistance in ovarian cancer cells in vitro and in vivo. Cancer Biol Ther. 2010;10(8):788–95.
73. Zeimet AG, Fiegl H, Goebel G, Kopp F, Allasia C, Reimer D, et al. DNA ploidy, nuclear size, proliferation index and DNA-hypomethylation in ovarian cancer. Gynecol Oncol. 2011;121(1):24–31.
74. Syed N, Coley HM, Sehouli J, Koensgen D, Mustea A, Szlosarek P, et al. Polo-like kinase Plk2 is an epigenetic determinant of chemosensitivity and clinical outcomes in ovarian cancer. Cancer Res. 2011; 71(9):3317–27.
75. de Groote ML, Kazemier HG, Huisman C, van der Gun BTF, Faas MM, Rots MG. Upregulation of endogenous ICAM-1 reduces ovarian cancer cell growth in the absence of immune cells. Int J Cancer. 2014;134(2):280–90.
76. Shen DW, Fojo A, Chin JE, Roninson IB, Richert N, Pastan I, et al. Human multidrug-resistant cell-lines – increased MDRL expression can precede gene amplification. Science. 1986;232(4750):643–5.
77. Bauerschlag DO, Ammerpohl O, Braeutigam K, Schem C, Lin Q, Weigel MT, et al. Progression-free survival in ovarian cancer is reflected in epigenetic DNA methylation profiles. Oncology. 2011; 80(1-2):12–20.
78. Zeller C, Dai W, Steele NL, Siddiq A, Walley AJ, Wilhelm-Benartzi CSM, et al. Candidate DNA methylation drivers of acquired cisplatin resistance in ovarian cancer identified by methylome and expression profiling. Oncogene. 2012;31(42):4567–76.
79. Gifford G, Paul J, Vasey PA, Kaye SB, Brown R, Scottish Gynaecological C. The acquisition of hMLH1 methylation in plasma DNA after chemotherapy predicts poor survival for ovarian cancer patients. Clin Cancer Res. 2004;10(13):4420–6.
80. Wang C, Cicek MS, Charbonneau B, Kalli KR, Armasu SM, Larson MC, et al. Tumor hypomethylation at 6p21.3 associates with longer time to recurrence of high-grade serous epithelial ovarian cancer. Cancer Res. 2014;74(11):3084–91.
81. Wrzeszczynski KO, Varadan V, Kamalakaran S, Levine DA, Dimitrova N, Lucito R. Integrative prediction of gene function and platinum-free survival from genomic and epigenetic features in ovarian cancer. In: Malek A, Tchernitsa O, editors. Ovarian cancer: methods and protocols. Methods Mol Biol. 2013;1049:35–51.
82. Wei SH, Brown R, Huang THM. Aberrant DNA methylation in ovarian cancer is there an epigenetic predisposition to drug response? In: Verma M, Dunn BK, Umar A, editors. Epigenetics in cancer prevention: early detection and risk assessment. Ann N Y Acad Sci. 2003;983:243–50.
83. Xiang Y, Ma N, Wang D, Zhang Y, Zhou J, Wu G, et al. MiR-152 and miR-185 co-contribute to ovarian cancer cells cisplatin sensitivity by targeting DNMT1 directly: a novel epigenetic therapy independent of decitabine. Oncogene. 2014;33(3):378–86.
84. Llaurado M, Majem B, Altadill T, Lanau L, Castellvi J, Luis Sanchez-Iglesias J, et al. MicroRNAs as prognostic markers in ovarian cancer. Mol Cell Endocrinol. 2014;390(1-2):73–84.
85. Chen X-P, Chen Y-G, Lan J-Y, Shen Z-J. MicroRNA-370 suppresses proliferation and promotes endometrioid ovarian cancer chemosensitivity to cDDP by negatively regulating ENG. Cancer Lett. 2014;353(2):201–10.
86. Swisher EM, Gonzalez RM, Taniguchi T, Garcia RL, Walsh T, Goff BA, et al. Methylation and protein

expression of DNA repair genes: association with chemotherapy exposure and survival in sporadic ovarian and peritoneal carcinomas. Mol Cancer. 2009;8.
87. Balch C, Fang F, Matei DE, Huang THM, Nephew KP. Epigenetic changes in ovarian cancer. Endocrinology. 2009;150(9):4003–11.
88. Suh DH, Kim M-K, Kim HS, Chung HH, Song YS. Epigenetic therapies as a promising strategy for overcoming chemoresistance in epithelial ovarian cancer. J Cancer Prev. 2013;18(3):227–34.
89. Matsumura N, Huang Z, Baba T, Lee PS, Barnett JC, Mori S, et al. Yin Yang 1 modulates taxane response in epithelial ovarian cancer. Mol Cancer Res. 2009;7(2):210–20.
90. Takai N, Narahara H. Histone deacetylase inhibitor therapy in epithelial ovarian cancer. J Oncol. 2010;2010:458431.
91. Li Y, Liu T, Ivan C, Huang J, Shen D-Y, Kavanagh JJ, et al. Enhanced cytotoxic effects of combined valproic acid and the aurora kinase inhibitor VE465 on gynecologic cancer cells. Front Oncol. 2013;3:58.
92. Wilson AJ, Cheng Y-Q, Khabele D. Thailandepsins are new small molecule class I HDAC inhibitors with potent cytotoxic activity in ovarian cancer cells: a preclinical study of epigenetic ovarian cancer therapy. J Ovarian Res. 2012;5.
93. Gu Y, Yang P, Shao Q, Liu X, Xia S, Zhang M, et al. Investigation of the expression patterns and correlation of DNA methyltransferases and class I histone deacetylases in ovarian cancer tissues. Oncol Lett. 2013;5(2):452–8.
94. Yap OWS, Bhat G, Liu L, Tollefsbol TO. Epigenetic modifications of the estrogen receptor beta gene in epithelial ovarian cancer cells. Anticancer Res. 2009;29(1):139–44.
95. Balch C, Huang THM, Brown R, Nephew KP. The epigenetics of ovarian cancer drug resistance and resensitization. Am J Obstet Gynecol. 2004;191(5):1552–72.
96. Matei DE, Nephew KP. Epigenetic therapies for chemoresensitization of epithelial ovarian cancer. Gynecol Oncol. 2010;116(2):195–201.
97. Fang F, Zuo Q, Pilrose J, Wang Y, Shen C, Li M, et al. Decitabine reactivated pathways in platinum resistant ovarian cancer. Oncotarget. 2014;5(11):3579–89.
98. Matei D, Fang F, Shen C, Schilder J, Arnold A, Zeng Y, et al. Epigenetic resensitization to platinum in ovarian cancer. Cancer Res. 2012;72(9):2197–205.
99. Candelaria M, Gallardo-Rincon D, Arce C, Cetina L, Aguilar-Ponce JL, Arrieta O, et al. A phase II study of epigenetic therapy with hydralazine and magnesium valproate to overcome chemotherapy resistance in refractory solid tumors. Ann Oncol. 2007;18(9):1529–38.
100. Falchook GS, Fu S, Naing A, Hong DS, Hu W, Moulder S, et al. Methylation and histone deacetylase inhibition in combination with platinum treatment in patients with advanced malignancies. Invest New Drugs. 2013;31(5):1192–200.
101. Karaca B, Atmaca H, Bozkurt E, Kisim A, Uzunoglu S, Karabulut B, et al. Combination of AT-101/cisplatin overcomes chemoresistance by inducing apoptosis and modulating epigenetics in human ovarian cancer cells. Mol Biol Rep. 2013;40(6):3925–33.
102. Du P, Zhang X, Liu H, Chen L. Lentivirus-mediated RNAi silencing targeting ERCC1 reverses cisplatin resistance in cisplatin-resistant ovarian carcinoma cell line. DNA Cell Biol. 2015;34(7):497–502.
103. Calcagno AM, Fostel JM, To KKW, Salcido CD, Martin SE, Chewning KJ, et al. Single-step doxorubicin-selected cancer cells overexpress the ABCG2 drug transporter through epigenetic changes. Br J Cancer. 2008;98(9):1515–24.
104. Paulikova S, Chmelarova M, Petera J, Palicka V, Paulik A. Hypermethylation of RAD51L3 and XRCC2 genes to predict late toxicity in chemoradiotherapy-treated cervical cancer patients. Folia Biol. 2013;59(6):240–5.
105. Institute NC. Cervix uteri cancer. SEER cancer statistics fact sheets. 2015.
106. Duenas-Gonzalez A, Lizano M, Candelaria M, Cetina L, Arce C, Cervera E. Epigenetics of cervical cancer. An overview and therapeutic perspectives. Mol Cancer. 2005;4.
107. At L. Cancer diagnostic classifiers based on quantitative DNA methylation. Expert Rev Mol Diagn. 2014;14(3):12.
108. Steenbergen RD, Snijders PJ, Heideman DA, Meijer CJ. Clinical implications of (epi)genetic changes in HPV-induced cervical precancerous lesions. Nat Rev Cancer. 2014;14(6):10.
109. Feng D, Cao Z, Li C, Zhang L, Zhou Y, Ma J, et al. Combination of valproic acid and ATRA restores RAR beta 2 expression and induces differentiation in cervical cancer through the PI3K/Akt pathway. Curr Mol Med. 2012;12(3):342–54.
110. Feng D, Wu J, Tian Y, Zhou H, Zhou Y, Hu W, et al. Targeting of histone deacetylases to reactivate tumour suppressor genes and its therapeutic potential in a human cervical cancer xenograft model. PLoS One. 2013;8(11):80657.
111. Khan MA, Hussain A, Sundaram MK, Alalami U, Gunasekera D, Ramesh L, et al. (−)-Epigallocatechin-3-gallate reverses the expression of various tumor-suppressor genes by inhibiting DNA methyltransferases and histone deacetylases in human cervical cancer cells. Oncol Rep. 2015;33(4):1976–84.
112. Khan MA, Sundaram MK, Hamza A, Quraishi U, Gunasekera D, Ramesh L, et al. Sulforaphane reverses the expression of various tumor suppressor genes by targeting DNMT3B and HDAC1 in human cervical cancer cells. Evid Based Complementary Altern Med. 2015;2015:Article ID 412149.
113. Narayan G, Goparaju C, Arias-Pulido H, Kaufmann AM, Schneider A, Duerst M, et al. Promoter hypermethylation-mediated inactivation of multiple Slit-Robo pathway genes in cervical cancer progression. Mol Cancer. 2006;5.

114. Chavez-Blanco A, Segura-Pacheco B, Perez-Cardenas E, Taja-Chayeb L, Cetina L, Candelaria M, et al. Histone acetylation and histone deacetylase activity of magnesium valproate in tumor and peripheral blood of patients with cervical cancer. A phase I study. Mol Cancer. 2005;4.
115. Takai N, Kira N, Ishii T, Nishida M, Nasu K, Narahara H. Novel chemotherapy using histone deacetylase inhibitors in cervical cancer. Asian Pac J Cancer Prev. 2011;12(3):575–80.
116. Smith NLD, Denning DW. Clinical implications of interferon-gamma genetic and epigenetic variants. Immunology. 2014;143(4):499–511.
117. Saha SK, Khuda-Bukhsh AR. Berberine alters epigenetic modifications, disrupts microtubule network, and modulates HPV-18 E6-E7 oncoproteins by targeting p53 in cervical cancer cell HeLa: A mechanistic study including molecular docking. Eur J Pharmacol. 2014;744:132–46.
118. Ying JM, Srivastava G, Hsieh WS, Gao ZF, Murray P, Liao SK, et al. The stress-responsive gene GADD45G is a functional tumor suppressor, with its response to environmental stresses frequently disrupted epigenetically in multiple tumors. Clin Cancer Res. 2005;11(18):6442–9.
119. Huang Y, Song H, Hu H, Cui L, You C, Huang L. Trichosanthin inhibits DNA methyltransferase and restores methylation-silenced gene expression in human cervical cancer cells. Mol Med Rep. 2012;6(4):872–8.
120. Woo HJ, Kim SJ, Song K-J, Kim SS, Yoon C-H, Choi B-S, et al. Hypermethylation of the tumor-suppressor cell adhesion molecule 1 in human papillomavirus-transformed cervical carcinoma cells. Int J Oncol. 2015;46(6):2656–62.
121. de la Cruz-Hernandez E, Perez-Cardenas E, Contreras-Paredes A, Cantu D, Mohar A, Lizano M, et al. The effects of DNA methylation and histone deacetylase inhibitors on human papillomavirus early gene expression in cervical cancer, an in vitro and clinical study. Virol J. 2007;4.
122. Sood S, Patel FD, Ghosh S, Arora A, Dhaliwal LK, Srinivasan R. Epigenetic alteration by DNA methylation of ESR1, MYOD1 and hTERT gene promoters is useful for prediction of response in patients of locally advanced invasive cervical carcinoma treated by chemoradiation. Clin Oncol. 2015;27(12):720–7.
123. Narayan G, Xie D, Ishdorj G, Scotto L, Mansukhani M, Pothuri B, Wright JD, Kaufmann AM, Schneider A, Arias-Pulido H, Murty VV. Epigenetic inactivation of TRAIL decoy receptors at 8p12-21.3 commonly deleted region confers sensitivity to Apo2L/trail-cisplatin combination therapy in cervical cancer. Genes Chromosomes Cancer. 2016;55:177–89.
124. Liu SSLR, Chan KY, Chiu PM, Cheung AN, Tam KF, Ng TY, Wong LC, Ngan HY. p73 expression is associated with the cellular radiosensitivity in cervical cancer after radiotherapy. Clin Cancer Res. 2004;10(10):7.
125. Liu N, Zhao L-J, Li X-P, Wang J-L, Chai G-L, Wei L-H. Histone deacetylase inhibitors inducing human cervical cancer cell apoptosis by decreasing DNA-methyltransferase 3B. Chin Med J (Engl). 2012;125(18):3273–8.
126. De la Cruz-Hernandez E, Perez-Plasencia C, Perez-Cardenas E, Gonzalez-Fierro A, Trejo-Becerril C, Chavez-Blanco A, et al. Transcriptional changes induced by epigenetic therapy with hydralazine and magnesium valproate in cervical carcinoma. Oncol Rep. 2011;25(2):399–407.
127. Duenas-Gonzalez A, Coronel J, Cetina L, Gonzalez-Fierro A, Chavez-Blanco A, Taja-Chayeb L. Hydralazine-valproate: a repositioned drug combination for the epigenetic therapy of cancer. Expert Opin Drug Metab Toxicol. 2014;10(10):1433–44.
128. Candelaria M, de la Cruz-Hernandez E, Taja-Chayeb L, Perez-Cardenas E, Trejo-Becerril C, Gonzalez-Fierro A, et al. DNA methylation-independent reversion of gemcitabine resistance by hydralazine in cervical cancer cells. PLoS One. 2012;7(3):29181.
129. Coronel J, Cetina L, Pacheco I, Trejo-Becerril C, Gonzalez-Fierro A, de la Cruz-Hernandez E, et al. A double-blind, placebo-controlled, randomized phase III trial of chemotherapy plus epigenetic therapy with hydralazine valproate for advanced cervical cancer. Preliminary results. Med Oncol. 2011;28:S540–6.
130. Candelaria M, Cetina L, Perez-Cardenas E, de la Cruz-Hernandez E, Gonzalez-Fierro A, Trejo-Becerril C, et al. Epigenetic therapy and cisplatin chemoradiation in FIGO Stage IIIB cervical cancer. Eur J Gynaecol Oncol. 2010;31(4):386–91.
131. Chen CC, Lee KD, Pai MY, Chu PY, Hsu CC, Chiu CC, Chen LT, Chang JY, Hsiao SH, Leu YW. Changes in DNA methylation are associated with the development of drug resistance in cervical cancer cells. Cancer Cell Int. 2015;15:98.
132. Roy M, Mukherjee S. Reversal of resistance towards cisplatin by curcumin in cervical cancer cells. Asian Pac J Cancer Prev. 2014;15(3):1403–10.
133. Mani E, Medina LA, Isaac-Olive K, Duenas-Gonzalez A. Radiosensitization of cervical cancer cells with epigenetic drugs hydralazine and valproate. Eur J Gynaecol Oncol. 2014;35(2):140–2.
134. Katoh M. Functional proteomics of the epigenetic regulators ASXL1, ASXL2 and ASXL3: a convergence of proteomics and epigenetics for translational medicine. Expert Rev Proteomics. 2015;12(3):317–28.
135. Wen WS, Yuan Z, Ma SJ, Xu J, Yuan DT. CRISPR-Cas9 systems: versatile cancer modelling platforms and promising therapeutic strategies. Int J Cancer. 2016.
136. Banno K, Yanokura M, Kawaguchi M, Kuwabara Y, Akiyoshi J, Kobayashi Y, et al. Epigenetic inactivation of the CHFR gene in cervical cancer contributes to sensitivity to taxanes. Int J Oncol. 2007;31(4):713–20.
137. Masuda K, Banno K, Yanokura M, Tsuji K, Kobayashi Y, Kisu I, et al. Association of epigenetic

inactivation of the WRN gene with anticancer drug sensitivity in cervical cancer cells. Oncol Rep. 2012;28(4):1146–52.
138. McLaughlin-Drubin ME, Park D, Munger K. Tumor suppressor p16(INK4A) is necessary for survival of cervical carcinoma cell lines. Proc Natl Acad Sci U S A. 2013;110(40):16175–80.
139. Froehlich LF, Mrakovcic M, Smole C, Lahiri P, Zatloukal K. Epigenetic silencing of apoptosis-inducing gene expression can be efficiently overcome by combined SAHA and TRAIL treatment in uterine sarcoma cells. PLoS One. 2014;9:3.
140. Liu Y, Broaddus RR, Zhang W. Identifying aggressive forms of endometrioid-type endometrial cancer: new insights into molecular subtyping. Expert Rev Anticancer Ther. 2015;15(1):1–3.
141. Banno K, Kisu I, Yanokura M, Masuda K, Ueki A, Kobayashi Y, et al. Epigenetics and genetics in endometrial cancer: new carcinogenic mechanisms and relationship with clinical practice. Epigenomics. 2012;4(2):147–62.
142. Theisen ER, Gajiwala S, Bearss J, Sorna V, Sharma S, Janat-Amsbury M. Reversible inhibition of lysine specific demethylase 1 is a novel anti-tumor strategy for poorly differentiated endometrial carcinoma. BMC Cancer. 2014;14.
143. Yang S, Thiel KW, De Geest K, Leslie KK. Endometrial cancer: reviving progesterone therapy in the molecular age. Discov Med. 2011;64: 205–12.
144. Jiang S-W, Li J, Podratz K, Dowdy S. Application of DNA methylation biomarkers for endometrial cancer management. Expert Rev Mol Diagn. 2008;8(5):607–16.
145. De Luca P, De Siervi A. Critical role for BRCA1 expression as a marker of chemosensitivity response and prognosis. Front Biosci (Elite Ed). 2016;8:11.
146. Ren J, Zhang J, Cai H, Li Y, Zhang Y, Zhang X, et al. HDAC as a therapeutic target for treatment of endometrial cancers. Curr Pharm Des. 2014; 20(11):1847–56.
147. Jones A, Teschendorff AE, Li Q, Hayward JD, Kannan A, Mould T, et al. Role of DNA methylation and epigenetic silencing of HAND2 in endometrial cancer development. PLoS Med. 2013;10(11), e1001551.
148. Hsu Y-T, Gu F, Huang Y-W, Liu J, Ruan J, Huang R-L, et al. Promoter hypomethylation of EpCAM-regulated bone morphogenetic protein gene family in recurrent endometrial cancer. Clin Cancer Res. 2013;19(22):6272–85.
149. Banno K, Nogami Y, Kisu I, Yanokura M, Umene K, Masuda K, et al. Candidate biomarkers for genetic and clinicopathological diagnosis of endometrial cancer. Int J Mol Sci. 2013;14(6):12123–37.
150. Banno K, Yanokura M, Kisu I, Yamagami W, Susumu N, Aoki D. MicroRNAs in endometrial cancer. Int J Clin Oncol. 2013;18(2):186–92.
151. Crea F, Sun L, Pikor L, Frumento P, Lam WL, Helgason CD. Mutational analysis of Polycomb genes in solid tumours identifies PHC3 amplification as a possible cancer-driving genetic alteration. Br J Cancer. 2013;109(6):1699–702.
152. Zhou XC, Dowdy SC, Podratz KC, Jiang S-W. Epigenetic considerations for endometrial cancer prevention, diagnosis and treatment. Gynecol Oncol. 2007;107(1):143–53.
153. Dong P, Kaneuchi M, Konno Y, Watari H, Sudo S, Sakuragi N. Emerging therapeutic biomarkers in endometrial cancer. Biomed Res Int. 2013;2013: Article ID 130362.
154. Yang S, Xiao X, Jia Y, Liu X, Zhang Y, Wang X, et al. Epigenetic modification restores functional PR expression in endometrial cancer cells. Curr Pharm Des. 2014;20(11):1874–80.
155. Xu S, Ren J, Bin Chen H, Wang Y, Liu Q, Zhang R, et al. Cytostatic and apoptotic effects of DNMT and HDAC inhibitors in endometrial cancer cells. Curr Pharm Des. 2014;20(11):1881–7.
156. Huber JC, Ott J. The dialectic role of progesterone. Maturitas. 2009;62(4):326–9.
157. Chu Y, Wang Y, Zhang G, Chen H, Dowdy SC, Xiong Y, et al. Chromatin composition alterations and the critical role of MeCP2 for epigenetic silencing of progesterone receptor-B gene in endometrial cancers. Cell Mol Life Sci. 2014;71(17):3393–408.
158. Yang S, Jia Y, Liu X, Winters C, Wang X, Zhang Y, et al. Systematic dissection of the mechanisms underlying progesterone receptor downregulation in endometrial cancer. Oncotarget. 2014;5(20):9783–97.
159. Xiong YN, Dowdy SC, Bosquet JG, Zhao Y, Eberhardt NL, Podratz KC, et al. Epigenetic-mediated upregulation of progesterone receptor B gene in endometrial cancer cell lines. Gynecol Oncol. 2005;99(1):135–41.
160. Janzen DM, Rosales MA, Paik DY, Lee DS, Smith DA, Witte ON, et al. Progesterone receptor signaling in the microenvironment of endometrial cancer influences its response to hormonal therapy. Cancer Res. 2013;73(15):4697–710.
161. McWhirter RE, Marthick JR, Boyle JA, Dickinson JL. Genetic and epigenetic variation in vulvar cancer: current research and future clinical practice. Aust N Z J Obstet Gynaecol. 2014;54(5):406–11.
162. Harris RM, Waring RH. Diethylstilboestrol—A long-term legacy. Maturitas. 2012;72(2):108–12.

# Part II

# Current Standard of Care for the Treatment of Gynecological Tumors

# Advances in Cervical Cancer and Ongoing Clinical Trials

3

Giuseppina D'Andrilli

**Abstract**

The big issue in the fight against cancer is to understand the molecular mechanisms underlying the carcinogenesis process and try to direct the knowledge acquired in the direction of new and hopefully efficient therapies. In recent years, numerous studies have greatly implemented the knowledge about cervical cancer. It is well known that human papillomavirus (HPV) types cause approximately 90 % of cervical cancer. This evidence led the scientists to focus on HPV infection in relationship with cervical cancer, thereby developing vaccines for the prevention of cervical cancer. Screening with HPV testing was introduced around 1990, and prophylactic HPV vaccination was licensed in 2006. The synergistic effect of cancer prevention and early detection of cancers has been shown to improve survival rates and decrease mortality by timely appropriate treatment. Unfortunately, prophylactic vaccines are not able to eradicate established HPV infections and their associated tumor lesions. Advances have been made also in the clinical and therapeutic management of patients affected by cervical cancer. Important immunotherapeutic studies in advanced cervical cancer have been recently reported. In addition, various classes of anti-angiogenesis agents are studied with great interest in order to improve the efficacy of the treatment for patients with cervical carcinoma.

**Keywords**

Human papillomavirus • Cervical cancer • DNA methylation • MicroRNA • Translational science • Vaccines • Clinical trials

G. D'Andrilli, PhD (✉)
Department of Biology, College of Science and Technology, Temple University, 1900 N 12th Street, Biolife Science Bld, Philadelphia, PA 19122, USA
e-mail: jdandrilli@yahoo.com; dandrill@temple.edu





A. Giordano, M. Macaluso (eds.), *Gynecological Cancers*, Current Clinical Oncology,
DOI 10.1007/978-3-319-32907-9_3

## Abbreviations

| | |
|---|---|
| CIN | Cervical intraepithelial neoplasia |
| DNMT | DNA methyltransferase |
| EGF | Epidermal growth factor |
| EGFR | Epidermal growth factor receptor |
| ERK1 | Extracellular signal-regulated kinase 1 |
| FGF | Fibroblast growth factor |
| GOG | Gynecologic Oncology Group |
| HDAC | Histone deacetylase |
| HER2 | Human epidermal growth factor receptor 2 |
| HPV | Human papillomavirus |
| IFN | Interferon |
| LNM | Lymph node metastasis |
| MAPK1 | Mitogen-activated protein kinase 1 |
| miRNA | MicroRNA |
| NCCN | National Comprehensive Cancer Network |
| NCI | National Cancer Institute |
| NIP | National Immunization Program |
| OS | Overall survival |
| PD | Programmed cell death |
| PD-L1 | Programmed cell death ligand 1 |
| PFS | Progression-free survival |
| PIK3CA | Phosphatidylinositol-45-bisphosphate 3-kinase, catalytic subunit alpha |
| RTK | Receptor tyrosine kinase |
| SCC | Squamous cell carcinoma |
| TIL | Tumor-infiltrating lymphocyte |
| VEGF | Vascular endothelial growth factor |

## Introduction

Cervical cancer is one of the most common types of cancer in women worldwide and is frequent in relatively young women. Cervical cancer being the fourth most diagnosed cancer among the females worldwide is the fourth leading cause of cancer-related mortality [1]. In the last decades, its incidence has decreased following the implementation of screening programs, mainly in developed countries. Cervical screening programs, while successful if properly carried out, are difficult and expensive to implement, especially in developing countries. Prophylactic human papillomavirus (HPV) vaccines and new HPV screening tests, combined with traditional Pap test screening, have greatly reduced cervical cancer. Yet, thousands of women (~470,000 new cases) continue to be diagnosed with and die (233,000 deaths per year) of this preventable disease annually. This critical situation has stimulated the scientists to find ways of evolving new strategies and settle novel treatment protocols.

Cervical cancer remains unique among solid tumor malignancies. Cervical carcinogenesis is a multistep process, which starts with viral infection and requires the establishment of persistent HPV infection. Persistent infection with oncogenic subtypes of the human papillomavirus (HPV) results in carcinogenesis, predominantly occurring at the cervical transformation zone where endocervical columnar cells undergo metaplasia to a stratified squamous epithelium. The molecular cascade involving viral oncoproteins, E6 and E7, and their degradative interactions with cellular tumor suppressor gene products, p53 and pRb respectively, has been precisely delineated. Functional inactivation of pRb by viral oncoprotein binding is shown in many neoplasias including cervical cancer [2]. In the early phases of carcinogenesis the three oncogenes of the virus E5, E6, and E7 play an important role in immune evasion. The precursor state of cervical neoplasia may last for years allowing for ready detection through successful screening programs in developed countries using cervical cytology and/or high-risk HPV DNA testing. HPV is one of the most common sexually transmitted infections worldwide and is associated with a wide spectrum of benign and malignant neoplasias.

Integration of high-risk HPV DNA into the host genome is also a crucial event in cervical carcinogenesis as it is found almost exclusively in high-grade lesions and invasive cancer often in association with progression and invasiveness [3].

Cancer development depends not only on efficient negative regulation of cell cycle control supporting the accumulation of genetic damage but also on immune evasion that allows the virus to live undetected for a long time. Several studies have described an increased prevalence and recurrence of both cervical HPV infection and invasive cervical cancer among HIV-1 positive women compared to HIV-1 negative cases. An upregulation of HPV E6 and E7 gene expressions by HIV-1 proteins such as Tat has been also documented. Some results suggest that HIV-1 may enhance cervical carcinogenesis by promoting cell cycle progression [4].

Smoking has also been linked to the development of cervical cancer [5, 6].

Women who lack access to healthcare and for those who undergo sporadic screening remain at risk. Although surgery (including fertility-sparing surgery) is available for patients with early-stage cancers, and chemoradiation plus high-dose-rate brachytherapy can cure the majority of those with locally advanced disease, patients with metastatic and non-operable recurrent cervical cancer constitute a high-risk population.

Squamous cell cervical carcinoma (SCC) represents approximately 80 % of cases, about 10 % are adenocarcinoma and a small number are other types. Cervical cancer develops through well-defined premalignant lesions, which are known as cervical intraepithelial neoplasia (CIN), ranging from grades I to III.

While screening programs have decreased the incidence of squamous cell cervical cancer, the incidence of adenocarcinoma of the cervix has risen from 5 to 24 % [7, 8]. Adenocarcinoma confers a worse prognosis with higher rates of nodal involvement, distant metastases, and decreased survival across stages, compared with SCC [9].

Cervical squamous cell carcinoma and adenocarcinoma have distinct molecular profiles, suggesting that clinical outcomes may be improved with the use of more tailored strategies.

## Genomic Alterations in Cervical Cancer

A number of studies discovered several recurrent genomic alterations in cervical carcinomas. A recent study investigated 80 cervical tumors for 1250 known mutations in 139 cancer genes. Data indicate that 60 % of patients carry somatic mutations, the most common of which were PIK3CA (Phosphatidylinositol-4, 5-Bisphosphate 3-Kinase, Catalytic Subunit Alpha) and KRAS (Kirsten rat sarcoma viral oncogene homolog). The highest mutation rates were PIK3CA (31.3 %), KRAS (8.8 %), and EGFR (3.8 %). PIK3CA (Phosphatidylinositol-4, 5-Bisphosphate 3-Kinase, Catalytic Subunit Alpha) mutation rates were not significantly different in adenocarcinoma and squamous cell carcinomas and were associated with decreased survival. In contrast, KRAS mutations were identified only in cervical adenocarcinoma, and a novel EGFR (epidermal growth factor receptor) mutation was detected only in squamous cell carcinomas. There were no associations between HPV-16 or HPV-18 and somatic mutations or overall survival [10]. In addition, E322K substitutions in the MAPK1 (mitogen-activated protein kinase 1)/ERK1 (extracellular signal-regulated kinase 1) gene appear recurrently in primary squamous cell carcinomas. SCC has higher frequencies of somatic nucleotide substitutions occurring at cytosines preceded by thymines (Tp*C sites) than adenocarcinomas [11].

HER2 (human epidermal growth factor receptor 2) aberrations (overexpression or gene amplification) occur in 1–21 % of cervical cancer patients. Recent advances in large-scale genomic analysis confirmed the existence of HER2 amplification across many tumor types [12]. HER2 overexpression has been rarely (<20 %) reported in invasive cervical cancer, and more frequently in adenocarcinoma than in squamous cell carcinoma [13].

The most important evidence emerging from these studies is that cervical squamous cell carcinoma and adenocarcinoma have distinct molecular profiles; this might explain the observed clinical differences. These studies encourage further efforts to identify and target distinct molecular subpopulations within cervical cancer providing an important opportunity to improve outcomes in women with both early and late-stage disease. Enhanced understanding of tumor heterogeneity will further enhance a multifaceted approach to cancer treatment with the hope of achieving a durable response.

## Epigenetic Alterations in Cervical Cancer

Epigenetic alterations, such as aberrant miRNA expression and changes in DNA methylation status, promote the expression of oncogenes and the silencing of tumor suppressor genes. Given that some miRNA genes can be regulated through epigenetic mechanisms, it has been proposed the alteration in methylation status of miRNA promoters could be the driving mechanism behind their aberrant expression in cervical cancer. For this reason, it is important to assess the relationship among HPV infection, cellular DNA methylation, and miRNA expression. The alterations in the methylation status of protein-coding genes and various miRNA genes are influenced by HPV infection, the viral genotype, the physical state of the viral DNA, and viral oncogenic risk.

HPV induces deregulation of miRNA expression, particularly at loci near fragile sites. This deregulation occurs through the E6 and E7 proteins, which target miRNA such as p53 [14].

## Dysregulated miRNAs Involved in Cervical Cancer

MicroRNAs (miRNAs) have become the center of interest in oncology. MiRNAs are short noncoding RNAs which function as oncogenes or tumor suppressor genes and regulate gene expression by controlling targets that play a role in cancer development and progression. Numerous recent studies have demonstrated that miRNAs regulate gene expression by influencing important regulatory genes and thus are responsible for causing cervical cancer. As miRNA deregulation plays a crucial role in malignant transformation of cervical cancer along with its targets that can be evaluated for both prognostic and therapeutic strategies. It has been stated that HPV infection and E6/E7 expression are essential but not sufficient to lead to cervical cancer development; hence other genetic and epigenetic factors have to be involved in this complex disease. Recent studies report an important level of interaction among E6/E7 viral proteins and cellular miRNA, and other noncoding RNAs. This interaction could affect therapeutic response in tumor cells [15].

## Circulating miRNA in Cervical Cancer

Circulating miRNAs have been proposed as diagnostic and prognostic biomarkers for gynecological malignancies, including cervical cancer.

A recent study demonstrated that the circulating miRNAs, miR-646, miR-141* and miR-542-3p, were differentially expressed in the serum of cervical squamous cell carcinoma (SCC) patients before and after surgery, and thus could potentially serve as noninvasive biomarkers and post-therapeutic monitors for cervical SCC [16]. The expression of miR-218 has been investigated in the sera from cervical cancer patients and its relationships with clinicopathological characteristics. MiR-218 was reduced significantly in the sera of cervical cancer patients. Moreover, decreased miR-218 was reported to be associated with later stages, cervical adenocarcinoma, and lymphatic node metastasis [17]. In another study, the authors found that the expression levels of miR-20a and miR-203 were both significantly higher in cervical cancer patients compared with healthy controls. Patients with lymph node metastasis (LNM) tended to have overexpression of miR-20a but downregulation of miR-203. These results suggested that the circulating miR-20a may be a potential biomarker for detecting the lymph node status of cervical cancer patients [18]. Since LNM is one of the crucial clinicopathological features of cervical SCC, numerous studies focused on the detection of LNM. Chen et al. evaluated the expression levels of miRNAs that dysregulated between LNM (+) and LNM (−) SCC samples, both in tissue samples and in sera of patients and healthy controls. They identified six serum miRNAs that can predict LNM in cervical SCC patients: miR-1246, miR-20a, miR-2392, miR-3147, miR-3162-5p, and miR-4484. Furthermore, they analyzed the prediction value of LNM using comprehensive set of these serum microRNAs. The predictive value of the serum miRNAs was inferior to that in tissue, but far superior to serum

SCC antigen (SCC-Ag) analysis, suggesting that serum miRNAs are potential novel predictors of LNM with clinical value in early-stage cervical SCC [19]. This is a new interesting field of cancer research but there *will be a long way* forward *before* these findings can be used in clinical practice.

## DNA Methylation and MicroRNA Expression in Cervical Cancer

DNA methylation of several human genes has been shown to be also a relevant event for cervical carcinoma development. DNA methylation is one of the epigenetic mechanisms that influence gene transcription, chromatin structure, genomic stability, and the inactivation of imprinted genes and X chromosome [20].

Epigenetic modifications are just as important as genetic modifications in terms of regulating gene expression and controlling disease onset. It has been shown that epigenetic silencing of some miRNA genes is functionally involved in cervical carcinogenesis [21, 22].

In normal tissues, epigenetic events such as DNA methylation, histone acetylation and expression of miRNAs, and other small RNAs regulate the expression of genes participating in the activation of differentiation processes as well as cellular functions that contribute to cellular homeostasis [23, 24]. Twenty-five years ago, it was discovered that epigenetic modifications participate in cancer development, leading to uncontrolled cell proliferation [23]. One of the most widely studied epigenetic mechanisms is DNA methylation, a reversible reaction catalyzed by DNA methyltransferase (DNMT) enzymes. Alterations to the DNA methylation pattern, which have also been described in cervical cancer, contribute to genomic instability, chromosomal rearrangements, and silencing of coding and noncoding genes, such as miRNAs [21, 25]. Silencing of tumor suppressor genes through DNA hypermethylation has been linked to the development of different types of cancers, including cervical cancer, and is frequently associated with poor clinical results.

In patients and cervical cancer cell lines, it has been observed that silencing of tumor suppressor miRNAs through aberrant promoter methylation enhances cervical carcinogenesis [26, 27]. It has been assumed that HR-HPV (high-risk HPV) can lead to modifications in the methylation pattern of miRNA promoters [28]. Evidence suggests that in cervical cancer, hypermethylation of miRNA promoters contributes to the decreased expression of miRNAs with tumor suppressor gene functions and leads to overexpression of miRNAs with oncogenic functions. Methylation is an important mechanism in the HPV viral cycle. Alterations to the methylation status of cellular DNA are influenced by HPV infection, the viral genotype, the physical state of the viral DNA, and oncogenic risk. The E6 and E7 oncoproteins of HPV 16 induce the overexpression of DNA methyltransferase enzymes, which can catalyze the aberrant methylation of protein-coding and miRNA genes that are susceptible to regulation by methylation [29].

## Advances in Translational Science

Since 1977, when Zur Hausen [30] discovered that the infection of human papillomavirus (HPV) is the major causative agent of cervical cancer, numerous studies have been conducted and are in progress. It has been determined that the relationship between cervical cancer and HPV infection is higher than the relationship between lung cancer and smoking, and also higher than the relationship between liver cancer and hepatitis B virus [31].

Advances in the understanding of the role of human papillomavirus (HPV) in the etiology of high-grade cervical lesions and cervical cancer have led to the development of two prophylactic HPV vaccines. Vaccination against the HPV, which is the major cause of cervical cancer, is a significant step forward and represents a century of successful translational research.

New biomarkers such as viral and cellular methylation profiles could represent the most accurate markers for cancer progression. Nevertheless, results on the novel promising biomarkers are in general based on small sample size, and additional clinical trials are needed to determine the real clinical value of these new treatments. The advent of pharmacogenomics and targeted therapy has provided the opportunity for tailored tumor treatment and with molecular profiling of gynecologic tumor types comes the added potential for discovering novel and improved therapeutic strategies aimed at a specific gene target.

## Human Papillomavirus Vaccines

Human papillomavirus (HPV) types cause approximately 90 % of cervical cancer worldwide [32]. In the last years, two new vaccines against two/four types of human papillomavirus (HPV) have been commercialized. Bivalent HPV 16 and 18 (Cervarix) and quadrivalent HPV 6, 11, 16, and 18 (Gardasil) vaccines are now extensively used in some countries. At least 40 countries had implemented HPV vaccination in their national immunization programs (NIPs) by the beginning of 2012. Among these countries, the United States, the UK, Canada, and Australia were the first countries to execute the implementation. In 2007, only three European countries had introduced HPV vaccine which then increased to 22 countries who had introduced the vaccine into their NIPs. While the target of most country programs is young adolescent girls, defined age groups vary by country to country. Such various implementation strategies are resulted from different healthcare infrastructure and systems. In general, HPV vaccinations are recommended for females aged minimum 11 to maximum 26 years [33].

The high efficacy of the two available cervical cancer vaccines and their proven ability to reduce the incidence of cervical cancer precursor lesions offer hope that the vaccine will have a significant worldwide impact and may dramatically reduce the cervical cancer incidence. The current vaccines protecting against HPV-16 and HPV-18 may prevent up to 70 % of new cervical cancers. Data from the trials together with postvaccine surveillance indicates that they have a good safety profile. Vaccine cross-reactivity for HPV-31, -33, -45, and -52 suggests that an even higher percentage of cervical cancers might be prevented with its use [34]. Currently, the prohibitive cost of the vaccine precludes its widespread implementation. Cooperation between governments, international health organizations, and the vaccine industry is needed to overcome this significant barrier so that women are no longer denied a potentially lifesaving advance. Worldwide HPV vaccination and cervical cancer screening should be an international priority [35].

Countries are now challenged by the rapid development of vaccines aimed at the primary prevention of infections. In the next future, several vaccines will need to be considered as potential candidates in routine immunization programs. The HPV vaccines will prevent infection and long-running complications, such as cervical cancer, other HPV-related cancers, and genital warts (for the quadrivalent vaccine). These vaccines are expected to significantly reduce HPV-associated morbidity and mortality. Unfortunately, the effect of HPV vaccination in the incidence of cervical cancer will not be perceived until about 20–30 years after a worldwide vaccination program is introduced.

Although prophylactic vaccination will provide significant advantages in the health system, cervical screening will need to be continued for the whole population of women that is already infected with HPV [36]. In the near future it is likely that human papillomavirus (HPV) vaccination and HPV-based screening will be complementary strategies.

## Antiangiogenic Therapy

In the last years, significant studies have been made in the antiangiogenic field.

Tumor neovascularization has been demonstrated to confer an aggressive course in cervical cancer. Vascular endothelial growth factor (VEGF) has emerged as an important therapeutic target to inhibit angiogenesis in many solid tumors [37]. Viral oncogenes E6 and E7 lead to altered p53 and retinoblastoma protein function, ultimately resulting in increased VEGF expression. Sequestration of VEGF using monoclonal antibody *bevacizumab* prevents tumor angiogenesis. The activity of *bevacizumab* in recurrent cervical cancer was demonstrated in the phase II study by the Gynecologic Oncology Group (GOG) (protocol 227C) [38].

Recently, in a randomized phase II study the protocol GOG240 was developed to evaluate anti-angiogenesis therapy using *bevacizumab* in advanced cervical cancer [39]. In 2013, the National Cancer Institute and the GOG jointly announced that GOG 240 demonstrated that compared to chemotherapy alone, the incorporation of the anti-angiogenesis agent *bevacizumab* led to significantly improved overall survival (OS), progression-free survival (PFS), and response rate without a significant worsening in quality of life [40, 41].

The *cisplatin-paclitaxel-bevacizumab* combination from GOG 240 was listed as Category 2A in the National Comprehensive Cancer Network (NCCN) Clinical Practice Guidelines for Cervical Cancer (NCCN Clinical Practice Guidelines in Oncology. Cervical Cancer Version 1.2014 NCCN.org). *Bevacizumab* is the first anti-angiogenesis agent to demonstrate an OS advantage in a gynecologic malignancy. On these bases, in the future other classes of anti-angiogenesis agents should be studied in the therapy of cervical cancer.

## Immunotherapy

The rationale for immunotherapy in cervical cancer is based on the causative role of HPV infection in this disease.

The immunologic aspect of cervical cancer induces some considerations regarding the function of T regulatory cells and other immunologic factors involved in the cellular immune response.

HPV infection triggers a cellular immune response involving regulatory T cells in HPV-associated malignancies [42].

The CTLA-4 receptor on T lymphocytes is a negative regulator of T-cell activation that outcompetes CD28 for binding to B7 on antigen-presenting cells, thus playing a role of immune checkpoint molecule. When programmed cell death 1 (PD-1) binds to its ligand PD-L1 present on tumor cells, the ability of the activated T cell to produce a strong immune response is decreased [43]. Each of these immunologic factors needs to be considered for the development of active immunotherapies.

Monoclonal antibodies targeting both PD-1 and PD-L1 currently are being developed to interrupt this pathway and to improve the antitumor immune response and may have a role in the treatment of cervical cancer.

The use of bacterial vectors directed against E7 has been shown to induce tumor regression in animal models [44], and a phase II trial with a live-attenuated Listeria monocytogenes vaccine suggests it may have activity in patients with cervical cancer. The results of this new strategy have been reported at the 2013 American Society of Clinical Oncology Annual meeting. More than 100 women with recurrent cervical cancer have been treated and 63 % were still alive at 6 months of follow-up, with evidence of both complete and partial responses in 12 patients.

These promising results opened the way to a trial in the United States using the same live-attenuated L. monocytogenes cancer vaccine.

A small phase II study used an approach called tumor-infiltrating lymphocyte (TIL) therapy, which has had some success in treating metastatic melanoma and B-cell malignancies. The researchers isolated T cells from patients' tumors and selected those with reactivity with HPV oncoproteins E6 and E7. The TILs were then expanded and infused back into each patient, along with IL2, a T-cell growth factor. All nine patients in the study had either HPV-16 or HPV-18 infections, which together cause about 80 % of cervical cancer. Two women with widespread metastases and chemotherapy-resistant disease achieved complete and lasting remissions of 11 and 18 months, respectively, at the time of analysis. The researchers are now exploring why this therapy was highly effective in only some women. However the study's results are limited but impressive considering that the patients treated are young women who failed multiple attempts at antitumor therapy [45].

In the early phases of viral carcinogenesis several different antiviral approaches have been considered, mainly acting through the inhibition of the oncoprotein E6 and E7 directly or by interfering with their related functions [46, 47]. *Lopinavir*, an antiviral agent employed in HIV disease, interacts with p53 and has shown activity in cervical cancer cell lines, suggesting a possible clinical use [48]. Finally, *cidofovir*, an acyclic nucleoside phosphonate with a broad spectrum antiviral activity, has been topically employed in CIN2/CIN3 lesions in a randomized trial, with encouraging results [49].

## The Importance of Alpha/Beta Interferon Receptors for the Treatment of Cervical Intraepithelial Neoplasias

Interferon-alpha/beta has been shown to play a key role in mediating immune responses.

Interferons (IFNs) are inducible glycoproteins that have immunomodulatory, antiviral, antiproliferative, and antiangiogenic effects. In particular, interferon-alpha (IFN-α) has been shown to inhibit the development and progression of cervical cancer [50].

Based on the antiviral and antitumor potential of IFNs, numerous studies have explored their effects on the immune system, in particular the ability of IFNs to enhance the treatment of different types of cancer. The presence of IFN receptors has been associated with an improved response to immunotherapies involving IFN-α. Both IFN-α and IFN-β bind the same receptors, and these receptors are expressed by many different type of cells [51].

Variations in the concentration and the number of receptors expressed by a cell can affect the intensity of the responses caused by the stimulation to IFN-α/β [52].

When expression of receptors in patients with different grades of CIN was analyzed versus a healthy control group, both lower local levels of IFN-α mRNA and reduced expression of IFN-α receptors were detected in the patients with CIN. These findings suggest that IFN-α immunotherapy can be ineffective if there is an inadequate number of receptors present on the cell surface, and may represent a mechanism by which HPV and neoplastic cells can elude the immune response [50].

The cervical intraepithelial neoplasias (CINs) are considered the precursors of cervical cancer; their early detection and subsequent intervention can potentially prevent tumor development.

A recent study demonstrated that immunotherapy with IFN-α 2b administrated intralesionally in patients with CIN II/III produces favorable results in patients who do not smoke [53].

## Ongoing Clinical Trials

Clinical trials are studies of new, innovative cancer treatments. Clinical trials are the instrument to find better ways to prevent, diagnose, and treat cancer. Each new treatment study goes through four phases. Patients join clinical trials at specific phases. A clinical research team selects women who are mostly likely to benefit from a particular investigational therapy and guide patients through the process of enrolling in the most appropriate clinical trial. If a patient is eligible to participate in a clinical trial, she may have access to new therapies that are not yet widely available. The aim of clinical trials is to improve treatment outcomes, which includes tumor response and quality of life.

## Antiangiogenetic Agents

Overexpression of the vascular endothelial growth factor (VEGF) family proteins is associated with poor prognosis in many cancers, including squamous and adenocarcinomas of the cervix, and usually correlates with advanced stages and lymph node metastases [54, 55].

Complex interactions occur among VEGF pathway and several growth factors, including epidermal growth factor receptor (EGFR), and other pathways involving receptor tyrosine kinases (RTKs) have also been implicated in the development and progression of cervical cancer [56, 57].

## Receptor Tyrosine Kinase (RTK) Inhibitors

Novel VEGF RTK inhibitors, such as *imatinib*, *sunitinib*, *cediranib*, *sorafenib*, and *pazopanib*, are being tested in phase I–II clinical trials in cervical cancer.

*Cediranib* is being tested in combination with *carboplatin*, *paclitaxel*, or *temsirolimus* in phase II (NCT01229930) and phase I trials (NCT01065662) in advanced cervical cancer.

Other compounds targeting angiogenesis, such as *brivanib*, an oral dual inhibitor of VEGF and the fibroblast growth factor (FGF) receptors, are currently under clinical evaluation (NCT01267253).

## Bevacizumab in Recurrent and Metastatic Cervical Cancer

*Bevacizumab*, a humanized monoclonal antibody directed against VEGF, was the first clinically available antiangiogenetic agent successfully tested in many solid tumors including cervical cancer [58].

Patients with advanced, recurrent, or persistent cervical cancer that was not curable with standard treatment who received the drug *bevacizumab* lived 3.7 months longer than patients who did not receive the drug according to findings from a large, randomized clinical trial. The clinical trial, known as GOG240, was sponsored by the National Cancer Institute (NCI), part of the National Institutes of Health, and conducted by a network of researchers led by the Gynecologic Oncology Group (GOG). The trial was designed to answer two questions: whether *topotecan* in combination with paclitaxel was superior to *cisplatin* and *paclitaxel* in combination, and whether the addition of *bevacizumab* to either regimen improved overall survival. The study achieved its primary endpoint of demonstrating improved overall survival in patients who received *bevacizumab*, which also means that it delayed the chance of dying from the disease. However, patients receiving *bevacizumab* experienced more side effects than those who did not. These side effects were consistent with side effects previously reported to be associated with *bevacizumab* and included hypertension, neutropenia, and thromboembolism, or formation of blood clots. Quality of life during the trial was not significantly different between the patients who received *bevacizumab* and those who received chemotherapy alone. The purpose of *bevacizumab* is to block the blood supply that feeds the tumor. The drug was designed to bind to and inhibit vascular endothelial growth factor (VEGF). VEGF is a protein that plays a crucial role in tumor blood vessel growth. A total of 452 patients in the United States and Spain with metastatic, recurrent, or persistent cervical cancer not curable with standard treatment were enrolled between 2009 and 2012 [40].

## Radiation, Cisplatin Chemotherapy, and Triapine Treatment

National Cancer Institute phase I and phase II clinical trials explored the safety and efficacy of *triapine* added to *cisplatin* radiochemotherapy in untreated patients with advanced-stage cervical cancer. The rationale for these two clinical trials in cervical cancer management is based on the ability of *triapine* to inhibit ribonucleotide reductase activity.

*Triapine* may stop the growth of tumor cells by blocking some of the enzymes needed for cell growth. *Cisplatin* works in different ways to stop the growth of tumor cell, either by killing the cells or by stopping them from dividing. Radiation therapy uses high-energy x-rays to kill tumor cells. Giving *triapine* together with *cisplatin* may make tumor cells more sensitive to radiation therapy.

Between 2006 and 2011, 24 untreated patients with cervical cancer met the criteria for enrolling these clinical trials. *Triapine* added to *cisplatin* radiochemotherapy resulted in a low treatment-related adverse event rate and produced a 3-year disease-free survival rate of 80 % [59]. The antitumor effect of ribonucleotide reductase inhibition by *triapine* represents an important advancement in cervical cancer treatment.

## Histone Deacetylase (HDAC) Inhibitors

*Trichostatin A*, an HDAC inhibitor, can compete with E6 for p53 binding, resulting in p53 hyperacetylation and increased apoptosis, and clinical trials in combination with chemoradiation are ongoing [60, 61].

Preliminary results of a phase III randomized trial of *hydralazine-valproate* versus placebo added to *cisplatin/topotecan* showed a significant advantage in PFS (progression-free survival) for epigenetic treatment over one of the current standard combination chemotherapies in cervical cancer [62]. The combination of *hydralazine* and *valproate*, a DNMT (DNA methyltransferase) and HDAC inhibitor, respectively, has been developed as epigenetic therapy.

## Antioxidants

Oxidative stress is receiving great interest for its role during the progression of neoplasias. Several risk factors of cervical cancer development, such as exposure to cigarette smoke and chronic inflammation, are well documented to increase oxidative stress, which could account for higher risk of cervical cancer in these two conditions [63, 64].

Among antioxidant agents, polyphenols demonstrated to inhibit the proliferation of HPV-positive cancer cells and have been found to be promising drugs for cervical cancer. Polyphenols, from natural and herbal extract, are raising great interest as powerful and safe anticancer strategy for their broad range targeting potential and low side effects [65].

Ongoing clinical trials show encouraging preliminary data. In a randomized clinical trial, antioxidant supplementation in patients treated with chemotherapy and radiotherapy apparently decreased oxidative stress; however, more studies are needed to study the long-term effect of this treatment [66].

## Conclusions

Because of the high incidence of cervical cancer worldwide, big efforts have been made by researchers to understand molecular mechanisms involved in cervical carcinogenesis and to develop new strategies of cure and prevention of this insidious disease. Advances in the understanding of the role of human papillomavirus (HPV) in the etiology of high-grade cervical lesions and cervical cancer have led to the development of two prophylactic HPV vaccines. Vaccination against the HPV, which is the major cause of cervical cancer, is a significant step forward. At least 40 countries had implemented HPV vaccination in their national immunization programs (NIPs) by the beginning of 2012. The current vaccines protecting against HPV-16 and HPV-18 may prevent up to 70 % of new cervical cancers. The high efficacy of the two available cervical cancer vaccines and their proven ability to reduce the incidence of cervical cancer precursor lesions offer hope that the vaccine will have a strong worldwide impact and may significantly reduce the cervical cancer incidence. There are several approaches for the prevention of cervical cancer, and in the near future it is likely that human papillomavirus (HPV) vaccination and HPV-based screening will be complementary strategies.

Cervical cancer harbors high rates of potentially targetable oncogenic mutations. Genomics investigations have documented gene mutations in important regulatory pathways.

Emerging data have suggested that there are molecular alterations present in cervical cancer that differ by histologic subtype. Distinct genomic alterations occur in squamous cell carcinoma and adenocarcinoma of the cervix, which encourage further studies to identify and target distinct molecular subpopulations within cervical cancer. Clinical outcomes may be improved with the use of more tailored treatment strategies, including PI3-Kinase and MEK inhibitors. The use of intracellular antibodies to inhibit protein function is a promising treatment for a large number of human diseases. Among the most investigated molecular targets are epidermal growth factor receptor (EGFR) and vascular epithelial growth factor (VEGF) signaling pathways, both playing a crucial role in cervical cancer development [67]. As a result of screening, most cervical cancers can be identified early and cured with surgery. Chemotherapy is reserved exclusively for the treatment of patients with metastatic or recurrent disease.

Early cervical cancer may be preventable, and when found is highly curable. Advanced and recurrent cervical cancer remain both a very rare challenge, with approximately 4000 cases diagnosed per year in the United States [68]. Moreover, there is also a clinical need for preneoplastic lesions. The biological behavior underlying CIN2–CIN3 is still uncertain, since only an unpredictable part of them will progress to invasive cancer when untreated. Thus, a therapeutic strategy able to interrupt the progression to malignancy for this wide subset of patients remains a significant challenge.

New frontiers in the treatment of cervical cancer are currently represented by antiangiogenic and immunologic therapies.

A number of clinical trials have been designed to validate new options of treatment for cervical cancer based on the use of antiangiogenic factors or novel immunotherapeutic approaches. Preliminary results on antiangiogenetic agents in cervical cancer are encouraging, and many other clinical studies are ongoing, but larger phase III trials are needed to better define the role of agents targeting angiogenesis in this disease. *Bevacizumab*, a humanized monoclonal antibody directed against VEGF, was the first clinically available antiangiogenetic agent successfully tested in many solid tumors, including cervical cancer [58].

Among antiangiogenetic agents, novel EGF RTK (receptor tyrosine kinase) is being tested in phase I–II clinical trials in cervical cancer [69].

Unfortunately, conducting clinical trials in patients with cervical cancer is becoming increasingly difficult depending on multiple factors. A small number of women are eligible for clinical trials, and the accessibility to these trials is poor for some of those women who are candidates because of limited resources. There are also logistical issues in the conduction of international collaborations.

Translational studies are currently focusing on understanding the key points involved in the malignant transformation and progression of cervical cancer, trying to better elucidate the mechanisms involved in this complex carcinogenesis and aiming to identify valid prognostic and predictive biomarkers for the selection of more personalized treatments.

## References

1. Stewart B, Wild CP, editors. World cancer report 2014. Chapter 5.12: cancers of the female reproductive organs. Lyon: World Health Organization; 2014.
2. Giacinti C, Giordano A. RB and cell cycle progression. Oncogene. 2006;25:5220–7.
3. Hopman AH, Smedts F, Dignef W, Ummelen M, Sonke G, Mravunac M, Vooijs GP, Speel EJ, Ramaekers FC. Transition of high-grade cervical intraepithelial neoplasia to micro-invasive carcinoma is characterized by integration of HPV 16/18 and numerical chromosome abnormalities. J Pathol. 2004;202:23–33.
4. Nyagol J, Leucci E, Onnis A, De Falco G, Tigli C, Sanseverino F, Torriccelli M, Palummo N, Pacenti L, Santopietro R, et al. The effects of HIV-1 Tat protein on cell cycle during cervical carcinogenesis. Cancer Biol Ther. 2006;5:684–90.
5. Luhn P, Walker J, Schiffman M, Zuna RE, Dunn ST, Gold MA, Smith K, Mathews C, Allen RA, Zhang R, et al. The role of co-factors in the progression from human papillomavirus infection to cervical cancer. Gynecol Oncol. 2013;128:265–70.
6. Remschmidt C, Kaufmann AM, Hagemann I, Vartazarova E, Wichmann O, Delere Y. Risk factors for cervical human papillomavirus infection and high-grade intraepithelial lesion in women aged 20 to 31 years in Germany. Int J Gynecol Cancer. 2013;23:519–26.
7. Wang SS, Sherman ME, Hildesheim A, Lacey Jr JV, Devesa S. Cervical adenocarcinoma and squamous cell carcinoma incidence trends among white women and black women in the United States for 1976–2000. Cancer. 2004;100:1035–44.

8. Galic V, Herzog TJ, Lewin SN, Neugut AI, Burke WM, Lu YS, Hershman DL, Wright JD. Prognostic significance of adenocarcinoma histology in women with cervical cancer. Gynecol Oncol. 2012;125:287–91.
9. Lee YY, Choi CH, Kim TJ, Lee JW, Kim BG, Lee JH, Bae DS. A comparison of pure adenocarcinoma and squamous cell carcinoma of the cervix after radical hysterectomy in stage IB-IIA. Gynecol Oncol. 2011;120:439–43.
10. Wright AA, Howitt BE, Myers AP, Dahlberg SE, Palescandolo E, Van Hummelen P, MacConaill LE, Shoni M, Wagle N, Jones RT, et al. Oncogenic mutations in cervical cancer: genomic differences between adenocarcinomas and squamous cell carcinomas of the cervix. Cancer. 2013;119:3776–83.
11. Ojesina AI, Lichtenstein L, Freeman SS, Pedamallu CS, Imaz-Rosshandler I, Pugh TJ, Cherniack AD, Ambrogio L, Cibulskis K, Bertelsen B, et al. Landscape of genomic alterations in cervical carcinomas. Nature. 2014;506:371–5.
12. Yan M, Parker BA, Schwab R, Kurzrock R. HER2 aberrations in cancer: implications for therapy. Cancer Treat Rev. 2014;40:770–80.
13. Fadare O, Zheng W. HER2 protein (p185(HER2)) is only rarely overexpressed in cervical cancer. Int J Gynecol Pathol. 2004;23:410–1. author reply 411-412.
14. Jimenez-Wences H, Peralta-Zaragoza O, Fernandez-Tilapa G. Human papilloma virus, DNA methylation and microRNA expression in cervical cancer (Review). Oncol Rep. 2014;31:2467–76.
15. Pedroza-Torres A, Lopez-Urrutia E, Garcia-Castillo V, Jacobo-Herrera N, Herrera LA, Peralta-Zaragoza O, Lopez-Camarillo C, De Leon DC, Fernandez-Retana J, Cerna-Cortes JF, et al. MicroRNAs in cervical cancer: evidences for a miRNA profile deregulated by HPV and its impact on radio-resistance. Molecules. 2014;19:6263–81.
16. Wang WT, Zhao YN, Yan JX, Weng MY, Wang Y, Chen YQ, Hong SJ. Differentially expressed microRNAs in the serum of cervical squamous cell carcinoma patients before and after surgery. J Hematol Oncol. 2014;7:6.
17. Yu J, Wang Y, Dong R, Huang X, Ding S, Qiu H. Circulating microRNA-218 was reduced in cervical cancer and correlated with tumor invasion. J Cancer Res Clin Oncol. 2012;138:671–4.
18. Zhao S, Yao D, Chen J, Ding N. Circulating miRNA-20a and miRNA-203 for screening lymph node metastasis in early stage cervical cancer. Genet Test Mol Biomarkers. 2013;17:631–6.
19. Chen J, Yao D, Li Y, Chen H, He C, Ding N, Lu Y, Ou T, Zhao S, Li L, et al. Serum microRNA expression levels can predict lymph node metastasis in patients with early-stage cervical squamous cell carcinoma. Int J Mol Med. 2013;32:557–67.
20. Bird A. DNA methylation patterns and epigenetic memory. Genes Dev. 2002;16:6–21.
21. Wilting SM, van Boerdonk RA, Henken FE, Meijer CJ, Diosdado B, Meijer GA, le Sage C, Agami R, Snijders PJ, Steenbergen RD. Methylation-mediated silencing and tumour suppressive function of hsa-miR-124 in cervical cancer. Mol Cancer. 2010;9:167.
22. Saavedra KP, Brebi PM, Roa JC. Epigenetic alterations in preneoplastic and neoplastic lesions of the cervix. Clin Epigenet. 2012;4:13.
23. Rouhi A, Mager DL, Humphries RK, Kuchenbauer F. MiRNAs, epigenetics, and cancer. Mamm Genome. 2008;19:517–25.
24. Bock C. Epigenetic biomarker development. Epigenomics. 2009;1:99–110.
25. Lopez-Serra P, Esteller M. DNA methylation-associated silencing of tumor-suppressor microRNAs in cancer. Oncogene. 2012;31:1609–22.
26. Yao T, Rao Q, Liu L, Zheng C, Xie Q, Liang J, Lin Z. Exploration of tumor-suppressive microRNAs silenced by DNA hypermethylation in cervical cancer. Virol J. 2013;10:175.
27. Wilting SM, Verlaat W, Jaspers A, Makazaji NA, Agami R, Meijer CJ, Snijders PJ, Steenbergen RD. Methylation-mediated transcriptional repression of microRNAs during cervical carcinogenesis. Epigenetics. 2013;8:220–8.
28. Botezatu A, Goia-Rusanu CD, Iancu IV, Huica I, Plesa A, Socolov D, Ungureanu C, Anton G. Quantitative analysis of the relationship between microRNA124a, -34b and -203 gene methylation and cervical oncogenesis. Mol Med Rep. 2011;4:121–8.
29. Au Yeung CL, Tsang WP, Tsang TY, Co NN, Yau PL, Kwok TT. HPV-16 E6 upregulation of DNMT1 through repression of tumor suppressor p53. Oncol Rep. 2010;24:1599–604.
30. zur Hausen H. Human papillomaviruses and their possible role in squamous cell carcinomas. Curr Top Microbiol Immunol. 1977;78:1–30.
31. Franco EL, Harper DM. Vaccination against human papillomavirus infection: a new paradigm in cervical cancer control. Vaccine. 2005;23:2388–94.
32. Bermudez-Humaran LG, Langella P. Perspectives for the development of human papillomavirus vaccines and immunotherapy. Expert Rev Vaccines. 2010;9:35–44.
33. Markowitz LE, Tsu V, Deeks SL, Cubie H, Wang SA, Vicari AS, Brotherton JM. Human papillomavirus vaccine introduction—the first five years. Vaccine. 2012;30 Suppl 5:F139–48.
34. D'Andrilli G, Bovicelli A, Giordano A. HPV vaccines: state of the art. J Cell Physiol. 2010;224:601–4.
35. Hakim AA, Dinh TA. Worldwide impact of the human papillomavirus vaccine. Curr Treat Options Oncol. 2009;10:44–53.
36. Arbyn M, Dillner J. Review of current knowledge on HPV vaccination: an appendix to the European guidelines for quality assurance in cervical cancer screening. J Clin Virol. 2007;38:189–97.
37. Ferrara N, Gerber HP, LeCouter J. The biology of VEGF and its receptors. Nat Med. 2003;9:669–76.
38. Monk BJ, Sill MW, Burger RA, Gray HJ, Buekers TE, Roman LD. Phase II trial of bevacizumab in the treatment of persistent or recurrent squamous cell carcinoma of the cervix: a gynecologic oncology group study. J Clin Oncol. 2009;27:1069–74.

39. Monk BJ, Chan JK. American Society of Clinical Oncology. Annual meeting update: summary of selected gynecologic cancer abstracts. Gynecol Oncol. 2010;2010(118):216–9.
40. Tewari KS, Sill MW, Long 3rd HJ, Penson RT, Huang H, Ramondetta LM, Landrum LM, Oaknin A, Reid TJ, Leitao MM, et al. Improved survival with bevacizumab in advanced cervical cancer. N Engl J Med. 2014;370:734–43.
41. NCI Press Release: Bevacizumab significantly improves survival for patients with recurrent and metastatic cervical cancer [Internet]. 2013. http://www.cancer.gov/news-events/press-releases/2013/GOG240.
42. Tewari KS. American Society of Clinical Oncology. Annual meeting: highlights from the gynecologic oncology track. Int J Gynecol Cancer. 2012; 2012(22):1634–9.
43. Karim R, Jordanova ES, Piersma SJ, Kenter GG, Chen L, Boer JM, Melief CJ, van der Burg SH. Tumor-expressed B7-H1 and B7-DC in relation to PD-1+ T-cell infiltration and survival of patients with cervical carcinoma. Clin Cancer Res. 2009;15:6341–7.
44. Radulovic S, Brankovic-Magic M, Malisic E, Jankovic R, Dobricic J, Plesinac-Karapandzic V, Maciag PC, Rothman J. Therapeutic cancer vaccines in cervical cancer: phase I study of Lovaxin-C. J BUON. 2009;14 Suppl 1:S165–8.
45. Hinrichs CS, Rosenberg SA. Exploiting the curative potential of adoptive T-cell therapy for cancer. Immunol Rev. 2014;257:56–71.
46. Baleja JD, Cherry JJ, Liu Z, Gao H, Nicklaus MC, Voigt JH, Chen JJ, Androphy EJ. Identification of inhibitors to papillomavirus type 16 E6 protein based on three-dimensional structures of interacting proteins. Antiviral Res. 2006;72:49–59.
47. Liu Y, Liu Z, Androphy E, Chen J, Baleja JD. Design and characterization of helical peptides that inhibit the E6 protein of papillomavirus. Biochemistry. 2004;43:7421–31.
48. Zehbe I, Richard C, Lee KF, Campbell M, Hampson L, Hampson IN. Lopinavir shows greater specificity than zinc finger ejecting compounds as a potential treatment for human papillomavirus-related lesions. Antiviral Res. 2011;91:161–6.
49. Van Pachterbeke C, Bucella D, Rozenberg S, Manigart Y, Gilles C, Larsimont D, Vanden Houte K, Reynders M, Snoeck R, Bossens M. Topical treatment of CIN 2+ by cidofovir: results of a phase II, double-blind, prospective, placebo-controlled study. Gynecol Oncol. 2009;115:69–74.
50. Montes L, Andrade CM, Michelin MA, Murta EF. The importance of alpha/beta (alpha/13) interferon receptors and signaling pathways for the treatment of cervical intraepithelial neoplasias. Eur J Gynaecol Oncol. 2014;35:368–72.
51. Kim SH, Cohen B, Novick D, Rubinstein M. Mammalian type I interferon receptors consists of two subunits: IFNaR1 and IFNaR2. Gene. 1997;196: 279–86.
52. Moraga I, Harari D, Schreiber G, Uze G, Pellegrini S. Receptor density is key to the alpha2/beta interferon differential activities. Mol Cell Biol. 2009;29:4778–87.
53. Machado FA, Abdalla DR, Montes L, Etchebehere RM, Michelin MA, Murta EF. An evaluation of immune system cell infiltrate in the cervical stroma of patients with grade III cervical intraepithelial neoplasia after treatment with intralesional alpha-2B interferon. Eur J Gynaecol Oncol. 2014;35:20–5.
54. Hashimoto I, Kodama J, Seki N, Hongo A, Yoshinouchi M, Okuda H, Kudo T. Vascular endothelial growth factor-C expression and its relationship to pelvic lymph node status in invasive cervical cancer. Br J Cancer. 2001;85:93–7.
55. Lee JS, Kim HS, Jung JJ, Lee MC, Park CS. Expression of vascular endothelial growth factor in adenocarcinomas of the uterine cervix and its relation to angiogenesis and p53 and c-erbB-2 protein expression. Gynecol Oncol. 2002;85:469–75.
56. del Campo JM, Prat A, Gil-Moreno A, Perez J, Parera M. Update on novel therapeutic agents for cervical cancer. Gynecol Oncol. 2008;110:S72–6.
57. Mathur RS, Mathur SP. Vascular endothelial growth factor (VEGF) up-regulates epidermal growth factor receptor (EGF-R) in cervical cancer in vitro: this action is mediated through HPV-E6 in HPV-positive cancers. Gynecol Oncol. 2005;97:206–13.
58. Shih T, Lindley C. Bevacizumab: an angiogenesis inhibitor for the treatment of solid malignancies. Clin Ther. 2006;28:1779–802.
59. Kunos CA, Sherertz TM. Long-term disease control with triapine-based radiochemotherapy for patients with stage IB2-IIIB cervical cancer. Front Oncol. 2014;4:184.
60. de la Cruz-Hernandez E, Perez-Cardenas E, Contreras-Paredes A, Cantu D, Mohar A, Lizano M, Duenas-Gonzalez A. The effects of DNA methylation and histone deacetylase inhibitors on human papillomavirus early gene expression in cervical cancer, an in vitro and clinical study. Virol J. 2007;4:18.
61. Lin Z, Bazzaro M, Wang MC, Chan KC, Peng S, Roden RB. Combination of proteasome and HDAC inhibitors for uterine cervical cancer treatment. Clin Cancer Res. 2009;15:570–7.
62. Coronel J, Cetina L, Pacheco I, Trejo-Becerril C, Gonzalez-Fierro A, de la Cruz-Hernandez E, Perez-Cardenas E, Taja-Chayeb L, Arias-Bofill D, Candelaria M, et al. A double-blind, placebo-controlled, randomized phase III trial of chemotherapy plus epigenetic therapy with hydralazine valproate for advanced cervical cancer preliminary results. Med Oncol. 2011;28 Suppl 1:540–6.
63. Moktar A, Singh R, Vadhanam MV, Ravoori S, Lillard JW, Gairola CG, Gupta RC. Cigarette smoke condensate-induced oxidative DNA damage and its removal in human cervical cancer cells. Int J Oncol. 2011;39:941–7.
64. Beevi SS, Rasheed MH, Geetha A. Evidence of oxidative and nitrosative stress in patients with cervical squamous cell carcinoma. Clin Chim Acta. 2007;375:119–23.
65. Di Domenico F, Foppoli C, Coccia R, Perluigi M. Antioxidants in cervical cancer: chemopreventive

and chemotherapeutic effects of polyphenols. Biochim Biophys Acta. 1822;2012:737–47.
66. Fuchs-Tarlovsky V, Rivera MA, Altamirano KA, Lopez-Alvarenga JC, Ceballos-Reyes GM. Antioxidant supplementation has a positive effect on oxidative stress and hematological toxicity during oncology treatment in cervical cancer patients. Support Care Cancer. 2013;21:1359–63.
67. Vici P, Mariani L, Pizzuti L, Sergi D, Di Lauro L, Vizza E, Tomao F, Tomao S, Mancini E, Vincenzoni C, et al. Emerging biological treatments for uterine cervical carcinoma. J Cancer. 2014;5:86–97.
68. Siegel R, Naishadham D, Jemal A. Cancer statistics, 2013. CA Cancer J Clin. 2013;63:11–30.
69. Mackay HJ, Tinker A, Winquist E, Thomas G, Swenerton K, Oza A, Sederias J, Ivy P, Eisenhauer EA. A phase II study of sunitinib in patients with locally advanced or metastatic cervical carcinoma: NCIC CTG Trial IND.184. Gynecol Oncol. 2010;116:163–7.

# 4 Advances in Ovarian Cancer and Ongoing Clinical Trials

Valeria Masciullo, Cristina Di Cesare, and Ida Paris


**Abstract**

Bevacizumab, a recombinant monoclonal antibody against vascular endothelial growth factor (VEGF), has gained European Medicine Agency approval for the frontline treatment of advanced epithelial ovarian cancer, fallopian tube cancer, or primary peritoneal cancer in combination with carboplatin and paclitaxel, and for the treatment of first recurrence of platinum-sensitive ovarian cancer in combination with carboplatin and gemcitabine. The addition of bevacizumab to standard chemotherapy as frontline treatment (GOG-0218 and ICON7) or in recurrent disease (OCEANS and AURELIA) shows significant efficiency. Promising data have been published for a number of emerging antiangiogenic agents.

Currently, single agent trabectedin is approved for treatment of patients with advanced soft tissue sarcoma after failure of anthracyclines and ifosfamide, and in association with pegylated liposomal doxorubicin for treatment of patients with relapsed partially platinum-sensitive ovarian cancer. In particular, its peculiar mechanisms of action suggest its potential activity in specific subsets of ovarian cancer patients endowed with BRCA mutation or the so-called BRCAness phenotype (i.e., serous, high-grade carcinomas; repeated response to platinum-based regimens); this is likely to enlarge in the future the clinical settings in which candidates can take advantage of even single agent trabectedin.

PARP inhibitors are proteins involved in the base excision repair of DNA single-strand breaks and represent one of the most promising targeted therapy demonstrating single-agent activity in BRCA-related and



V. Masciullo, MD, PhD (✉) • C. Di Cesare, MD
I. Paris, MD
Division of Gynecologic Oncology, Agostino Gemelli Hospital, Catholic University of Sacred Heart, Largo Agostino Gemelli, 8, Rome 00168, Italy
e-mail: valeriamasciullo@yahoo.com; cristinadicesare9@gmail.com; ida_paris@yahoo.it





A. Giordano, M. Macaluso (eds.), *Gynecological Cancers*, Current Clinical Oncology,
DOI 10.1007/978-3-319-32907-9_4

sporadic high grade serous ovarian cancer. Active search is ongoing in order to define biomarkers predictive of response to these novel treatments, and also to help clarify the biological mechanisms sustaining the achievement of long-lasting stable disease.

**Keywords**
Epithelial ovarian cancer • Chemotherapy • Bevacizumab • Trabectedin • PARP-inhibitors • Ipilimumab • Selumetinib • Binimetinib • Cediranib • Farletuzumab • Lurbinectin • Nivolumab • Catumaxomab

Epithelial ovarian cancer (EOC) is diagnosed at an advanced stage in most patients due to the lack of effective screening tests for early detection. The worldwide incidence is 225,500 diagnoses per year; in the USA in 2014, 21,980 women have been diagnosed with ovarian cancer. Global mortality of this cancer remains high, with 140,200 deaths per year, and minimal improvement in mortality rate has been observed over the past decade [1, 2].

Primary debulking surgery (PDS) remains the cornerstone in the surgical approach for women with advanced disease. After surgical cytoreduction, the treatment of choice for patients with advanced EOC (FIGO stage IIB-IIIC) is platinum-based chemotherapy (six cycles of carboplatin plus paclitaxel [CP] given every 3 weeks). Recently a modified CP regimen with weekly paclitaxel resulted in better long-term outcome than the 3-weekly regimen in a phase III study in Japanese women with advanced ovarian cancer [3], with confirmatory findings reported in European women in the randomized, multicenter phase III MITO-7 study [4], and in the chemotherapy arm of the phase III GOG-0262 trial [5]. This regimen has now been included in the NCCN treatment guidelines [6].

Although approximately 80 % of patients respond to frontline chemotherapy, more than 70 % of patients with advanced stage disease recur within 5 years and develop drug resistance.

Neoadjuvant chemotherapy (NACT) followed by interval debulking surgery (IDS) has been recognized as a valuable therapeutic option in patients unsuitable for complete PDS because of their general performance status or of extensive disease [7].

For recurrent disease, the treatment choice is based on the timing and nature of the recurrence and the extent of prior chemotherapy. Most patients with advanced ovarian cancer will recur according to two patterns: the subgroup with platinum-sensitive recurrence (defined as cancer recurring 6 months after the last platinum), and patients with recurrent platinum-resistant disease (defined as cancer recurring <6 months after last platinum). Patients that recur between 6 and 12 months of initial treatment may respond to a rechallenge with a platinum plus taxane therapy, whereas those who relapse earlier or develop significant toxicity may be given pegylated liposomal doxorubicin, gemcitabine (in combination with platinum), etoposide, Alkeran, topotecan, and/or hexamethylmelamide [8]. Unfortunately, the response rate to these agents is generally less than 30 %, and survival benefits have not yet been reported.

More effective treatment strategies, particularly molecular targeted agents, are required to improve outcomes for women with advanced ovarian cancer.

## Antiangiogenetic Inhibitors

The vascular endothelial growth factor (VEGF)-mediated angiogenesis plays a vital role in the development and progression of ovarian cancer. Several studies found VEGF serum levels to be an independent prognostic factor for OS in multivariate analysis [9]. Thus, a number of antiangiogenic agents are currently in development as potential treatment options for patients with advanced disease.

## Bevacizumab

It is a recombinant, humanized, monoclonal antibody that binds to all isoforms of VEGF and is indicated for treatment of several solid tumors (such as metastatic colorectal cancer, non-small-cell lung cancer, metastatic renal cell carcinoma, and glioblastoma) in combination with cytotoxic chemotherapy. Recently, the European Agency has approved bevacizumab, in combination with CP, for the frontline treatment of patients with advanced EOC, fallopian tube cancer or primary peritoneal cancer and, in combination with carboplatin and gemcitabine (CG), for the treatment of first recurrence of platinum-sensitive ovarian cancer. Efficacy data are available from four randomized, double-blind, phase III trials of bevacizumab in advanced ovarian cancer: GOG-0218 [10] and ICON7 [11, 12] in the frontline treatment setting and OCEANS [13, 14] and AURELIA [15] in patients with recurrent disease. The GOG-0218 enrolled 1873 women with newly diagnosed stage III or stage IV EOC to receive CP with placebo or CP with bevacizumab from cycles 2–6 and placebo from cycles 7–22 (bevacizumab initiation) or CP with bevacizumab (bevacizumab throughout). Compared with the control arm, the primary endpoint of PFS was longer in the bevacizumab initiation arm and significantly longer in the bevacizumab throughout arm (median 14.1 vs 10.3 months; $p<0.001$). In the ICON7 study, 1528 women with high risk early stage ovarian cancer were randomized to receive frontline CP or CP plus bevacizumab followed by bevacizumab for a maximum of 12 months. A statistically significant increase in PFS was noted in the bevacizumab arm compare to the CP arm (median 19.0 vs 17.3 months, $p=0.004$). In the OCEAN study a total of 484 patients whose disease had recurred ≥6 months after frontline platinum-containing chemotherapy were randomized 1:1 to receive gentamicin plus bevacizumab or gentamicin plus placebo. The addition of bevacizumab to gemcitabine significantly increased PFS compared with placebo ($p<0.0001$). The AURELIA trial is investigating the combination of bevacizumab and chemotherapy in platinum-resistant recurrent ovarian cancer cells. A statistically significant and clinically meaningful improvement in PFS ($p<0.001$) and in overall response rate ($p=0.001$) was observed in the bevacizumab plus chemotherapy group compared with the chemotherapy alone group.

Bevacizumab is actually being evaluated in a large number of ongoing, randomized, phase III trials in ovarian cancer (National Cancer Institute. http://www.clinicaltrialsgov/show/NCT00565851; and NCT01462890 and NCT01167712). Safety results from these studies are awaited. Furthermore, several trials are assessing the efficacy and safety of bevacizumab in combination with novel targeted agents.

## Cediranib

Antiangiogenic agents in recurrent ovarian cancer have not demonstrated OS benefits until just recently. In ICON6, combination of the oral VEGFR tyrosine kinase inhibitor cediranib [16] with platinum-based chemotherapy in platinum-sensitive recurrent ovarian cancer, followed by cediranib maintenance, improved OS in a preliminary analysis [17]. PFS improved from 9.4 months of the arm with chemotherapy alone to 12.6 months of the cediranib/chemotherapy arm, while OS increased from 17.6 to 20.3 months, respectively (hazard ratio, 0.70; *p* ¼ 0.0419). Although trials of various antiangiogenetic agents have demonstrated progression-free survival (PFS) benefit in randomized trials [18], only recently, the addition of cediranib to platinum-based chemotherapy in patients with platinum-sensitive recurrent ovarian cancer resulted in a significant increase in OS [19].

## Trabectedin (ET-743)

Among the pharmaceutical options currently available for the medical treatment of ovarian cancer, much emphasis has been progressively placed on trabectedin (ET-743, Yondelis®; Zeltia, Madrid, Spain, and Johnson & Johnson, New Brunswick, NJ, USA), which had gained much attention because of its unique mechanism of action and the demonstration of clinical activity in ovarian cancer as well as other solid malignancies. Since 2007, trabectedin represents the first anticancer marine-derived drug that has obtained marketing authorization from the European Medicines Agency (EMA), and from many other countries worldwide for treatment of patients with advanced soft tissue sarcoma. Moreover, based on the reported results of OVA-301 Phase III randomized study [20], in 2009 EMEA granted marketing authorization for trabectedin combined with pegylated liposomal doxorubicin (PLD) for treatment of patients with relapsed partially platinum-sensitive ovarian cancer [21]. In the USA the New Drug Application (NDA) for trabectedin when administered in combination with Doxil (doxorubicin HCI liposome injection) for the treatment of women with relapsed ovarian cancer has been submitted to Food and Drug Administration (FDA) in 2008. However, the agency has requested additional information, including overall survival data from the company's ongoing pivotal trial and additional clinical pharmacology studies.

Trabectedin is a marine-derived tetrahydroisoquinoline alkaloid with antitumor activity, originally isolated from the tunicate *Ecteinascidia turbinata* and currently synthetically produced [22]. In particular, its peculiar structure might allow the drug to interact with DNA through a covalent binding at the N2-guanine at the minor DNA groove, This binding induces a bend of the helix toward the major groove and a DNA damage; this is recognized by the nucleotide excision repair (NER) system, and results in the accumulation of ternary DNA–trabectedin protein repair complexes which lead, after collision with the replication fork, to the formation of double-strand DNA breaks, block of cell cycle, and induction of p53-independent apoptosis (Fig. 4.1). Besides these direct effects on the DNA helix, trabectedin is able to interfere with transcription regulatory pathways in a promoter- and gene-dependent manner, as well as in a cell-dependent fashion; in particular, trabectedin has been shown to inhibit binding of transcription factors to DNA, thus blocking their transactivating effects. Very recent studies have also high-

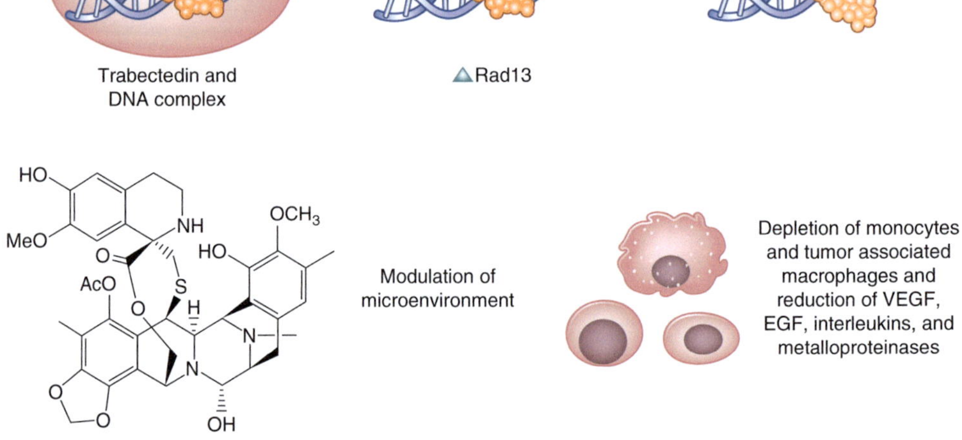


**Fig. 4.1** Mechanism of action of trabectedin. *EGF* epidermal growth factor, *VEGF* vascular endothelial growth factor

**Table 4.1** Phase II studies with trabectedin single agent or in combination

| Author | Type of study | Patients (no.) | Dose, schedule | Patients with ≤2 previous lines (%) | Platinum-resistant patients (%) | Response rate (%) | Median PFS (mts) | Median OS (mts) |
|---|---|---|---|---|---|---|---|---|
| Sessa et al. [60] | Phase II | All 59<br>Res 19<br>Sen 30 | 1.3 mg/m$^2$, q21-d | 37 | 32.0 | All 22<br>Res 7<br>Sen 43 | na | na |
| Krasner et al. [61] | Phase II | All 147 | 0.58 mg/m$^2$ (3-h), weekly for 3 weeks, q28-d | All 31 | 55.0 | All 16.3 | | |
| | | Res 81 | | Res 35 | | Res 6.3 | 2.0 | 11.1 |
| | | Sen 66 | | Sen 26 | | Sen 29.0 | 5.1 | nr |
| Del Campo et al. [62] | Randomized phase II | Arm I 55 | 1.5 mg/m$^2$ (24 h), q21-d vs 1.3 mg/m$^2$ (3-h), q21-d | 40.7 | 9.2 | Arm I 38.9 | 6.1 | na |
| | | Arm 2 53 | | 28.3 | 3.8 | Arm 2 35.8 | 6.8 | |
| Lo Russo et al. [63] | Phase II | All 94 | Trabectedin 1.3 mg/mq i.v. q 3 weeks | 10.1 | 51.0 | All 39.4 | | 18 |
| | | Res 48 | | | | Res 31.2 | 3.0 | |
| | | Sen 46 | | | | Sen 47.8 | 6.0 | |

lighted that trabectedin could exert its antitumor activity by targeting some normal host cells. In particular, trabectedin has been shown to selectively deplete blood monocytes and tumor-associated macrophages in tumor-bearing mice as well as in tissue biopsies from soft tissues sarcoma and ovarian cancer patients [23].

Phase 1 studies reported neutropenia and thrombocytopenia as the most frequent dose-limiting toxicities (DLT). Hepatotoxicity consisted mainly of elevation of transaminases; this toxicity was consistently reported to increase with trabectedin area under the curve (AUC), although it was always reversible (duration between 3 and 4 weeks), and not dose limiting. Moreover, hepatotoxicity was even lower when the dose was divided over 5 days compared to the single-dose schedule. Earlier preclinical studies have demonstrated a synergistic effect of the combination of trabectedin with platinum [24]. The rationale relies on the available evidences about the molecular target of the two drugs. Platinum agents hit the major groove of DNA, thus inducing DNA damage which is repaired by the HRR system. On the other hand, trabectedin activity requires an efficient NER machinery. Overall, the combination of trabectedin with the most commonly used agent in ovarian cancer (PLD, paclitaxel, or gemcitabine) was demonstrated to be feasible and endowed with some antitumor activity [25].

A summary of Phase II studies using trabectedin as a single agent in ovarian cancer is presented in Table 4.1. The whole series in each study shows a response rate ranging between 16.3 and 38.9 %. As expected, in the subgroup of platinum-resistant patients, the rate of response was low (6.3–7 %), while in patients with platinum-sensitive disease trabectedin was able to induce objective response between 29.0 and 43.0 %. A pooled analysis of the available phase II studies reported an objective response rate of 26 %, a median duration of response of 5.5 months, and a very encouraging rate of stable disease in almost 30 % of cases [26]. Interestingly enough, patients administered the 3-weekly schedule exhibited a higher response rate compared to cases administered the weekly regimen (36.0 % vs 16.0 %, $p=0.0001$). Finally, it has to be emphasized that trabectedin activity does not seem to be related to the amount of previous chemotherapy lines [27]. All phase II studies highlighted the promising activity of trabectedin single agent, especially in patients with platinum-sensitive disease, as well as a manageable and noncumulative toxicity profile of the drug.

The Phase III trial OVA-301 (NCT00113607), planned in 2005, aimed at comparing trabectedin 1.1 mg/m$^2$/PLD 30 mg/m$^2$ every 21 days versus PLD 50 mg/m$^2$ every 28 days in ovarian, peritoneal, and tubal cancer recurring/progressing after first-line chemotherapy, with the exclusion of refractory cases [28]. Overall, 672 patients were enrolled (337 allocated to trabectedin/PLD versus 335 allocated to PLD). In the whole series, the response rate, as assessed by independent radiology review by RECIST (Response Evaluation Criteria in Solid Tumors), was significantly higher in trabectedin/PLD than PLD alone group (27.6 % vs 18.8 %, $p=0.008$). In platinum-resistant cases ($n=242$), no difference in response rate was observed in the combination versus PLD alone (13.4 % vs 12.2 %, respectively), while platinum-sensitive patients showed a higher response rate to trabectedin/PLD compared to PLD (35.3 % vs 22.6 %; $p=0.0042$). A very recent cost-effectiveness analysis based on the final survival data of the OVA-301 study confirmed a significant improvement of OS, and an increased cost-effectiveness ratio per quality-adjusted life-year compared to the original evaluation [29].

Based on these data, novel clinical trials are ongoing. The Inovatyon (International Ovarian Cancer Patients Trial with Yondelis) study (NCT01379989) investigates the superiority of trabectedin/PLD versus carboplatin/PLD in partially platinum-sensitive disease. Moreover, due to the strong rationale sustaining the role of BRCA 1/2 mutation or BRCAness in conditioning responsiveness to trabectedin, the MITO-15 (Multicenter Italian Trials in Ovarian Cancer and Gynecology) study (NCT01772979) has been conducted to investigate the efficacy of single agent trabectedin in relapsed ovarian cancer with BRCA mutation or exhibiting the BRCAness phenotype. The trial has recently closed patient accrual, and analysis of data is ongoing. Recently, a Phase II study (NCT01735071) is assessing the efficacy and safety of the combination trabectedin and bevacizumab with or without carboplatin in partially platinum-sensitive recurrent ovarian cancer patients. Active search is also ongoing in order to define biomarkers predictive of response to trabectedin treatment, and also to help clarify the biological mechanisms sustaining one of the special features of trabectedin activity, namely the achievement of long-lasting stable disease.

## Poly(ADP-Ribose) Polymerase (PARP) Inhibitors

PARP inhibitors are the most interesting new class of targeted therapy in ovarian cancer demonstrating single-agent activity in BRCA-related and sporadic high grade serous ovarian cancer. PARP proteins are involved in the base excision repair of DNA single-strand breaks (Fig. 4.2).

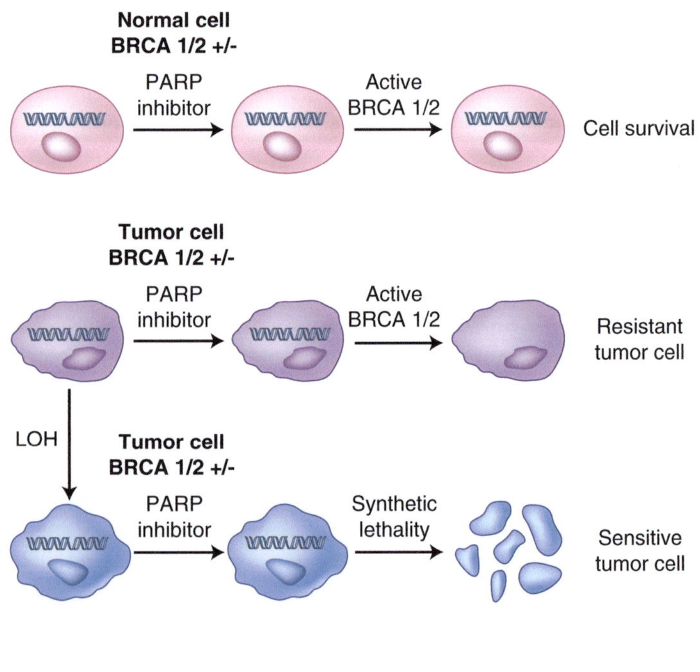


**Fig. 4.2** Mechanism of action of PARP inhibitors in normal and cancer ovarian cells. *SSB* single strand break, *DSB* double strand break, *LOH* loss of heterozygosis

Cells lacking BRCA show defects in DNA repair by homologous recombination and are 1000-fold more sensitive to PARP inhibitors [30]. The sensitivity to PARP inhibitors is also evident in high grade serous ovarian cancer. Phase III PARP inhibitor studies are ongoing for treatment of newly diagnosed germ line BRCA-mutated cancers and of platinum-sensitive recurrent ovarian cancer. Maintenance monotherapy with the PARP inhibitor olaparib significantly prolonged progression-free survival (PFS) than placebo (8.4 vs 4.8 months) in patients with platinum-sensitive relapsed high grade serous ovarian cancer [31]. The presence of a *BRCA* mutation was not required for study entry, although a significant number of patients carried a *BRCA* mutation (97 out of 265 patients (36.6 %)). A recent study has shown that patients with germ line or tumor BRCA mutation have a median PFS significantly longer in the olaparib maintenance group than in the placebo group (11.2 vs 4.3 months). Overall survival did not significantly differ between the groups [32]. These results lead to a phase III trial named SOLO1 (Olaparib Monotherapy in Patients with BRCA Mutated Ovarian Cancer Following First Line Platinum Based Chemotherapy; http://clinicaltrials.gov/show/NCT01844986) based on olaparib 300 mg as maintenance therapy in platinum-sensitive patients after first line chemotherapy. Actually, Olaparib is also being evaluated in BRCA mutated, platinum-sensitive, recurrent ovarian cancer in a phase III trial named SOLO2 (Olaparib Treatment in BRCA Mutated Ovarian Cancer Patients After Complete or Partial Response to Platinum Chemotherapy; http://clinicaltrials.gov/show/ NCT01874353).

The efficacy of olaparib has also been tested in an open-label, randomized, phase II study, for BRCA1/2 mutated patients with recurrent ovarian cancer (within 12 months of prior platinum therapy). Median PFS was 6.5 months (95 % CI, 5.5–10.1 months), 8.8 months (95 % CI, 5.4–9.2 months), and 7.1 months (95 % CI, 3.7–10.7 months) for the olaparib 200 mg twice per day, the olaparib 400 mg twice per day, and pegylated liposomal doxorubicin (PLD) 50 mg/m$^2$ administered intravenously, respectively. However, differences among groups were not statistically significant [33]. Evidence of efficacy of olaparib in combination therapy with carboplatinum/paclitaxel and subsequent maintenance treatment derived from a phase II trial recently published by Oza et al. [34] demonstrating that median progression-free survival was significantly longer in the arm with olaparib plus chemotherapy group (12.2 months) than in the arm with chemotherapy alone (9.6 months) (HR 0.51 [95 % CI, 0.34–0.77]; $p=0.0012$), especially in patients with BRCA mutations (HR 0.21 [0.08–0.55]; $p=0.0015$). Results from the SOLO1 and SOLO2 trials will help to clarify the role of olaparib in treatment of primary and recurrent ovarian cancer.

*Rucaparib* (AG-014699) is a PARP inhibitor with a similar action to olaparib, actually tested in two trials: (1) ARIEL2 aimed to evaluate specific biomarkers to predict sensitivity to rucaparib (A Study of Rucaparib in Patients With Platinum-Sensitive, Relapsed, High-Grade Epithelial Ovarian, Fallopian Tube, or Primary Peritoneal Cancer; http://clinicaltrials.gov/show/NCT01891344) and (2) ARIEL3, a randomized, double-blind phase III study comparing rucaparib to placebo in ovarian cancer patients platinum sensitive (A Study of Rucaparib as Switch Maintenance Following Platinum-Based Chemotherapy in Patients With Platinum-Sensitive, High-Grade Serous or Endometrioid Epithelial Ovarian, Primary Peritoneal or Fallopian Tube Cancer; http://clinicaltrials.gov/show/NCT01968213).

*Niraparib (MK-4827)* is a potent PARP inhibitor with efficacy in both germ line BRCA mutated and BRCA negative high grade serous ovarian cancer patients. Recently, a phase I study has established the dose well tolerated was a recommended phase 2 dose of 300 mg/day [35]. Actually a phase III study, ENGOT-OV16/NOVA trial, is ongoing on maintenance therapy with niraparib versus placebo in ovarian cancer platinum-sensitive patients [36].

*Veliparib*: In a phase 2 study of 50 ovarian cancer patients with *BRCA* mutation, treatment with veliparib at a dose of 400 mg resulted in a

26 % objective response rate, according to RECIST criteria. Two of these women had a complete response, and 24 had disease stabilization for more than 4 months [37]. Actually, several trials are ongoing testing veliparib in monotherapy (Veliparib Monotherapy for Relapsed Ovarian Cancer With BRCA Mutation; http://clinicaltrials.gov/show/ 01472783) or in combination with chemotherapy (Carboplatin, Paclitaxel, Bevacizumab, and Veliparib in Treating Patients With Newly Diagnosed Stage II–IV Ovarian Epithelial, Fallopian Tube, or Primary Peritoneal Cancer; http://clinicaltrials.gov/show/NCT00989651) in ovarian cancer patients BRCA mutated or with BRCA status unknown (Veliparib and Topotecan for Relapsed Ovarian Cancer With Negative or Unknown BRCA Status.NCT 01690598).

Combinations in clinical testing include PARPis and PI3K inhibitors; preclinical results combining olaparib and the PI3K inhibitor BKM120 demonstrated synergy [38, 39].

## MAPK Kinase (MEK-1 and -2) Inhibitors

*Selumetinib* (AZD6244): Selumetinib is a mitogen-activated protein kinase inhibitor that shows preclinical benefit in targeting the MEK oncogenic pathway. The small molecular agent is a protein regulator in activated oncogenic pathways expressed in ovarian cancer patients. Results from a phase II study indicate positive activity in the treatment of ovarian cancer. Fifty-two women received two doses of selumetinib (100 mg daily) in the clinical trial, and grade 4 adverse events were only observed in three patients (6 %). Thirty-four (63 %) of the women in the study had a PFS of more than 6 months, with a median OS of 11 months [40, 41].

*Binimetinib (MEK 162)* is an oral inhibitor of MEK-1 and MEK-2, both of which play an important role in cancer cell proliferation and survival via the RAS/RAF/MEK/ERK signal cascade. Inhibiting this pathway is believed to interrupt growth-factor mediated cell signaling as well as inhibit the production of inflammatory cytokines. A phase III study, MILO, is underway on recurrent or persistent low grade serous ovarian cancer [42].

## VEGF Receptor, Platelet-Derived and Fibroblast Growth Factor Receptor

*Nintedanib* (BIBF 1120). Nintedanib is a triple angiokinase inhibitor that simultaneously blocks the VEGF, platelet-derived, and fibroblast growth factor receptors [43, 44]. A randomized, placebo-controlled phase II trial evaluated nintedanib maintenance therapy (250 mg for 36 weeks), after chemotherapy in patients with relapsed ovarian cancer. Eighty-three women were enrolled, and the 63-week PFS rate was 16.3 % for nintedanib and 5 % for placebo groups, respectively. Nintedanib patients experienced a much higher rate of grade 3 or 4 hepatotoxicity (51.2 %), compared to that of the placebo group (7.5 %) [45]. The potential effect of nintedanib nearly tripling PFS, when compared to the placebo, has warranted a 1300 patient, phase III study of this drug in the LUME-Ovar 1 trial (Nintedanib (BIBF 1120) or Placebo in Combination With Paclitaxel and Carboplatin in First Line Treatment of Ovarian Cancer; http://clinicaltrials.gov/show/NCT01015118).

## Chemotherapy

The DNA hypomethylating agent 5-aza-2′-deoxycytodine (decitabine) can reverse resistance to carboplatin in women with relapsed ovarian cancer [46].

*Lurbinectedin (PM01183)*: It is a new compound that binds covalently to DNA preventing the transactivated transcription and inducing the formation of double-strand breaks in several cancer cell lines, including platinum-resistant ovarian cancer cell [47]. At ASCO 2014 it has been presented a phase II study of Lurbinectedin in resistant/refractory pretreated ovarian cancer showing statistically significant superiority of PM01183 over Topotecan in terms of ORR, PFS, and OS [48].

## Anti-programmed Death-1 (PD-1)

PD-1 is a co-inhibitory receptor expressed on activated T cells which regulates antitumor immunity. Ovarian cancer cell expression of PD-L1 correlates with prognosis, thus PD-1 and PD-L1 pathways may be a viable target in ovarian cancer [49]. Nivolumab is a fully humanized IgG4 that blocks the engagement of PD-1 by PD-1 ligands (PDL-1). Preliminary data from an ongoing clinical trial show that Nivolumab at 1 mg/kg cohort is well tolerated and has encouraging clinical efficacy for advanced or relapsed, platinum-resistant ovarian cancer patients [50].

*Farletuzumab* is a humanized monoclonal antibody to folate receptor-α, which is overexpressed in most epithelial ovarian cancers but absent in normal tissue. A recent clinical study demonstrated that farletuzumab combined with carboplatin and taxane may enhance the response rate and duration of response in platinum-sensitive ovarian cancer patients with first relapse of disease after remission of 6–18 months [51]. A randomized, double-blind, placebo-controlled, phase 2 study is ongoing.

## COMBO Target Therapy

### VEGFBlockade/PARP Inhibition (Cediranib-Olaparib)

Provocative results from a phase II study of the combination of olaparib and cediranib were reported in patients with platinum-sensitive recurrent ovarian cancer [52]. Ninety patients were randomized to either olaparib alone versus the combination of cediranib/olaparib; median PFS was significantly longer with the combination cediranib/olaparib than with olaparib alone (17.7 vs 9 months; hazard ratio, 0.42; 95 % CI 0.23–0.76, $p=0.005$). Subset analysis by germ line BRCA mutation status revealed a significant improvement in PFS in germ line BRCA wild-type or unknown patients receiving cediranib/olaparib compared with olaparib alone (16.5 vs 5.7 months; $p=0.008$) with no significant improvement in PFS observed in the germ line BRCA patients (19.4 vs 16.5 months; $p=0.16$). These results raise the possibility that combining targeted therapies may result in enhanced clinical effect, warranting studies in a phase 3 trial.

### PARPi/PI3Ki (Olaparib/BKM120)

Preclinical results combining olaparib and the PI3K inhibitor BKM120 demonstrated synergy of the two compounds [38, 39]. A phase I study with the two agents has demonstrated anticancer activity of the combination in patients with recurrent high grade serous ovarian cancer or triple-negative breast cancer [53].

### Therapeutic Vaccines

Ipilimumab was administered in recurrent ovarian cancer following administration of a GM-CSF–BKM120 based vaccine [54]; a phase II study is ongoing in recurrent ovarian cancer (NCT01611558).

### EpCAM, CD3, and Fc Receptor Antibody

Catumaxomab is a trifunctional antibody composed of an anti-EpCAM antibody and an anti-CD3 antibody. This allows catumaxomab to bind to the antigen EpCAM on tumor cells, the CD3 molecules on T cells, and to the Fc receptor on accessory cells, thus triggering an antitumor immune response [55]. Catumaxomab has been approved in Europe in 2009 for the intraperitoneal treatment of malignant ascites in EpCAM-positive cancer patients, and it is currently in clinical trials in the USA. An open-label, phase II study of catumaxomab in patients with malignant ascites enrolled 32 women and resulted in almost one-fourth (22.6 %) of patients having at least a fourfold increase in their platinum-free interval following catumaxomab treatment. The median OS was 3.6 months, with toxicities that were tolerable and consistent with the expectation for this type of antibody [56]. Another single-arm phase

II study administered one intraoperative (10 μg) and four postoperative (10, 20, 50, 150 μg) doses of catumaxomab on days 7, 10, 13, and 16. The study demonstrated a 3-year survival benefit in patients who received catumaxomab when compared to a match-pair control group (survival rates of 85.4 and 63.4 %, respectively) [57]. This favorable survival data warranted a phase III trial of 258 EpCAM-positive cancer patients with malignant ascites (Study in EpCAM Positive Patients with Symptomatic Malignant Ascites Using Removab Versus an Untreated Control Group. http://clinicaltrials.gov/ct2/show/NCT00836654).

Several clinical studies are ongoing targeting different pathway involved in ovarian cancer proliferation or in angiogenesis in high grade serous carcinoma (HGSC) and in low grade carcinomas. High grade serous carcinomas are characterized by several mutations. Indeed, TP53, NOTCH, PI3K, RAS/MEK, BRCA, and FOXM1 pathway signaling are defective in HGSC [58].

Mucinous carcinoma is a distinct disease presenting platinum intermediate sensitivity with RAS mutations [59], and mutations in ARID1A, PIK3CA, PTEN, and CTNNB1.

## References


1. Siegel R, Ma J, Zou Z, Jemal A. Cancer statistics 2014. CA Cancer J Clin. 2014;64:9–29.
2. Jayson GC, Kohn EC, Kitchener H, Ledermann JA. Ovarian cancer. Lancet. 2014;384(9951):1376–88.
3. Katsumata N, Yasuda M, Isonishi S, Takahashi F, Michimae H, Kimura E, et al. Long-term results of dose-dense paclitaxel and carboplatin versus conventional paclitaxel and carboplatin for treatment of advanced epithelial ovarian, fallopian tube, or primary peritoneal cancer (JGOG 3016): a randomised, controlled, open-label trial. Lancet Oncol. 2014;14(10):1020–6.
4. Pignata S, Scambia G, Katsaros D, Gallo C, Pujade-Lauraine E, De Placido S, et al. Carboplatin plus paclitaxel once a week versus every 3 weeks in patients with advanced ovarian cancer (MITO-7): a randomised, multicentre, open-label, phase 3 trial. Lancet Oncol. 2014;15:396–405.
5. Chan J, Brady M, Penson R, Monk B, Boente M, Walker J, et al. Phase III trial of every-3-weeks paclitaxel versus dose dense weekly paclitaxel with carboplatin +/− bevacizumab in epithelial ovarian, peritoneal, fallopian tube cancer: GOG 262 (NCT0116712) (Oral presentation). 18th international meeting of the European Society of Gynecological Oncology; 19–22 Oct 2013; Liverpool.
6. National Comprehensive Cancer Network (NCCN). Clinical practice guidelines in Ovarian Cancer, 2014. http://www.nccn.org/professionals/physician_gls/f_guidelines.asp#ovarian. Accessed 28 Nov 2014.
7. Vergote I, Tropé CG, Amant F, Kristensen GB, Ehlen T, Johnson N, et al. Neoadjuvant chemotherapy or primary surgery in stage IIIC or IV ovarian cancer. N Engl J Med. 2012;363:943–53.
8. Colombo N, Peiretti M, Parma G, Lapresa M, Mancari R, Carinelli S, et al. ESMO Guidelines Working Group. Newly diagnosed and relapsed epithelial ovarian carcinoma: ESMO clinical practice guidelines for diagnosis, treatment and follow-up. Ann Oncol. 2010;21 Suppl 5:v23–30.
9. Bandiera E, Franceschini R, Specchia C, Bignotti E, Trevisiol C, Gion M, et al. Prognostic significance of vascular endothelial growth factor serum determination in women with ovarian cancer. Obstet Gynecol. 2012;2012:245756.
10. Burger RA, Brady MF, Bookman MA, Fleming GF, Monk BJ, Huang H, et al. Incorporation of bevacizumab in the primary treatment of ovarian cancer. N Engl J Med. 2011;365:2473–83.
11. Perren TJ, Swart AM, Pfisterer J, Ledermann JA, Pujade-Lauraine E, Kristensen G, et al. A phase 3 trial of bevacizumab in ovarian cancer. N Engl J Med. 2011;365:2484–96.
12. Oza AM, Perren TJ, Swart AM, Schroder W, Pujade-Lauraine E, Havsteen H, et al. ICON7: final overall survival results in the GCIG phase III randomized trial of bevacizumab in women with newly diagnosed ovarian cancer [abstract]. Eur J Cancer. 2013;49(2):6.
13. Aghajanian C, Blank SV, Goff BA, Judson P, Teneriello MG, Husain A, et al. OCEANS: a randomized, double-blind, placebo-controlled phase III trial of chemotherapy with or without Bevacizumab in patients with platinum-sensitive recurrent epithelial ovarian, primary peritoneal, or fallopian tube cancer. J Clin Oncol. 2012;30:2039–45.
14. Aghajanian C, Goff B, Nycum LR, Wang Y, Husain A, Blank S, et al. Independent radiologic review: bevacizumab in combination with gemcitabine and carboplatin in recurrent ovarian cancer. Gynecol Oncol. 2014;133(1):105–10.
15. Pujade-Lauraine E, Hilpert F, Weber B, Reuss A, Poveda A, Kristensen G, et al. Bevacizumab combined with chemotherapy for platinum-resistant recurrent ovarian cancer: the AURELIA open-label randomized phase III trial. J Clin Oncol. 2014;32:1302–8.
16. Matulonis UA, Berlin S, Ivy P, Tyburski K, Krasner C, Zarwan C, et al. Cediranib, an oral inhibitor of vascular endothelial growth factor receptor kinases, is an active drug in recurrent epithelial ovarian, fallopian tube and peritoneal cancer. J Clin Oncol. 2009;27:5601–6.
17. Ledermann J, Perren TJ, Raja FA, Embleton A, Rustin G, Jayson GC et al. Randomised double-blind phase

III trial of cediranib (AZD 2171) in relapsed platinum sensitive ovarian cancer: results of the ICON6 trial [abstract]. 13th Annual European cancer congress; 27 Sept to 1 Oct 2013; Amsterdam.
18. Monk BJ, Poveda A, Vergote I, Raspagliesi F, Fujiwara K, Bae DS, et al. Anti-angiopoietin therapy with trebananib for recurrent ovarian cancer (TRINOVA-1): a randomised, multicentre, double-blind, placebo-controlled phase 3 trial. Lancet Oncol. 2014;15:799–808.
19. Ledermann J, Perren TJ, Raja FA, Embleton A, Rustin G, Jayson GC, et al. Randomised double-blind phase III trial of cediranib (AZD 2171) in relapsed platinum sensitive ovarian cancer: results of the ICON6 trial [abstract]. Eur J Cancer. 2013;49(2):10.
20. Monk BJ, Herzog TJ, Kaye SB, Krasner CN, Vermorken JB, Muggia FM, et al. Trabectedin plus pegylated liposomal Doxorubicin in recurrent ovarian cancer. J Clin Oncol. 2010;28(19):3107–14.
21. European Medicines Agency (EMA). Assessment Report for Yondelis. International non-proprietary name/common name; Trabectedin procedure. No EMEA/H/C/000773/11/0008. 2009. http://www.ema.europa.eu/humandocs/PDFs/EPAR/Yondelis/EMEA-H-773-II-08-AR.pdf.
22. Vincenzi B, Napolitano A, Frezza AM, Schiavon G, Santini D, Tonini G. Wide-spectrum characterization of trabectedin: biology, clinical activity and future perspectives. Pharmacogenomics. 2010;11(6):865–78.
23. Allavena P, Signorelli M, Chieppa M, Erba E, Bianchi G, Marchesi F, et al. Anti-inflammatory properties of the novel antitumor agent yondelis (trabectedin): inhibition of macrophage differentiation and cytokine production. Cancer Res. 2005;65(7):2964–71.
24. Sessa C, Cresta S, Noberasco C, Capri G, Gallerani E, De Braud F, et al. Phase I clinical and pharmacokinetic study of trabectedin and cisplatin in solid tumours. Eur J Cancer. 2009;45(12):2116–22.
25. Von Mehren M, Schilder RJ, Cheng JD, Temmer E, Cardoso TM, Renshaw FG, et al. A phase I study of the safety and pharmacokinetics of trabectedin in combination with pegylated liposomal doxorubicin in patients with advanced malignancies. Ann Oncol. 2008;19(10):1802–9.
26. Del Campo JM, Sessa C, Krasner CN, Vermorken JB, Colombo N, Kaye S, et al. Trabectedin as single agent in relapsed advanced ovarian cancer: results from a retrospective pooled analysis of three phase II trials. Med Oncol. 2013;30(1):435.
27. Ferrandina G, Salutari V, Vincenzi B, Marinaccio M, Naglieri E, Loizzi V, et al. Trabectedin as single agent in the salvage treatment of heavily treated ovarian cancer patients: a retrospective, multicenter study. Gynecol Oncol. 2013;130(3):505–10.
28. Poveda A, Vergote I, Tjulandin S, Kong B, Roy M, Chan S, Filipczyk-Cisarz E, Hagberg H, Kaye SB, Colombo N, Lebedinsky C, Parekh T, Gómez J, Park YC, Alfaro V, Monk BJ. Trabectedin plus pegylated liposomal doxorubicin in relapsed ovarian cancer: outcomes in the partially platinum-sensitive (platinum-free interval 6-12 months) subpopulation of OVA-301 phase III randomized trial. Ann Oncol. 2011;22(1):39–48.
29. Fisher M, Gore M. Cost-effectiveness of trabectedin plus pegylated liposomal doxorubicin for the treatment of women with relapsed platinum-sensitive ovarian cancer in the UK: analysis based on the final survival data of the OVA-301 trial. Value Health. 2013;16(4):507–16.
30. Fong PC, Boss DS, Yap TA, Tutt A, Wu P, Mergui-Roelvink M, et al. Inhibition of poly (ADP-ribose) polymerase in tumors from BRCA mutation carriers. N Engl J Med. 2009;361:123–34.
31. Ledermann J, Harter P, Gourley C, Friedlander M, Vergote I, Rustin G, et al. Olaparib maintenance therapy in platinum sensitive relapsed ovarian cancer. N Engl J Med. 2012;366:1382–92.
32. Ledermann J, Harter P, Gourley C, Friedlander M, Vergote I, Rustin G, et al. Olaparib maintenance therapy in patients with platinum-sensitive relapsed serous ovarian cancer: a preplanned retrospective analysis of outcomes by BRCA status in a randomised phase 2 trial. Lancet Oncol. 2014;15(8):852–61.
33. Kaye SB, Lubinski J, Matulonis U, Ang JE, Gourley C, Karlan BY, et al. Phase II, open-label, randomized, multicenter study comparing the efficacy and safety of olaparib, a poly (ADP-ribose) polymerase inhibitor, and pegylated liposomal doxorubicin in patients with BRCA1 or BRCA2 mutations and recurrent ovarian cancer. J Clin Oncol. 2012;30(4):372–9.
34. Oza AM, Cibula D, Benzaquen AO, Poole C, Mathijssen RH, Sonke GS, et al. Olaparib combined with chemotherapy for recurrent platinum-sensitive ovarian cancer: a randomised phase 2 trial. Lancet Oncol. 2015;16(1):87–97.
35. Sandhu SK, Schelman WR, Wilding G, Moreno V, Baird RD, Miranda S, et al. The poly (ADP-ribose) polymerase inhibitor niraparib (MK4827) in BRCA mutation carriers and patients with sporadic cancer: a phase 1 dose-escalation trial. Lancet Oncol. 2013;14:882–92.
36. Mirza MR, Monk BJ, Ledermann JA, Oza AM, Del Campo JM, Berek JS, et al. Engot-OV16/NOVA: a phase 3 randomized double-blind trial of maintenance with PARP inhibitor Niraparib versus placebo in patients with platinum-sensitive ovarian cancer. Int J Gynecol Cancer. 2014;24(9):33–4.
37. Coleman RL, Sill M, Bell-McGuinn K, Aghajanian C, Gray HJ, Tewari KS et al. A phase II evaluation of the potent, highly selective PARP inhibitor veliparib in the treatment of persistent or recurrent epithelial ovarian, fallopian tube, or primary peritoneal cancer in patients who carry a germline BRCA1 or BRCA2 mutation [abstract]. 45th Annual meeting on women's cancer (SGO); 22–25 Mar 2014; Tampa, FL.
38. Juvekar A, Burga LN, Hu H, Lunsford EP, Ibrahim YH, Balmana J, et al. Combining a PI3K inhibitor with a PARP inhibitor provides an effective therapy for BRCA1-related breast cancer. Cancer Discov. 2012;2:1048–63.

39. Ibrahim YH, García-García C, Serra V, He L, Torres-Lockhart K, Prat A, et al. PI3K inhibition impairs BRCA1/2 expression and sensitizes BRCA-proficient triple-negative breast cancer to PARP inhibition. Cancer Discov. 2012;2:1036–47.
40. Farley J, Brady WE, Mirrer BJ, Lankes H, Coleman R, et al. A phase II trial of Selumetinib (AZD6244; ARRY-142886) in women with recurrent low-grade serous carcinoma of the ovary or peritoneum. American Association for Cancer Research annual meeting, 31 Mar to 4 Apr 2012; Chicago, IL.
41. Farley J, Brady WE, Vathipadiekal V, Lankes HA, Coleman R, Morgan MA, et al. Selumetinib in women with recurrent low-grade serous carcinoma of the ovary or peritoneum: an open-label, single-arm, phase 2 study. Lancet Oncol. 2013;14:134–40.
42. Monk BJ, Grisham RN, Marth C, Banerjee SN, Hilpert F, Coleman RL, et al. The MEK inhibitor in low-grade serous ovarian cancer (MILO)/ENGOT-ov11 study: a multinational, randomized, open-label phase 3 study of binimetinib (MEK162) versus physician's choice chemotherapy in patients with recurrent or persistent low-grade serous carcinomas of the ovary, fallopian tube, or primary peritoneum. J Clin Oncol. 2014;32:5.
43. McCormack PL. Nintedanib: first global approval. Drugs. 2015;75(1):129–39.
44. Hilberg F, Roth GJ, Krssak M, Kautschitsch S, Sommergruber W, Tontsch-Grunt U, et al. BIBF 1120: triple angiokinase inhibitor with sustained receptor blockade and good antitumor efficacy. Cancer Res. 2008;68:4774–82.
45. Ledermann JA, Hackshaw A, Kaye S, Jayson G, Gabra H, McNeish I, et al. Randomized phase II placebo-controlled trial of maintenance therapy using the oral triple angiokinase inhibitor BIBF 1120 after chemotherapy for relapsed ovarian cancer. J Clin Oncol. 2011;29:3798–804.
46. Glasspool RM, Brown R, Gore ME, Rustin GJ, McNeish IA, Wilson RH, et al. A randomised, phase II trial of the DNA-hypomethylating agent 5-aza-20-deoxycytidine (decitabine) in combination with carboplatin vs carboplatin alone in patients with recurrent, partially platinum-sensitive ovarian cancer. Br J Cancer. 2014;110:1923–9.
47. Vidal A, Muñoz C, Guillén MJ, Moretó J, Puertas S, Martínez-Iniesta M, et al. Lurbinectedin (PM01183), a new DNA minor groove binder, inhibits growth of orthotopic primary graft of cisplatin-resistant epithelial ovarian cancer. Clin Cancer Res. 2012;18(19):5399–411.
48. Poveda A, Berton-Rigaud D, Ray-Coquard IL, Kong B, Provansal M, Soto A, et al. Lurbinectedin (PM01183), an active compound in platinum-resistant/refractory ovarian cancer (PRROC) patients: results of a two-stage, controlled phase II study. J Clin Oncol. 2014;32:5s. Abstract no. 5505.
49. Hamanishi J, Mandai M, Iwasaki M, Okazaki T, Okazaki T, Tanaka y Y, et al. Programmed cell death 1 ligand 1 and tumor-infiltrating CD8+ T lymphocytes are prognostic factors of human ovarian cancer. Proc Natl Acad Sci U S A. 2007;104(9):3360–5.
50. Hamanishi J, Mandai M, Ikeda T, Minami M, Kawaguchi A, Matsumura N, et al. Efficacy and safety of anti-PD-1 antibody (Nivolumab: BMS-936558, ONO-4538) in patients with platinum-resistant ovarian cancer. J Clin Oncol. 2014;32:5s. Abstract no. 5511.
51. Armstrong DK, White AJ, Weil SC, Philips M, Coleman RL. Farletuzumab (a monoclonal antibody against folate receptor alpha) in relapsed platinum-sensitive ovarian cancer. Gynecol Oncol. 2013; 129(3):452–8.
52. Liu JF, Barry WT, Birrer M, Lee JM, Buckanovich RJ, Fleming GF. Combination cediranib and olaparib versus olaparib alone for women with recurrent platinum-sensitive ovarian cancer: a randomised phase 2 study. Lancet Oncol. 2014;11:1207–14.
53. Matulonis U, Wulf GM, Birrer MJ, Westin SN, Torres-Lockhart K, Prat A, et al. Phase I of oral BKM120 and oral olaparib for high grade serous ovarian cancer or triple negative breast cancer. J Clin Oncol. 2014;32:5. Abstract no. 2510.
54. Hodi FS, Butler M, Oble DA, Seiden MV, Quy P, Bell-McGuinn KM, et al. Immunologic and clinical effects of antibody blockade of cytotoxic T lymphocyte-associated antigen 4 in previously vaccinated cancer patients. Proc Natl Acad Sci U S A. 2008;105:3005–10.
55. Chelius D, Ruf P, Gruber P, Plöscher M, Haluska FG, Kruse A, et al. Structural and functional characterization of the trifunctional antibody catumaxomab. MAbs. 2010;2:309–19.
56. Berek JS, Edwards RP, Parker L, De Mars LR, Herzog TJ, Lentz SS, et al. Catumaxomab treatment of malignant ascites in patients with chemotherapy-refractory ovarian cancer: a phase II study. J Clin Oncol. 2011;29:5048.
57. Pietzner K, Chekerov R, Reinthaller A, Reimer D, Reimer T, Angleitner-Boubenizek L, et al. A matched pair analysis of intra- and postoperative catumaxomab in patients with ovarian cancer from a multicenter, single- arm phase II trial versus a consecutive single-center collective of ovarian cancer patients without immunotherapy. J Clin Oncol. 2012;30:5080.
58. Cancer Genome Atlas Research Network. Integrated genomic analyses of ovarian carcinoma. Nature. 2011;474:609–15.
59. Brown J, Frumovitz M. Mucinous tumors of the ovary: current thoughts on diagnosis and management. Curr Oncol Rep. 2014;16:389.
60. Sessa C, De Braud F, Perotti A, et al. Trabectedin for women with ovarian carcinoma after treatment with platinum and taxanes fails. J Clin Oncol. 2005; 23(9):1867–74.
61. Krasner CN, McMeekin DS, Chan S, et al. A phase II study of trabectedin single agent in patients with recurrent ovarian cancer previously treated with

platinum-based regimens. Br J Cancer. 2007; 97(12):1618–24.

62. Del Campo JM, Roszak A, Bidzinski M, et al. Yondelis Ovarian Cancer Group. Phase II randomized study of trabectedin given as two different every 3 weeks dose schedules (1.5 mg/m$^2$ 24 h or 1.3 mg/m$^2$ 3 h) to patients with relapsed, platinum-sensitive, advanced ovarian cancer. Ann Oncol. 2009; 20(11):1794–802.

63. Lorusso D, Scambia G, Pignata L, et al. Prospective phase II trial of trabectedin in BRCA-mutated and/or BRCAness phenotype recurrent ovarian cancer patients: the MITO 15 trial. Ann Oncol. 2015;17 [Epub ahead of print].

# 5 Novel Methods for Prevention and Early Diagnosis of Ovarian and Endometrial Cancers

Roberto Piccoli, Nicoletta De Rosa, and Selina Davis


## Abstract

Because of the high incidence of endometrial cancer and the to poor prognosis of ovarian cancer establish a standardized practice method in early detection and diagnosis of these gynecological tumors is nowadays a primary goal in oncology research. Genomics and proteomics advances and new discoveries about tumor behavior and its specific characteristics bring the attention on several emerging factors that in the next future could become specific diagnostics tool in gynecologic oncology.

The interaction between the genetic predisposition and the environment exposure has been recognized as one of the main pathogenic moments of tumor's development and growth. Clarify the exact mechanism that regulates these interactions and the cellular pathways involved in tumor growth can substantially contribute in identify "high-risk" populations. To target diagnostic investigations, to selected populations maximizing health benefits of screening programs and, of great importance, to allow the early detection of cancers remain main positive prognostic factors in tumor survivors.

On the other hand, the second area of study, which benefits gynecologic oncology, is the constant improvement of imaging techniques. The tumor growth is early recognized observing specific changes in tissue morphology. Future innovations in gynecologic-oncology imaging will go beyond anatomy to focus on function.



R. Piccoli, MD (✉) • N. De Rosa, MD
Department of Gynecology, Outpatient Clinic Center "Piccoli", Via Petrarca 129 n, 80122 Naples, Italy
e-mail: rpiccoli1954@gmail.com

S. Davis, MD
Department of Obstetrics and Gynecology, Albert Einstein Medical Center, Philadelphia, PA, USA




A. Giordano, M. Macaluso (eds.), *Gynecological Cancers*, Current Clinical Oncology,
DOI 10.1007/978-3-319-32907-9_5

**Keywords**

Ovarian cancer • Endometrial cancer • Biomarkers • Genetic markers • BRCA1 • BRCA2 • MLH1 • MSH2 • MSH6 • PMS2 • TP53 • PTEN • CA125 • HE4 • Inhibins • Lysophosphatidic acid • Mesothelin osteopontin • CA72.4 • Interleukin 13 • B7-H4 • Exosome • MiRNAs • Prolactin • Macrophage inhibitory factor • Macrophage-colony stimulating factor • OVA1 algorithm • IOTA • Dynamic contrast-enhanced (DCE) MRI • Diffusion weighted imaging

The age at the time of diagnosis, the stage of the disease, the histological subtype, and tumor grade are common prognostic factors in gynecological malignancies.

Identifying specific molecules and establishing a standardized practice method in early detection and diagnosis of gynecological tumors is nowadays both a primary goal and a key discovery challenge in oncology.

Ovarian cancer (OC) remains, over the recent years, the major cause of death due to gynecological malignancies. About 22,000 new cases and 14,000 deaths are expected in the United States alone in 2014 [1]. Because of the lack of obvious and specific symptoms at the onset of the disease, the majority of the cases are diagnosed at a late stage.

Endometrial cancer (EC) is the most common gynecologic malignancy, with a lifetime risk of one in 38, and is the fourth most prevalent female neoplasm, with over 42,000 US cases annually. Despite an overall 5-year survival rate of 83 %, EC ranks second in mortality among female genital tract cancers, causing an estimated 7780 US deaths in 2009, with the death rate steadily increasing over the past 20 years [2].

## Endometrial and Ovarian Cancer Susceptibility and Primary Prevention: Genetic and Environmental Factors

It is now thought that up to 25 % of all OCs has a heritable component [3]. A familial risk has been identified also in EC development.

The two main syndromes associated with familial OC are hereditary breast ovarian cancer syndrome (HBOC) and Lynch syndrome (also known as heritable non-polyposis colorectal cancer syndrome, HNPCC). Other much rare syndromes associated with hereditary ovarian or EC include Li-Fraumeni, Cowden, and Peutz-Jeghers syndromes [4].

Gene mutations in BRCA1 and BRCA2 account for the majority of familial hereditary OC syndrome. BRCA1 and BRCA2 encode proteins that are involved in DNA repair; specifically, they are involved in homologous recombination, a highly accurate mechanism of double-stranded DNA break repair [5].

It is unclear why these mutations are predominantly associated with breast and OCs. Because these tissues share the property of being hormonally regulated, some researchers have speculated that there may be an interaction between hormones and BRCA1/BRCA2 signaling while others speculate that hormonal signaling may increase oxidative stress on DNA therefore increasing the susceptibility to mutations [6].

The risk of developing OC in a woman with a BRCA1 mutation is 39–46 %, while it is 12–27 % in a woman with a BRCA2 mutation [7]. Despite substantial improvement in managing OC risks owing to BRCA1/BRCA2 mutations, the guidelines recommend prophylactic bilateral salpingo-oophorectomy (PO) by age 40 years [8].

The association between germ line mutations in BRCA genes and the risk of EC remains controversial [9].

Actually, advances in genomic technologies quicken the finding of other cancer susceptibility genes. To date, various genes, including, RAD51C, RAD51D, BRIP1, BARD1, CHEK2, MPE11A, NBN, PALB2, RAD50, MLH1, MSH2, MSH6,

PMS2, and TP53, have been associated with ovarian and endometrial cancer [10].

Lynch syndrome is an autosomal dominant condition that is characterized by the presence of synchronous or metachronous colorectal tumors. It is also associated with an increased frequency of extracolonic tumors including endometrial, ovarian, urogenital, brain, renal, gastric, and biliary cancers. Several genes encoding DNA mismatch repair (MMR) proteins have been implicated in Lynch syndrome: MLH1, MSH2, MSH6, and PMS2. MMR proteins recognize and correct short insertions and deletions as well as single base mismatches [11]. Lynch syndrome is the second commonest cause of hereditary OC, accounting for 10–15 % of such familial presentations [11]. In women affected by Lynch syndrome the estimated cumulative risk of developing EC by age 70 is 54 % for MLH1, 21 % for MSH2, and 16 % for MSH6 mutations [12]. This risk of EC rises significantly after the age of 40, with a mean age of diagnosis of 46 years [13].

The majority of patients diagnosed with ovarian or endometrial cancer is considered to have a "sporadic" form of these malignancies. Both for endometrial and ovarian cancer on the basis of a series of morphologic and molecular genetic studies, a dualistic model has been proposed that groups tumors into two broad categories, nominated type I and type II.

Type I OC includes low-grade serous, low-grade endometrioid, mucinous, and clear cell carcinomas. These neoplasms typically present as large cystic masses restricted to one ovary; have a relatively indolent course; and are associated with mutations in KRAS, BRAF, PTEN, PIK3CA, CTNNB1, ARID1A, and PPP2R1A that disturb signaling pathways. These molecular alterations result in morphologic changes, which are reflected by a stepwise progression from benign through varying degrees of atypia (borderline tumor), then to noninvasive and finally to invasive and metastatic carcinoma.

Type I ECs were described as tumors associated with a constellation of clinical findings (obesity, hypertension, and diabetes), which included a hyperestrogenic state. The tumors were in general of endometrioid (endometrial-like) histology, low-grade (i.e., well to moderately differentiated), low-stage (confined to the uterus), indolent lesions often, and associated with endometrial hyperplasia.

Type II OCs are collected of high-grade serous, high-grade endometrioid, undifferentiated carcinomas, and malignant mixed mesodermal tumors (carcinosarcomas). These tumors are aggressive and typically present at an advanced stage, which adds to their high mortality rate. Unlike type I tumors, which are relatively genetically stable, type II tumors demonstrate several chromosomal aberrations at diagnosis, but these remain relatively stable over the course of the disease. The commonest mutation is that of TP53 followed by somatic inactivation of BRCA1/BRCA2 [14].

Type II ECs, approximately 2–5 %, were associated with aging and unique genetic/molecular changes, were not associated with estrogen stimulation and instead arouse in the setting of atrophy, were poorly differentiated tumors, and behaved in an aggressive manner. It often have a serous (fallopian tube-like) morphology. Somatic mutations in the PTEN gene are common in sporadic ECs [15].

The main risk factor for EC is exposure to endogenous and exogenous estrogens associated with obesity, diabetes, early age at menarche, nulliparity, late-onset menopause, older age (≥55 years), and use of tamoxifen [16]. The relation between diabetes and EC is controversial [17, 18].

Compared to EC, adult BMI and postmenopausal hormone use are weaker and less consistent risk factors for OC, suggesting that endogenous estrogens may play a lesser role in the etiology of OC [19–21]. Only one prospective study has been conducted to date, and women with the highest levels of circulating estradiol had three times the risk of OC (OR = 3.0, 95 % CI: 0.6–14.9) compared to women with the lowest estradiol levels [22].

The incessant ovulatory damage is the major hypothesis involved in OC pathogenesis. Ovulation creates a proinflammatory state at the ovarian surface epithelium and distal fallopian tube through the release of cytokines, reactive oxygen species, and steroids; repeated ovulation may therefore increase risk of damage to DNA in these areas [23]. So that, age and reproductive factors such as low parity and infertility, or other pathologic factor such as endometriosis increase risk of developing OC [24].

On the contrary, that use of the oral contraceptive pill (OCP) is a protective factor for OC in patients with BRCA1/BRCA2 mutations. A meta-analysis looking at OCP use in BRCA1/BRCA2 mutation carriers demonstrated significant risk reduction (OR 0.57; 95 % CI 0.47–0.70); this effect was more notable with longer duration of OCP use [25, 26]. Indeed, similar trends were seen in a recent meta-analysis of OCP use for the general population (OR 0.73; 95 % CI 0.66–0.81), with a reduction in incidence of OC of more than 50 % with 10 or more years of use [27].

Understanding the hormonal microenvironment of ovulation is critical to establishing a molecular link between incessant ovulation and early OC pathogenesis. It has been demonstrated that follicular fluid (FF) exposure led to DNA double-stranded breaks and, consequently, the stabilization of the tumor suppressor TP53. Early precursors of high-grade serous OCs are also defined by their high expression of TP53 and high levels of DNA damage, although in the vast majority of these cases TP53 is also mutated, often with a gain of function mutation. Understanding the link between the temporary induction of TP53 in response to FF exposure and the acquisition of mutations in P53 in early precursor lesions will be key in the future of OC research [28].

A complete comprehension of ovarian and EC pathogenesis and of risk factors associated with their development was still today an object of study and improvement. New findings in these fields may influence significantly the future clinicians behavior and the cancer patient's management. The identification and better characterization of "high-risk" populations, for genetic or environmental factors, indeed, represent the best target to control cancer morbidity and mortality.

## Endometrial and Ovarian Screening and Diagnosis

OC is the second gynecological malignancy after cervical cancer that may meet the criteria of a disease for which population screening is justified. The disease is usually diagnosed in advanced stages when chances for long-term survival are poor; effective treatment is available for early-stage disease. Conversely, EC is a symptomatic disease in early stage, but due to its high incidence, screening of "high-risk" population (about 30 %) is recommended. So that, patients with HNPCC, Cowden syndrome, obesity, diabetes, or breast cancer patients on tamoxifen would certainly benefit from the advent of a reliable screening strategy to aid early diagnosis of EC.

Screening strategy is based on detection of tumors markers. Markers may be biochemical substance produced by or in response to the tumor or any cytological, molecular, cytogenetic, or architectural abnormalities detected in the presence of malignancy. Ideally, tumor markers should be tumor specific, allow detection of minimal disease, and quantitatively reflect tumor burden.

A true precursor lesion for OC has not yet been identified, limiting the effectiveness of OC screening. The early diagnosis of OC is still in the research stage, and there are no definite markers, which can be used in the clinical setting. Biochemical, morphological, vascular, and cytological tumor markers have all been explored with varying success. Currently, traditional methods for screening or diagnosing OC mainly include serum CA-125, color Doppler ultrasound, laparoscopy, and cytological examination.

Clinical symptoms and imaging results are currently the main pillars to detect ECs development, progression, or recurrence. Indeed, the standard diagnostic evaluation for EC includes pelvic ultrasonography, office endometrial biopsy, or dilatation and curettage (D&C) with or without hysteroscopy. In EC currently no assays are available to be included in the clinical algorithms that can facilitate monitoring of disease, such as CA-125 in OC.

## Biochemical Markers

The best-known biochemical marker of OC is *CA-125*, an antigen expressed by fetal amniotic and coelomic epithelium. About 80 % of patients with advanced OC have the elevation of CA-125. But it has some limitations: indeed, only 50–60 % of patients with early-stage OC have the increased CA-125. In addition, single CA-125 detection may cause false positive, infact the increase of CA-125 have also been found in other cancers, such as pancreatic, breast, bladder, liver, or lung cancer. Other benign diseases such as diverticulitis, cirrhosis, endometriosis, or physiologic condition (menstruation or pregnancy) may also produce a high level of CA-125 [29, 30].

A serum CA125 of 35 U/mL is usually accepted as the arbitrary cutoff of normal. In postmenopausal women or in patients after hysterectomy CA125 levels tend to be lower than general population so a lower cutoff of 20 and 26 U/mL respectively seem to be more appropriate [31].

CA-125 is the established biomarker for detecting OC recurrence and monitoring therapeutic response. In addition, recent guidelines recommend its measurement in the primary care setting in women with suggestive symptoms or at high risk for OC, in combination with pelvic ultrasound [32, 33], even though some authors have discouraged this application because of the low sensitivity of the test, which is even worse in early-stage tumors (<50 %) [34]. However, according to the current guidelines measurement of serum CA125 antigen remains the gold standard in the follow-up OC [35].

Fewer studies have been performed to evaluate the efficacy of CA-125 for EC detection and/or monitoring. Although CA-125 is elevated in EC patients relative to healthy control, serum concentrations of CA-125 are elevated in only 10–20 % of women with early-stage EC, and only 25 % of asymptomatic patients with recurrences will present with elevated CA-125 levels [36, 37].

The intrinsic limitations of CA-125 have greatly stimulated the search of additional biomarkers sought to improve the accuracy for identifying malignancy in women with a pelvic tumor. In the new era of proteomics there has been a great deal of interest in identifying global pattern of serum proteins and peptides that relate to cancer risk and prognosis. Other biomolecules, including human epididymis protein 4 (HE4), the inhibins, the lysophosphatidic acid, and other, are also elevated in the serum of OC patients and may be of diagnostic value in various combinations with one another and/or with CA-125 [38].

Even if no accurate biomarkers for EC detection are currently available some molecules have been proposed; among them the most significant are HE4, prolactin, and miRNAs.

*HE4* is a secretory protein originally identified in the distal human epididymis. The function of HE4 has not been definitely demonstrated; however, HE4 shows significant structural similarity to proteinase inhibitors and is proposed to have a function in sperm maturation [39, 40].

A prominent upregulation of HE4 expression was seen in epithelial OC tissue, especially in serous and endometrioid adenocarcinomas. No expression was detected in normal ovarian tissue, and a lower expression was observed in both benign and borderline ovarian tumors compared with protein expression levels in epithelial OC. In combination with serum marker CA125, a significant increase in sensitivity and specificity was revealed in differentiating between benign gynecologic conditions and epithelial OC.

Upregulation of HE4 was also demonstrated in malignancies of the gastrointestinal canal, urinary tract, bladder, and breast. HE4 could potentially be a tumor marker in primary lung adenocarcinomas. The widespread upregulation of HE4 seen in a range of malignancies implies that HE4 is neither organ nor tumor specific. Moreover, a potential role of HE4 as a tumor marker in EC has been reported, because HE4 measured in serum from patients with EC was significantly elevated compared with serum levels in healthy individuals and women with benign uterine disease [41].

HE4 levels in healthy subjects increased with age and smoking habits, but its serum levels are not affected by the menstrual cycle, oral contraceptive use, or endometriosis [42–45].

No optimal cutoff exists, as well as there is no consensus for correct parameters to include in the examination. Two recent studies [46, 47] have suggested reference intervals of serum HE4 in healthy women at 65.87 pmol/L for premenopausal and 90.76 pmol/L for postmenopausal. In women with pelvic masses, Fujirebio Diagnostics [48] has defined the normal range below 150 pmol/L, whereas Abbott Diagnostics [49] defined normal ranges below 70 pmol/L for premenopausal women and 140 pmol/L for postmenopausal women. However, both the manufacturers recommend that reference intervals are determined for each population investigated yielding the highest sensitivity and specificity possible.

Subsequent to the discovery of serum HE4, researches have focused on its role in differentiating between epithelial OC and benign masses. HE4 was combined in two formulas evaluating high-risk disease, called "risk of malignancy algorithm" (ROMA) formulated for premenopausal and for postmenopausal women with adnexal mass. ROMA combines the diagnostic power of the CA125 and HE4 markers with menopausal status. This algorithm has been approved by the FDA as a useful indicator for differentiating malignant from benign pelvic masses. Although this index has been enhanced as a diagnostic instrument, high ROMA scores have been also reported to be independently associated with a negative prognosis in some patients with OC [50].

Many studies report that ROMA algorithm implements better in the premenopausal population than in the postmenopausal women. A predicted probability (PP) greater than 13.1 % suggests a high risk in the premenopausal women, whereas PP value higher than 27.7 % indicates a high risk in the postmenopausal women. Using this algorithm, 93.8 % of epithelial OCs were correctly defined as high risk [51, 52]. ROMA sensitivity and specificity suggest its use for the triage of woman with an adnexal mass to gynecologic oncologist.

HE4's efficacy as a serum marker for endometrial malignancies has been investigated. Data from these studies indicate a promising value for HE4 as a component of the biomarker panel in EC detection. Moore et al. measured preoperative serum samples from patients with endometrioid adenocarcinoma [53]. The ROC-AUC values for HE4 were higher than all other markers (CA72-4 and CA-125) investigated for stage I, stages II–IV, and all stages combined (ROC-AUC: 76.7, 83.6, and 78.7 %, respectively). The sensitivity of the HE4 assay was also highest of all other single markers regardless of stage (sensitivity at 90 % specificity for stage I, stages II–IV and all stages combined: 48.4, 71.4, and 55.0 %, respectively). The addition of CA-125 to the HE4 assay considerably increased the sensitivity compared with that achievable by CA-125 alone (50.1 vs 24.6 % at 95 % specificity, respectively) [54]. These results suggest that in the future HE4 could be considered an EC specific diagnostic tumor marker.

The *Inhibins* were initially isolated from gonadal fluids based on their relevant abilities to inhibit follicle stimulating hormone (FSH) secretion from the pituitary. Successively, these proteins were recognized as members of a family of growth factors, the transforming growth factor-beta (TGFb) superfamily, with multiple functions as confined regulators of gonadal biology. Inhibin A and Inhibin B act as antagonists and are structural homologues of activins, including the activin b-subunit and a unique a-subunit. It has been validated that the alteration of the inhibin/activin pathway may contribute to the development of epithelial OC due to the alteration of the crosstalk between granulosa and epithelial cells. In a recent study, Walentowicz et al. propose the association of high levels of inhibin A with a poor prognosis and a low survival at 5 years [55].

The *mesothelin* gene encodes a 71-kDa precursor protein that undergoes physiological cleavage by a furin like protease to produce two main proteins, the first is the 31-kDa NH2-terminal megakaryocyte potentiation factor (MPF), which is secreted into the blood, the second COOH-terminal product is a 40-kDa fragment referred to as mesothelin, which is attached to the cell membrane and is overexpressed in several cancers, including mesothelioma, ovarian and pancreatic cancers, and some squamous cell carcinomas.

In patients with OC, Scholler et al. [56] have described a 42- to 44-kDa protein termed soluble mesothelin-related peptide (SMRP). A high expression of mesothelin in both tissue and serum indicates a poor prognosis. The mechanism of release of mesothelin from the cell surface is not clear. Many studies showed that serum mesothelin levels are related to the FIGO surgical pathological staging and pathological grade in OC patients. Patients with advanced stage and low differentiation tumors showed higher levels of SMRP. The most recent study reported the expression of mesothelin in ovarian tissue correlated to chemotherapy resistance and poor prognosis suggesting a role for mesothelin in diagnosis and disease staging [57].

*Osteopontin* (OPN) is a secreted, integrin-binding phosphoprotein that has been associated with cancer and is overexpressed in different tumor types. Physiologically, OPN is secreted by osteoblasts and the epithelial cells of multiple organs as well as by activated T lymphocytes, macrophages, and leukocytes at the site of inflammation. Some authors showed that OPN-c, an OPN splicing variant, contributed to the increased proliferation, migration, and invasion of OC cells. However, this glycoprotein is strongly associated with progressive tumor stage, poor patient prognosis, and metastasis formation. Although several studies have focused on the role of OPN in OC screening, the utility of OPN for differentiating between malignant and benign ovarian tumors has not been sufficiently elucidated [58].

*Carbohydrate antigen 72-4* (CA72.4) is another biomarker for OC; the level of this 200–400 kDa glycoprotein rises in gastric, cholic, breast, and ovarian adenocarcinomas. It can be used alone or in association with CA125. The sensitivity of CA72.4 is lower than CA125 in detecting OC, but the levels of this marker are not affected by pregnancy or the menstrual period. There is evidence in the literature that CA72.4 levels can be found slightly increased with endometriosis, benign ovarian tumors, or inflammatory conditions. Some authors have demonstrated the role of the biomarker CA72.4 combined with CA125 as a predictive factor of epithelial OC recurrence [59]. The combination of more tumor markers including HE4 together with CA72.4 increased the sensitivity and specificity in the diagnosis of OC in patients with pelvic masses [60].

*Interleukin 13* (IL13) is a cytokine with an inflammatory activity that plays important roles in many biological activities. The level of this cytokine has been measured and found more elevated in cancerous tissues. IL13 receptor is composed of two strands (ILA3Ra1 and IL13Ra2) and the second one has been found in high levels in 44 of 53 OC samples [61]. A cytotoxic therapy mediated by IL-13 has been designed and tested in phase I/II clinical trial. This therapy showed an antitumor activity and was very efficient when administered intraperitoneally, since it blocks the spread of OC cells through the peritoneum in late stages of OC [62].

The serum *macrophage inhibitory factor* (MIF) has also been tested for its presence in the blood of OC patients and a sensitivity of 77.8 % and a specificity of 53.3 % were measured for this marker [63].

*Macrophage-colony stimulating factor* (M-CSF) [64] has been used alone and detected OC with a specificity of around 61–68 % and 93 % specificity, but the results for the detection were better when used in conjunction with CA-125 [65]. Indeed, the use of either CA-125 or M-CSF enabled the identification of 96–98 % of OCs and 81 % in early stages.

*Lysophosphatidic acid* (LPA) in plasma is a recently discovered tumor marker. The LPA has been reported to have a sensitivity of 100 % for high-stage cancers and 90 % for low-stage cancers [66]. Its plasma concentration is significantly different between benign and malignant tumors. LPA has three subtypes: LPA1, LPA2, and LPA3. Wang et al. identified that LPA was highly expressed in OC and LPA can stimulate growth and metastasis of OC cells [67]. Others have found that the plasma level of LPA in patients with stage I OC was nearly three times higher than that in patients with benign ovarian tumors and seven times higher than that in healthy control group, which further confirmed the reliability of LPA as a tumor marker [68–70].

*B7-H4* is a new member of T cell costimulatory molecule B7 family, which has been recently discovered. B7-H4 can reduce T cell immunity by inhibiting proliferation of T cells, synthesis of cytokines, and cell cycle progression [71]. The expression of B7-H4 was significantly higher in OC while in normal ovarian tissue B7-H4 was hardly expressed [72–76]. Therefore, it can be considered as an important marker for early-stage OC diagnosis [77].

*Exosomes* appear to be a new and powerful signal mediator between cancer cells and their microenvironment [78]. In OC, tumor-derived exosomes could activate adipose tissue-derived mesenchymal stem cells to tumor-supporting myofibroblasts, contributing to tumor progression [79, 80]. Thus exosomes could be an important mediator between tumor and their microenvironment in the establishment of premetastatic niche.

Exosomes in plasma of patients with OC were found to express immunosuppressive factors such as IL-10 and TGFβ1 to promote T regulatory cell function and impair antitumor immunity. More recently, malignant ascites-derived exosomes of OC patients have been observed to induce apoptosis of peripheral blood lymphocytes and dendritic cells, suggesting another mechanism of impairing the antitumor immunity by these tumor-derived exosomes.

Exosomes, which are rich reservoirs of tumor-specific proteins, have been especially important in the discovery of biomarkers. Exosomes possess several unique advantages, including (1) being extremely stable (under various conditions of freezing, cold storage, and thawing for many years), (2) abundant (108–113 exosomes/ml plasma), (3) tumor specific, and (4) their content correlates with tumor staging and treatment outcome. The presence of exosomes in blood and other body fluids such as urine also suggests an important advantage over invasive biopsies. By comparing exosomes captured in OC patients with those in healthy individuals, there was a significant difference in both number and protein content [81]. TGFβ1 and MAGE3/6 are significantly more prevalent in malignant ovarian tumors than in benign lesions [81]. For screening biomarkers, claudin 4-positive exosomes were present in the plasma samples from 32 out of 63 OC patients but only one out of 50 healthy individuals, raising the possibility that it could be used as a highly sensitive and specific indicator [82].

There also seems to be a correlation between exosome content and clinical outcome. A recent study that examines OC patients' exosomal proteins before and after chemotherapy has shown that the exosome levels were relatively unchanged in patients who were irresponsive to chemotherapy, whereas significantly altered levels were observed in responders, suggesting that the protein content of exosomes may be useful in predicting treatment response [81].

Exosome has also been proposed as a biomarker in EC. Indeed, exosomes are microRNA (miRNA) carriers, released from cells into blood. *MiRNAs* are small RNA molecules of about 22 nucleotides that induce gene silencing. miRNAs are implicated in cancer development and progression, and expression patterns of miRNAs in normal tissues differ from those of cancer tissues. Lawrie et al. first showed that cancer-specific miRNAs were effective biomarkers, and subsequently development of biomarkers using miRNAs has increased [83]. Torres et al. found that the expression of miRNAs (miR-99a, miR-100, and miR-199b) was upregulated in serum of patients with endometrioid adenocarcinoma. Analysis of miRNAs in serum in a genome-wide study showed that a combination of four serum miRNAs, miR-222, miR-223, miR-186, and miR-204, can be used to diagnose endometrioid adenocarcinoma with high probability [84]. Expression of miR-125b in type II EC cells is significantly upregulated compared to that in type I cells. Tumor protein p53 inducible nuclear protein 1 (TP53INP1) gene, a target of miR-125b, may be related to malignancy of type II EC because cancer cells proliferate when this gene is not regulated [85].

Yurkovetsky et al. firstly showed evidence of EC screening potential for *prolactin*, a single-chain peptide from the growth hormone family.

The primary source of prolactin is the anterior pituitary gland, yet endometrial stroma also produces the protein during the secretory phase of the menstrual cycle. Prolactin's main function is the regulation of breast development and lactation [86]. It also acts as a cytokine with central roles in the immune and inflammatory processes. It is a paracrine/autocrine hormone, thereby influencing local angiogenic responses [87, 88]. Recent data from Yurkovetsky et al. has also suggested that prolactin's diagnostic power in discriminating EC from healthy controls is superior to all other biomarkers examined to date. In their study involving 115 EC patients and 135 healthy control females, prolactin serum marker assays were able to identify EC with a sensitivity of 98.3 % and a specificity of 98 % [89].

The use of multiple markers may increase the sensitivity for early detection of OC. However increased sensitivity is usually associated with decreased specificity. The use of the combination of 5 markers (CA 125, OVX1, LASA, CA 15-3, CA 72-4) showed sensitivity of 90.6 % and specificity of 93.2 %, when included in CART analysis (classification and regression tree analysis), which is a marker-based classification algorithm of the disease [90].

CA 125, CA72-4, CA 15-3, and PLA when combined were found to have a sensitivity from 68 to 87 % and the same specificity as for CA 125 [91].

The *OVA1 algorithm* is based on several serum biomarkers (CA-125, β2-microglobulin, transferrin, apolipoprotein A1, and transthyretin) combined with menopausal status. This algorithm was developed on the basis of proteomic studies with the exception of CA-125. It was approved by the FDA to differentiate benign and malignant adnexal lesions. In post- and premenopausal patients, the sensitivity and specificity of this algorithm are 96 % and 28 % and 85 % and 40 %, respectively. The cutoff value is 5.0 for premenopausal and 4.4 for postmenopausal females [92]. Miller et al. [93] and Ueland et al. [94] demonstrated that specificity of the OVA1 test for epithelial malignancy was 99 %. Specificity in non-epithelial malignant ovarian, borderline epithelial and metastatic ovarian tumors was 82, 75, and 76 %, respectively. Moreover, the OVA1 test detected 76 % of OCs in which CA-125 was normal. Despite improved sensitivity in differentiating ovarian tumors from 78 % to as high as 99 %, the OVA1 test caused a fairly large decrease in specificity, i.e., from 75 to 26 %.

Visintin et al. proposed the use of six markers (leptin, prolactin, osteopontin, IGFII, MIF, and CA 125) to discriminate OC and benign tissues with an accuracy of 89 % for early stage cancers and 100 % for late stage disease [95]. However, none of these markers used alone was able to discriminate properly diseased and unaffected samples. Recently, the association of the markers mesothelin, osteopontin, and HE4 has been selected by the Specialized Program of Research Excellence (SPORE) committee for their good sensitivity and specificity values [96]. However, the applications of all these tumor markers in clinical laboratories for early-stage OC screening need to be further confirmed.

## Morphological and Cytological Markers

Transvaginal ultrasonography (TVS) is a relatively simple and noninvasive diagnostic method that provides clinicians with useful information relevant for identifying and characterizing ovarian masses. Moreover, endometrial thickness measured using TVS is the most commonly used tumor marker of EC.

Screening studies using conventional and color Doppler US in apparently healthy postmenopausal women have established that EC can be detected at a preclinical stage and that TVS is more sensitive than blind endometrial biopsy. A review of data from approximately 2900 patients collected from 13 published studies demonstrated that an endometrial thickness cutoff of 5 mm on TVS resulted in a sensitivity of 90 % and a specificity of 54 % compared to 98 and 35 %, respectively, if the cutoff was reduced to 3 mm. In addition, the 3-mm cutoff could reduce the pretest probability of EC from 10 to 0.7 % in women with negative results. The reviewers concluded that a 3-mm endometrial thickness cutoff on TVS might reliably exclude EC in women with postmenopausal bleeding [97].

TVS can observe morphology of ovarian clearly; many studies suggested TVS can be used as a method for screening early-stage OC. TVS can accurately characterize about 90 % of adnexal masses and the reported sensitivity and specificity of US for detecting ovarian malignancies is 88–96 % and 90–96 %, respectively [98–101]. Various approaches have been used to characterize ovarian masses, including pattern recognition approach, simple scoring systems, statistically derived scoring systems, probability predictors based on logistic regression analysis, and complex mathematical models such as neural networks [102, 103].

## International Ovarian Tumor Analysis (IOTA)

The *International Ovarian Tumor Analysis* (IOTA) framework is a pattern recognition approach that has been frequently used to present large-scale multicenter-based consensus results. It includes a standardized methodology for the US evaluation of ovarian masses and definitions of the ultrasonographic parameters of ovarian masses [104–106]. In the IOTA six categories, from "certainly malignant" to "certainly benignant," have been proposed for the subjective US assessment of adnexal masses [107]. The simple rules developed by the IOTA are based on five ultrasound features of malignancy (irregular solid tumor; presence of ascites; at least four papillary structures; irregular multilocular solid tumor with largest diameter >100 mm; very strong blood flow with color score = 4) and five ultrasound features suggestive of a benign lesion (unilocular tumor; presence of solid components where the largest solid component has a largest diameter <7 mm; presence of acoustic shadows; smooth multilocular tumor with largest diameter <100 mm; no blood flow with color score = 1) [50, 108]. An adnexal mass is classified as malignant if at least one malignant feature (M-features) and no benign features (B-features) are present and vice versa. When no B- or M-features are present, or if both B- and M-features are present, then simple rules are considered inconclusive (uncertain), and a different diagnostic method should be used. So far, these simple rules have been externally validated in five studies in 17 clinical centers [108]. In these studies, the rules could be applied to 79–89 % of all adnexal masses [109–112].

Only a small proportion (6–8 %) of masses cannot be confidently classified as benign or malignant when using subjective assessment by experienced ultrasound examiners [113]. Unclassifiable adnexal tumors have certain typical morphological features. These tumors were larger than classifiable masses, more often had a unilocular-solid or multilocular-solid appearance, and more frequently had irregular walls and papillary projections than classifiable masses. Multilocular cysts, with more than ten cyst locules, were also more often observed among unclassifiable masses. An absence of color Doppler signals was less common in these masses, whereas a moderate amount of color Doppler signals (color score 3) was more common.

Unfortunately, ultrasound imaging, such as biomarkers, is equivocal in some cases. So that, in the last years, other algorithms have been proposed as alternative approach to triage women as being at low or high risk of cancer combining diagnostic imaging with biomarkers or other parameters. The most frequent are: Risk of Malignancy Index (RMI), the IOTA LR1 and LR2.

The *RMI*, a widely used algorithm, involves specific ultrasound parameters, measurement of CA-125 and hormonal status to assign patients to a low or a high OC risk [114–116]. Using a 200 cutoff value, the sensitivity and specificity of this algorithm are 64–94 % and 82–92 %, respectively, while the area under the receiver operating characteristics (ROC) curve (AUC) range is 0.931–0.945 [117, 118].

The *IOTA logistic regression model LR2* (IOTA LR2) was a risk prediction model based on ultrasound imaging [119–121] and other parameters that include age, presence of ascites, presence of abnormal flow in papillary lesions, maximum dimension of the solid structure, presence of irregular cystic lesions, and presence of an acoustic shadow. Using a cutoff value of 10 % sensitivity was 93.8 %, specificity was 81.9 %, and the AUC was 0.952. What is particularly interesting is that diagnostic test performance was better for pre- vs postmenopausal women.

The *logistic regression model* based on 12 variables (*IOTA LR1*) has a performance that is at least as good as that of LR2. However, LR2 is based on six variables only (see below), which facilitates its use in clinical practice.

A group of tumors have proven difficult to classify with transvaginal ultrasound and remain a diagnostic challenge for which accurate second-stage tests would be of value. Other imaging techniques in addition to TVU are available that may be used to provide an assessment of a tumor before treatment (i.e., magnetic resonance imaging, computed tomography, and positron emission tomography combined with computed tomography).

Some studies suggest that magnetic resonance imaging (MRI), compared with other imaging modalities, may play a role in the assessment of the cohort of "difficult to classify" adnexal masses. MRI is, also, an accurate imaging technique for preoperative assessment of EC and for evaluating the depth of myometrial invasion [122, 123]. The depth of myometrial invasion in patients with EC correlates strongly with the prevalence of lymph node metastasis and with patient survival.

A recent meta-analysis demonstrated that contrast-enhanced T1-weighted (T1WI) MRI was substantially better than ultrasonography, CT, or noncontrast MRI for EC evaluation [124]. Moreover, dynamic contrast-enhanced MRI (DCE-MRI) is considered more accurate than T2-weighted imaging (T2WI) in tumor detection and in assessing myometrial invasion due to greater contrast and clearer demonstration of the border between the tumor and myometrium in the early phase [125–127].

Both conventional and contrast-enhanced MRI protocols are now well established in guidelines provided by the European Society of Urogenital Radiology for characterizing "difficult" ovarian masses. These protocols use straightforward decision trees that divide "difficult" masses into three distinct groups on the basis of findings on standard T1-weighted and T2-weighted sequences: the T1-weighted high-signal intensity mass, the T2-weighted solid mass, and the cystic-solid mass. Additional sequences might be of interest in defining the site of origin and the nature of the mass [128]. The T1 "bright" masses may require additional fat-suppressed T1-weighted (FST1W) imaging to distinguish fat in teratomas from mucinous or hemorrhagic cyst content.

T2 solid masses may require oblique imaging to identify their relationship with the uterus to distinguish between uterine leiomyoma and ovarian fibroma. In addition, solid masses with inhomogeneous low T2 signal or intermediate T2 signal require assessment of the degree of contrast (gadolinium) enhancement. All cystic-solid masses with suspected solid elements require gadolinium-enhanced T1-weighted sequences to determine the presence of malignancy [129].

Dynamic contrast-enhanced (DCE) MRI with semi-quantitative analysis provides information on tissue vascularization by measuring changes in signal intensity before, during, and after intravenous contrast administration, and helps differentiate some complex benign and malignant lesions.

Combined DCE MRI in addition to conventional morphologic assessment has been shown to improve the overall accuracy of MRI for depicting OC [130, 131].

DWI is a recent prevailing technique that enables distinction between cancerous and normal tissues, determines lesion aggressiveness, and monitors responses to therapy by providing information on extracellular space tortuosity and tissue cellularity [132]. It characterizes tissues by probing differences in the random mobility of water molecules related to tissue cellularity and cellular membrane integrity [133].

Besides evaluating adnexal pathology, DWI is a particularly powerful diagnostic tool for identifying peritoneal metastases and recurrent invasive disease [134, 135].

Both functional sequences DCE MRI and DWI provided new criteria to those already being commonly used with conventional MRI protocols to describe indeterminate adnexal masses after TVS, and resulted in the development of a novel $A_{DNEx}MR_{SCORING}$ system [136] to improve standardization of MRI reports in these adnexal tumors. Using a score of ≥4 to define a malignant tumor, the $A_{DNEx}MR_{SCORING}$ system predicted malignancy with 93.5 % sensitivity and 96.6 % specificity. DW-MRI offers potential advantages over DCE-MRI because it does not involve intravenous administration of a contrast agent and entails a shorter imaging time.

Multiple studies have shown DWI combined with T2 or with the application of fused image to be effective in assessing deep myometrial invasion for EC. A recent meta-analysis showed that DWI has excellent accuracy in the diagnosis of deep myometrial invasion, with an area under the ROC curve of 0.91. The pooled PLR of 8 suggests that patients with deep myometrial invasion have approximately eightfold chance of having DWI positive compared to patients with superficial or no myometrial invasion. On the other hand, the pooled NLR of 0.1 suggests that if the DWI was negative, the probability that this patient has deep myometrial invasion was 0.1 %, which is low enough to rule out deep myometrial invasion [137].

Cytological tumor markers for ovarian and endometrial cancer screening have not been actually introduced in clinical practice. The conventional Pap test has been thought to be unreliable in the detection of endometrial lesions. However, the presence of atypical endometrial cells has been reported to be associated with a higher rate of significant endometrial pathology and should lead to additional evaluation for the presence of endometrial disease.

In addition, in asymptomatic noncycle premenopausal and postmenopausal women, benign endometrial cells in Pap smears might also be an indicator of endometrial pathology. The 2001 Bethesda System recommended the reporting of endometrial cells in women 40 years of age or older, regardless of menstrual status or clinical history. Lai et al introduced new finding that leads to a reconsideration of cytology for early diagnosis of EC. The degenerative necrotic endometrial debris in the background of Pap smears was composed of histiocytes, degenerative inflammatory and individual necrotic cells. Necrotic debris and phagocytosis were also frequent findings in endometrial adenocarcinoma. Lay et al. have shoved that when benign-appearing endometrial cells are present in the Pap smear, degenerative necrotic debris is a significant risk factor for endometrial pathology, regardless of menopausal status [138]. Moreover, other studies have shown that liquid-based Pap test technology increased the detection of endometrial adenocarcinoma. Two studies specific to ThinPrep (Hologic, Bedford, MA) technology reported endometrial adenocarcinoma detection sensitivity rates of 65.2 and 88.3 % compared with 38.6 % with conventional smears [139, 140].

## References

1. Siegel R, Ma J, Zou Z, et al. Cancer statistics, 2014. CA Cancer J Clin. 2014;64(1):9–29.
2. Sorosky JI. Endometrial cancer. Obstet Gynecol. 2008;111(2 Pt 1):436–47.
3. Weissman SM, Weiss SM, Newlin AC. Genetic testing by cancer site: ovary. Cancer J. 2012;18:320–7.
4. Pruthi S, Gostout BS, Lindor NM. Identification and management of women with BRCA mutations or hereditary predisposition for breast and ovarian cancer. Mayo Clin Proc. 2010;85:1111–20.
5. Roy R, Chun J, Powell SN. BRCA1 and BRCA2: different roles in a common pathway of genome protection. Nat Rev Cancer. 2012;12:68–78.
6. Karlan BY, Berchuck A, Mutch D. The role of genetic testing for cancer susceptibility in gynecologic practice. Obstet Gynecol. 2007;110:155–67.
7. Struewing JP, Hartge P, Wacholder S, et al. The risk of cancer associated with specific mutations of BRCA1 and BRCA2 among Ashkenazi Jews. N Engl J Med. 1997;336:1401–8.
8. Kurian AW, Munoz DF, Rust P, et al. Online tool to guide decisions for BRCA1/2 mutation carriers. J Clin Oncol. 2012;30:497–506.
9. Levine DA, Lin O, Barakat RR, et al. Risk of endometrial carcinoma associated with BRCA mutation. Gynecol Oncol. 2001;80(3):395–8.
10. Mutch D, Denny L, Quinn M. FIGO committee on gynecologic oncology. Hereditary gynecologic cancers. Int J Gynaecol Obstet. 2014;124:189–92.
11. Lynch HT, Casey MJ, Snyder CL, et al. Hereditary ovarian carcinoma: heterogeneity, molecular genetics, pathology, and management. Mol Oncol. 2009;3:97–137.
12. Bonadona V, Bonaïti B, Olschwang S, et al. Cancer risks associated with germline mutations in MLH1,

MSH2, and MSH6 genes in Lynch syndrome. JAMA. 2011;305(22):2304–10.
13. Katabathina VS, Prasad SR. Genetics of susceptibility to sporadic ovarian cancer, in e LS. Oxford: Wiley; 2013.
14. Sherman ME, Sturgeon S, Brinton LA, et al. Risk factors and hormone levels in patients with serous and endometrioid uterine carcinomas. Mod Pathol. 1997;10:963–8.
15. Zhou XP, Kuismanen S, Nystrom-Lahti M, et al. Distinct PTEN mutational spectra in hereditary non-polyposis colon cancer syndrome-related endometrial carcinomas compared to sporadic microsatellite unstable tumors. Hum Mol Genet. 2002;11(4): 445–50.
16. Karageorgi S, Hankinson SE, Kraft P, et al. Reproductive factors and postmenopausal hormone use in relation to endometrial cancer risk in the Nurses' Health Study cohort 1976–2004. Int J Cancer. 2010;126(1):208–16.
17. Amankwah EK, Friedenreich CM, Magliocco AM, et al. Anthropometric measures and the risk of endometrial cancer, overall and by tumor microsatellite status and histological subtype. Am J Epidemiol. 2013;177(12):1378–87.
18. Gunter MJ, Hoover DR, Yu H, et al. A prospective evaluation of insulin and insulin-like growth factor I as risk factors for endometrial cancer. Cancer Epidemiol Biomarkers Prev. 2008;17(4):921–9.
19. Lukanova A, Kaaks R. Endogenous hormones and ovarian cancer: epidemiology and current hypotheses. Cancer Epidemiol Biomarkers Prev. 2005; 14(1):98–107.
20. Danforth KN, Tworoger SS, Hecht JL, et al. A prospective study of postmenopausal hormone use and ovarian cancer risk. BJC. 2007;96:151–6.
21. Leitzmann MF, Koebnick C, Danforth KN, et al. Body mass index and risk of ovarian cancer. Cancer. 2009;115(4):812–22.
22. Helzlsouer KJ, Alberg AJ, Gordon GB, et al. Serum gonadotropins and steroid hormones and the development of ovarian cancer. JAMA. 1995;274(24): 1926–30.
23. Fathalla MF. Incessant ovulation and ovarian cancer—a hypothesis re-visited. Facts Views Vis Obgyn. 2013;5:292–7.
24. Doufekas K, Olaitan A. Clinical epidemiology of epithelial ovarian cancer in the UK. Int J Womens Health. 2014;6:537–45.
25. Cibula D, Zikan M, Dusek L, et al. Oral contraceptives and risk of ovarian and breast cancers in BRCA mutation carriers: a meta-analysis. Expert Rev Anticancer Ther. 2011;11:1197–207.
26. Havrilesky LJ, Moorman PG, Lowery WJ, et al. Oral contraceptive pills as primary prevention for ovarian cancer: a systematic review and meta-analysis. Obstet Gynecol. 2013;122:139–47.
27. Lee Y, Miron A, Drapkin R, et al. A candidate precursor to serous carcinoma that originates in the distal fallopian tube. J Pathol. 2007;211:26–35.
28. Sasieni PD, Adams J. Standardized lifetime risk. Am J Epidemiol. 1999;149(9):869–75.
29. Partridge EE, Greenlee RT, Riley TL, et al. Assessing the risk of ovarian malignancy in asymptomatic women with abnormal CA 125 and transvaginal ultrasound scans in the prostate, lung, colorectal, and ovarian screening trial. Obstet Gynecol. 2013;121:25–31.
30. Dong X, Men X, Zhang W, et al. Advances in tumor markers of ovarian cancer for early diagnosis. Indian J Cancer. 2014;51 Suppl 3:e72–6.
31. National Collaborating Centre for Cancer (UK). Cardiff, UK; 2011.
32. Sturgeon CM, Duffy MJ, Stenman UH, et al. National academy of clinical biochemistry laboratory medicine practice guidelines for use of tumor markers in testicular, prostate, colorectal, breast, and ovarian cancers. Clin Chem. 2008;54:e11–79.
33. Bast Jr RC. Status of tumor markers in ovarian cancer screening. J Clin Oncol. 2003;21:S200–5.
34. Urban N, McIntosh MW, Andersen M, et al. Ovarian cancer screening. Hematol Oncol Clin North Am. 2003;17:989–1005.
35. Rustin GJ, Bast Jr RC, Kelloff GJ, et al. Use of CA-125 in clinical trial evaluation of new therapeutic drugs for ovarian cancer. Clin Cancer Res. 2004;10:3919–26.
36. Duk JM, Aalders JG, Fleuren GJ, et al. CA 125: a useful marker in endometrial carcinoma. Am J Obstet Gynecol. 1986;155:1097–102.
37. Moore RG, MacLaughlan S, Bast Jr RC. Current state of biomarker development for clinical application in epithelial ovarian cancer. Gynecol Oncol. 2010;116(2):240–5.
38. Kirchhoff C. Molecular characterization of epididymal proteins. Rev Reprod. 1998;3:86–95.
39. Hellstrom I, Raycraft J, Hayden-Ledbetter M, et al. The HE4 (WFDC2) protein is a biomarker for ovarian carcinoma. Cancer Res. 2003;63:3695–700.
40. Karlsen NS, Karlsen MA, Høgdall CK, et al. HE4 tissue expression and serum HE4 levels in healthy individuals and patients with benign or malignant tumors: a systematic review. Cancer Epidemiol Biomarkers Prev. 2014;23(11):2285–95.
41. Moore RG, Miller MC, Eklund EE, et al. Serum levels of the ovarian cancer biomarker HE4 are decreased in pregnancy and increase with age. Am J Obstet Gynecol. 2012;206:349.
42. Huhtinen K, Suvitie P, Hiissa J, et al. Serum HE4 concentration differentiates malignant ovarian tumours from ovarian endometriotic cysts. Br J Cancer. 2009;100:1315–9.
43. Holcomb K, Vucetic Z, Miller MC, et al. Human epididymis protein 4 offers superior specificity in the differentiation of benign and malignant adnexal masses in premenopausal women. Am J Obstet Gynecol. 2011;205:358.e1–6.
44. Park Y, Lee JH, Hong DJ, et al. Diagnostic performances of HE4 and CA125 for the detection of ovarian cancer from patients with various gynecologic

and non- gynecologic diseases. Clin Biochem. 2011;44:884–8.

45. Hallamaa M, Huhtinen K, Suvitie P, et al. Serum concentrations of HE4 change little during in vitro fertilization. Acta Obstet Gynecol Scand. 2014; 93:640–6.
46. Mokhtar N, Thevarajah M, Ma N, et al. Human epididymis protein 4 reference intervals in a multiethnic asian women population. Asian Pac J Cancer Prev. 2012;13:6391–5.
47. Yang J, Sa M, Huang M, Yang J, et al. The reference intervals for HE4, CA125 and ROMA in healthy female with electrochemiluminescence immunoassay. Clin Biochem. 2013;46:1705–8.
48. Fujirebio Diagnostics [homepage on the Internet]. HE4 EIA—Instructions for Use [24 p.]; c2008–06. http://www.fdi.com/documents/products/inserts/eia/HE4%20EIA%20404-10US%202008-06%20%20F5908%20r1%20r0%20(3).pdf.
49. Abbott Diagnostics. HE4 and CA125 Information. https://www.abbottdiagnostics.com/en-int/HE4-CA125.
50. Kaijser J, Sayasneh A, Van Hoorde K, et al. Presurgical diagnosis of adnexal tumours using mathematical models and scoring systems: a systematic review and meta-analysis. Hum Reprod Update. 2014;20(3):449–62.
51. Bandiera E, Romani C, Specchia C, et al. Serum human epididymis protein 4 and risk for ovarian malignancy algorithm as new diagnostic and prognostic tools for epithelial ovarian cancer management. Cancer Epidemiol Biomarkers Prev. 2011;20(12):2496–506.
52. Chen WT, Gao X, Han XD, et al. HE4 as a serum biomarker for ROMA prediction and prognosis of epithelial ovarian cancer. Asian Pac J Cancer Prev. 2014;15(1):101–5.
53. Sood AK, Buller RE, Burger RA, et al. Value of preoperative CA 125 level in the management of uterine cancer and prediction of clinical outcome. Obstet Gynecol. 1997;90:441–7.
54. Li J, Dowdy S, Tipton T, et al. HE4 as a biomarker for ovarian and endometrial cancer management. Expert Rev Mol Diagn. 2009;9(6):555–66.
55. Walentowicz P, Krintus M, Sadlecki P, et al. Serum inhibin A and inhibin B levels in epithelial ovarian cancer patients. PLoS One. 2014;9(3), e90575.
56. Scholler N, Crawford M, Sato A, et al. Bead-based ELISA for validation of ovarian cancer early detection markers. Clin Cancer Res. 2006;12(7 Pt 1):2117–24.
57. Wu X, Li D, Liu L, et al. Serum soluble mesothelin-related peptide (SMRP): a potential diagnostic and monitoring marker for epithelial ovarian cancer. Arch Gynecol Obstet. 2014;289(6):1309–14.
58. Tilli TM, Bellahcène A, Castronovo V, et al. Changes in the transcriptional profile in response to overexpression of the osteopontin-c splice isoform in ovarian (OvCar-3) and prostate (PC-3) cancer cell lines. BMC Cancer. 2014;14:433.
59. Lenhard MS, Nehring S, Nagel D, et al. Predictive value of CA 125 and CA 72-4 in ovarian borderline tumors. Clin Chem Lab Med. 2009;47(5):537–42.
60. Moore RG, Brown AK, Miller MC, et al. The use of multiple novel tumor biomarkers for the detection of ovarian carcinoma in patients with a pelvic mass. Gynecol Oncol. 2008;108:402–8.
61. Kioi M, Kawakami M, Shimamura T, et al. Interleukin-13 receptor alpha2 chain: a potential biomarker and molecular target for ovarian cancer therapy. Cancer. 2006;107:1407–18.
62. Longuespée R, Boyon C, Desmons A, et al. Ovarian cancer molecular pathology. Cancer Metastasis Rev. 2012;31(3-4):713–32.
63. Agarwal R, Whang DH, Alvero AB, et al. Macrophage migration inhibitory factor expression in ovarian cancer. Am J Obstet Gynecol. 2007; 196:348e1–5.
64. Suzuki M, Ohwada M, Aida I, et al. Macrophage colony-stimulating factor as a tumor marker for epithelial ovarian cancer. Obstet Gynecol. 1993;82:946–50.
65. Chechlinska M, Kaminska J, Markowska J, et al. Peritoneal fluid cytokines and the differential diagnosis of benign and malignant ovarian tumors and residual/recurrent disease examination. Int J Biol Markers. 2007;22:172–80.
66. Xu Y, Shen Z, Wiper DW, et al. Lysophosphatidic acid as a potential biomarker for ovarian and other gynecologic cancers. JAMA. 1998;280(8):719–23.
67. Wang P, Wu X, Chen W, et al. The lysophosphatidic acid (LPA) receptors their expression and significance in epithelial ovarian neoplasms. Gynecol Oncol. 2007;104:714–20.
68. Sedláková I, Vávrová J, Tošner J, et al. Lysophosphatidic acid (LPA) – a perspective marker in ovarian cancer. Tumour Biol. 2011;32:311–6.
69. Pua TL, Wang FQ, Fishman DA. Roles of LPA in ovarian cancer development and progression. Future Oncol. 2009;5:1659–73.
70. Tanyi J, Rigó Jr J. Lysophosphatidic acid as a potential target for treatment and molecular diagnosis of epithelial ovarian cancers. Orv Hetil. 2009;150: 1109–18.
71. Smith JB, Stashwick C, Powell Jr DJ. B7-H4 as a potential target for immunotherapy for gynecologic cancers: a closer look. Gynecol Oncol. 2014;134: 181–9.
72. Salceda S, Tang T, Kmet M, et al. The immunomodulatory protein B7-H4 is overexpressed in breast and ovarian cancers and promotes epithelial cell transformation. Exp Cell Res. 2005;306:128–41.
73. Tringler B, Liu W, Corral L, et al. B7-H4 overexpression in ovarian tumors. Gynecol Oncol. 2006;100:44–52.
74. Simon I, Katsaros D, Rigault de la Longrais I, et al. B7-H4 is over-expressed in early-stage ovarian cancer and is independent of CA125 expression. Gynecol Oncol. 2007;106:334–41.
75. Simon I, Liu Y, Krall KL, et al. Evaluation of the novel serum markers B7-H4, Spondin 2, and DcR3

for diagnosis and early detection of ovarian cancer. Gynecol Oncol. 2007;106:112–8.

76. Cheng L, Jiang J, Gao R, et al. B7-H4 expression promotes tumorigenesis in ovarian cancer. Int J Gynecol Cancer. 2009;19:1481–6.
77. Tang MK, Wong AS. Exosomes: emerging biomarkers and targets for ovarian cancer. Cancer Lett. 2015;367(1):26–33.
78. Cho JA, Park H, Lim EH, et al. Exosomes from ovarian cancer cells induce adipose tissue-derived mesenchymal stem cells to acquire the physical and functional characteristics of tumor-supporting myofibroblasts. Gynecol Oncol. 2011;123:379–86.
79. Lis R, Touboul C, Raynaud CM, et al. Mesenchymal cell interaction with ovarian cancer cells triggers pro-metastatic properties. PLoS One. 2012;7, e38340.
80. Szajnik M, Derbis M, Lach M, et al. Exosomes in plasma of patients with ovarian carcinoma: potential biomarkers of tumor progression and response to therapy. Gynecol Obstet. 2013;4:3.
81. Li J, Sherman-Baust CA, Tsai-Turton M, et al. Claudin-containing exosomes in the peripheral circulation of women with ovarian cancer. BMC Cancer. 2009;9:244.
82. Im H, Shao H, Park YI, et al. Label-free detection and molecular profiling of exosomes with a nano-plasmonic sensor. Nat Biotechnol. 2014;32:490–5.
83. Lawrie CH, Gal S, Dunlop HM, et al. Detection of elevated levels of tumour-associated microRNAs in serum of patients with diffuse large B-cell lymphoma. Br J Haematol. 2008;141:672–5.
84. Torres A, Torres K, Pesci A, et al. Deregulation of miR-100, miR-99a and miR-199b in tissues and plasma coexists with increased expression of mTor kinase in endometrioid endometrial carcinoma. BMC Cancer. 2012;12:369.
85. Jiang F, Liu T, He Y, et al. MiR-125b promotes proliferation and migration of type II endometrial carcinoma cells through targeting TP53INP1 tumor suppressor in vitro and in vivo. BMC Cancer. 2011;11:425.
86. Clapp C, Lopez-Gomez FJ, Nava G, et al. Expression of prolactin mRNA and of prolactin-like proteins in endothelial cells: evidence for autocrine effects. J Endocrinol. 1998;158:137–44.
87. Corbacho AM, Martinez De La Escalera G, Clapp C. Roles of prolactin and related members of the prolactin/growth hormone/placental lactogen family in angiogenesis. J Endocrinol. 2002;173:219–38.
88. Yurkovetsky Z, Ta'asan S, Skates S, et al. Development of multimarker panel for early detection of endometrial cancer. High diagnostic power of prolactin. Gynecol Oncol. 2007;107:58–65.
89. Woolas RP, Conaway MR, Xu F, et al. Combinations of multiple serum markers are superior to individual assays for discriminating malignant from benign pelvic masses. Gynecol Oncol. 1995;59:111–6.
90. Zhang Z, Barnhill SD, Zhang H, et al. Combination of multiple serum markers using an artificial neural network to improve specificity in discriminating malignant from benign pelvic masses. Gynecol Oncol. 1999;73:56–61.
91. Zhang Z, Chan DW. The road from discovery to clinical diagnostics: lessons learned from the first FDA-cleared in vitro diagnostic multivariate index assay of proteomic biomarkers. Cancer Epidemiol Biomarkers Prev. 2010;19:2995–9.
92. Bast RC, Skates S, Lokshin A, et al. Differential diagnosis of a pelvic mass: improved algorithms and novel biomarkers. Int J Gynecol Cancer. 2012;22(Suppl):5–8.
93. Ware Miller R, Smith A, Desimone CP, et al. Performance of the American Collage of Obstetricians and Gynecologists' ovarian tumor referral guidelines with multivariate index assay. Obstet Gynecol. 2011;117:1298–306.
94. Ueland FR, Desimone CP, Seamon LG, et al. Effectiveness of multivariate index assay in the preoperative assessment of ovarian tumors. Obstet Gynecol. 2011;117:1289–97.
95. Visintin I, Feng Z, Longton G, et al. Diagnostic markers for early detection of ovarian cancer. Clin Cancer Res. 2008;14:1065–72.
96. Moore RG, Maclaughlan S. Current clinical use of biomarkers for epithelial ovarian cancer. Curr Opin Oncol. 2010;22:492–7.
97. Timmermans A, Opmeer BC, Khan KS, et al. Endometrial thickness measurement for detecting endometrial cancer in women with postmenopausal bleeding: a systematic review and meta-analysis. Obstet Gynecol. 2010;116(1):160–7.
98. Timmerman D, Schwarzler P, Collins WP, et al. Subjective assessment of adnexal masses with the use of ultrasonography: an analysis of interobserver variability and experience. Ultrasound Obstet Gynecol. 1999;13:11–6.
99. Valentin L. Prospective cross-validation of Doppler ultrasound examination and gray-scale ultrasound imaging for discrimination of benign and malignant pelvic masses. Ultrasound Obstet Gynecol. 1999;14:273–83.
100. Valentin L. Pattern recognition of pelvic masses by gray-scale ultrasound imaging: the contribution of Doppler ultrasound. Ultrasound Obstet Gynecol. 1999;14:338–47.
101. Brown DL, Dudiak KM, Laing FC. Adnexal masses: US characterization and reporting. Radiology. 2010;254:342–54.
102. Geomini P, Kruitwagen R, Bremer GL, et al. The accuracy of risk scores in predicting ovarian malignancy: a systematic review. Obstet Gynecol. 2009;113:384–94.
103. Valentin L. Use of morphology to characterize and manage common adnexal masses. Best Pract Res Clin Obstet Gynaecol. 2004;18:71–89.
104. Testa AC. Malignant ovarian neoplasms: the sonographic voyage of discovery. Ultrasound Obstet Gynecol. 2008;31:611–4.
105. Timmerman D, Valentin L, Bourne TH, et al. Terms, definitions and measurements to describe the sono-

graphic features of adnexal tumors: a consensus opinion from the International Ovarian Tumor Analysis (IOTA) Group. Ultrasound Obstet Gynecol. 2000;16:500–5.
106. Valentin L, Ameye L, Savelli L, et al. Adnexal masses difficult to classify as benign or malignant using subjective assessment of gray-scale and Doppler ultrasound findings: logistic regression models do not help. Ultrasound Obstet Gynecol. 2011;38:456–65.
107. Timmerman D, Testa AC, Bourne T, et al. Simple ultrasound-based rules for the diagnosis of ovarian cancer. Ultrasound Obstet Gynecol. 2008; 31:681–90.
108. Timmerman D, Ameye L, Fischerova D, et al. Simple ultrasound rules to distinguish between benign and malignant adnexal masses before surgery: prospective validation by IOTA group. BMJ. 2010;341:c6839.
109. Fathallah K, Huchon C, Bats AS, et al. External validation of simple ultrasound rules of Timmerman on 122 ovarian tumors. Gynecol Obstet Fertil. 2011;39:477–81.
110. Sayasneh A, Wynants L, Preisler J, et al. Multicenter external validation of IOTA prediction models and RMI by operators with varied training. Br J Cancer. 2013;108:2448–54.
111. Alcázar JL, Pascual MA, Olartecoechea B, et al. IOTA simple rules for discriminating between benign and malignant adnexal masses: prospective external validation. Ultrasound Obstet Gynecol. 2013;42:467–71.
112. Hartman CA, Juliato CR, Sarian LO, et al. Ultrasound criteria and CA 125 as predictive variables of ovarian cancer in women with adnexal tumors. Ultrasound Obstet Gynecol. 2012;40:360–6.
113. Jacobs I, Oram D, Fairbanks J, et al. A risk of malignancy index incorporating CA 125, ultrasound and menopausal status for the accurate preoperative diagnosis of ovarian cancer. Br J Obstet Gynecol. 1990;97:922–9.
114. Morgante G, Ia Marca A, Ditto A, et al. Comparison of two malignancy risk indices based on serum CA125, ultrasound score and menopausal status in the diagnosis of ovarian masses. Br J Obstet Gynaecol. 1999;106:524–7.
115. Tinglustad S, Hagen B, Skjeldestad FE, et al. The risk of malignancy index to evaluate potential ovarian cancers in local hospitals. Obstet Gynecol. 1999;93:448–52.
116. Havrilesky LJ, Whitehead CM, Rubatt JM, et al. Evaluation of biomarker panels for early stage ovarian cancer detection and monitoring for disease recurrence. Gynecol Oncol. 2008;110:374–82.
117. Anton C, Carvalho FM, Oliveira EI, et al. A comparison of CA125, HE4, risk ovarian malignancy algorithm (ROMA), and risk malignancy index (RMI) for the classification of ovarian masses. Clinics. 2012;67:437–41.
118. Van Gorp T, Veldman J, Van Calster B, et al. Subjective assessment by ultrasound is superior to the risk of malignancy index (RMI) or the risk of ovarian malignancy algorithm (ROMA) in discriminating benign from malignant adnexal masses. Eur J Cancer. 2012;48:1649–56.
119. Kaijser J, Van Gorp T, Van Hoorde K, et al. A comparison between an ultrasound based prediction model (LR2) and the risk of ovarian malignancy algorithm (ROMA) to assess the risk of malignancy in women with adnexal mass. Gynecol Oncol. 2013;129:377–83.
120. Kaijser J, Van Gorp T, Smet ME, et al. Are serum HE4 or ROMA scores useful to experienced examiners for improving characterization of adnexal masses after transvaginal ultrasonography? Ultrasound Obstet Gynecol. 2014;43:89–97.
121. Kijser J. Differentiating stage I epithelial ovarian cancer from benign disease in women with adnexal tumor s using biomarkers or the ROMA algorithm. Gynecol Oncol. 2013;130:398–400.
122. Manfredi R, Mirk P, Maresca G, et al. Local-regional staging of endometrial carcinoma: role of MR imaging in surgical planning. Radiology. 2004;231:372–8.
123. Hricak H, Rubinstein L, Gherman G, et al. MR imaging evaluation of endometrial carcinoma: results of an NCI cooperative study. Radiology. 1991;179:829–32.
124. Sironi S, Colombo E, Villa G, et al. Myometrial invasion by endometrial carcinoma: assessment with plain and gadolinium enhanced MR imaging. Radiology. 1992;185:207–12.
125. Kinkel K, Kaji Y, Yu KK, et al. Radiologic staging in patients with endometrial cancer: a meta-analysis. Radiology. 1999;212:711–8.
126. Yamashita Y, Harada M, Sawada T, et al. Normal uterus and FIGO stage I endometrial carcinoma: dynamic gadolinium-enhanced MR imaging. Radiology. 1993;186:495–501.
127. Seki H, Kimura M, Sakai K. Myometrial invasion of endometrial carcinoma: assessment with dynamic MR and contrast-enhanced T1-weighted images. Clin Radiol. 1997;52:18–23.
128. Savci G, Ozyaman T, Tutar M, et al. Assessment of depth of myometrial invasion by endometrial carcinoma: comparison of T2-weighted SE and contrast-enhanced dynamic GRE MR imaging. Eur Radiol. 1998;8:218–23.
129. Spencer JA, Forstner R, Cunha TM, et al. ESUR Female Imaging Sub-Committee. ESUR guidelines for MR imaging of the sonographically indeterminate adnexal mass: an algorithmic approach. Eur Radiol. 2010;20:25–35.
130. Kinkel K, Lu Y, Mehdizade A, et al. Indeterminate ovarian mass at US: incremental value of second imaging test for characterization: meta-analysis and Bayesian analysis. Radiology. 2005;236:85–94.
131. Hricak H, Chen M, Coakley FV, et al. Complex adnexal masses: detection and characterization with

MR imaging d multivariate analysis. Radiology. 2000;214:39–46.
132. Patterson DM, Padhani AR, Collins DJ. Technology insight: water diffusion MRI – a potential new biomarker of response to cancer therapy. Nat Clin Pract Oncol. 2008;5:220–33.
133. Le Bihan D. Molecular diffusion, tissue microdynamics and microstructure. NMR Biomed. 1995;8:375–86.
134. Fujii S, Matsusue E, Kanasaki Y, et al. Detection of peritoneal dissemination in gynecological malignancy: evaluation by diffusion-weighted MR imaging. Eur Radiol. 2008;18:18–23.
135. Sala E, Rockall A, Rangarajan D, et al. The role of dynamic contrast enhanced and diffusion weighted magnetic resonance imaging in the female pelvis. Eur J Radiol. 2010;76:367–85.
136. Thomassin-Naggara I, Aubert E, Rockall A, et al. Adnexal masses: development and preliminary validation of an MR imaging scoring system. Radiology. 2013;267:432–43.
137. Das SK, Niu XK, Wang JL, et al. Usefulness of DWI in preoperative assessment of deep myometrial invasion in patients with endometrial carcinoma: a systematic review and meta-analysis. Cancer Imaging. 2014;14:32.
138. Lai CR, Hsu CY, Li AF. Degenerative necrotic endometrial debris in Papanicolaou smears. The role in the prediction of endometrial pathology. Am J Clin Pathol. 2012;137(2):290–4.
139. Zhou J, Tomashefski Jr J, Khiyami A. Diagnostic value of the thin-layer, liquid based Pap test in endometrial cancer: a retrospective study with emphasis on cytomorphological features. Acta Cytol. 2007;51:735–41.
140. Schorge JO, Saboorian MH, Hynan L, et al. ThinPrep detection of cervical and endometrial adenocarcinoma: a retrospective cohort study. Cancer. 2002;96:338–43.

# Part III

# Gynecological Cancers: New Therapies, Drug Development, and Challenges

# Developmental Therapeutics for Gynecologic Cancers: An Overview

6

Jennifer L. Brown and Christina S. Chu

**Abstract**

Traditionally, gynecologic cancers are approached in a multimodal fashion, employing surgery, chemotherapy, and radiation. These important therapies, while often very effective at treating malignancy, often result in difficult multisystem toxicities for patients. Identification of genomic and molecular differences between normal and cancer cells has allowed development of targeted therapies that focus on inhibition of pathways involved in cancer proliferation and metastasis. These therapies ideally provide a more directed approach by selectively acting on targets that are expressed on or in close proximity to tumor cells, thereby limiting toxicity and allowing administration at minimum effective dose rather than maximum tolerated dose, as is standard for traditional cytotoxics. Pathways involving DNA damage repair, angiogenesis, signal transduction, cell proliferation, survival, and metabolism are under active investigation in gynecologic malignancies. Immune therapies involving vaccination and adoptive T-cell infusion are also under evaluation to augment innate tumor-specific immunity.

**Keywords**

Immunotherapy • Targeted therapy • Ovarian cancer • Endometrial cancer • Cervical cancer • Angiogenesis • mTOR • EGFR • Tumor vaccination • Adoptive immunotherapy

J.L. Brown, MD (✉) • C.S. Chu, MD
Division of Gynecologic Oncology, Fox Chase Cancer Center, 333 Cottman Avenue, Philadelphia, PA 19111, USA
e-mail: jenniferbrown0683@me.com; Christina.Chu@fccc.edu



A. Giordano, M. Macaluso (eds.), *Gynecological Cancers*, Current Clinical Oncology,
DOI 10.1007/978-3-319-32907-9_6

## Introduction

Traditionally, gynecologic cancers are approached in a multimodal fashion, employing surgery, chemotherapy, and radiation. Chemotherapy primarily focuses on killing rapidly dividing cells and thus does not discriminate between normal and cancer cells. Radiation affects all cells in the treated field, which often includes normal tissues as well. These important therapies, while very effective at treating malignancy, often result in undesirable effects on the gastrointestinal, hepatic, renal, hematologic, and integumentary systems.

Identification of genomic and molecular differences between normal and cancer cells has allowed development of targeted therapies that focus on inhibition of pathways involved in cancer proliferation and metastasis [1]. These therapies ideally provide a more directed approach by selectively acting on targets that are expressed on or in close proximity to tumor cells, thereby limiting toxicity and allowing administration at minimum effective dose rather than maximum tolerated dose, as is standard for traditional cytotoxics. Pathways involving DNA damage repair, angiogenesis, signal transduction, cell proliferation, survival, and metabolism are under active investigation in gynecologic malignancies. Immune therapies involving vaccination and adoptive T cell infusion are also under evaluation to augment innate tumor-specific immunity. This chapter will review existing and emerging data surrounding new biologic agents for the treatment of gynecologic malignancies.

## Targeted Therapeutic Approaches

### Angiogenesis

Angiogenesis is the formation of new blood vessels from preexisting vessels. Angiogenesis is a normal process necessary for growth and development as well as for wound healing [2]. However, angiogenesis is also instrumental in tumorigenesis. In the early 1800s, Virchow identified increased blood vessels within tumors, and as early as the 1930s, Ide and associates documented the ability of cancers to induce blood vessel formation, noting a potent response after implanting a tumor in a rabbit's ear [3]. In 1971, Folkman proposed angiogenesis as not just a byproduct of tumor growth, but as a key step in tumor growth and development [4]. Indeed, formation of a new blood supply is essential for the development and maintenance of tumor cells [5, 6]. Because endothelial cells within tumor vessels are disorganized and express imbalanced surface molecules, a molecular basis exists for selective inhibition or even destruction of tumor vessels by angiogenesis inhibitors [7].

#### VEGF

Vascular endothelial growth factor (VEGF), also known as vascular permeability factor, was first identified in 1989. VEGF is a signal protein produced by normal cells to allow vasculogenesis and angiogenesis. However, VEGF and its receptors play an essential role in tumor angiogenesis as well [8, 9]. Inhibition of this pathway is a promising therapeutic strategy for preventing angiogenesis and tumor growth [10].

VEGF also functions to facilitate several biologic processes in endothelial cells such as cell proliferation, migration, differentiation, survival, and cell-to-cell communication [11, 12]. The activities of VEGF are mediated through the VEGF-specific tyrosine-kinase receptors [13]. Downstream signaling effects of the interaction between VEGF and its receptor result in increased endothelial cell proliferation and decreased apoptosis [14], which aids survival of immature tumor blood vessels [10, 15–17]. VEGF-mediated enhanced vascular and endothelial cell permeability helps facilitate tumor cell dissemination via circulation, and also allows greater delivery of oxygen and nutrients to the primary tumor [10, 15–17]. Many studies have shown that elevated levels of pro-angiogenic proteins such as VEGF and platelet-derived growth factor (PDGF) are often poor prognostic factors in patients with solid tumors such as cervical, endometrial, and ovarian cancer [18–22]. Conversely, Alvarez et al. showed that a low microvessel count was associated with better 5-year survival in patients with ovarian cancer in both early and advanced stage disease [23].

### Bevacizumab for Ovarian Cancer

Bevacizumab (Avastin™), a humanized monoclonal antibody targeted against VEGF-A, was the first anti-angiogenesis agent in wide clinical use. It has been approved by the U. S. Food and Drug Administration (FDA) for the treatment of metastatic colorectal, non-small cell lung, renal cell, and most recently in 2014, for cervical and ovarian cancers as well [24]. A great majority of the research done on bevacizumab in gynecologic cancers has focused on ovarian cancer. The Gynecologic Oncology Group (GOG) conducted a phase II trial evaluating patients with recurrent or persistent ovarian and primary peritoneal cancer to assess the efficacy and tolerability of bevacizumab as a single agent. Patients received a dose of 15 mg/kg every 3 weeks based on a 17- to 21-day half-life [25]. Thirteen patients (21.0 %) experienced clinical responses (two complete, 11 partial). Twenty-five patients (40.3 %) survived progression free for a minimum of 6 months. One patient developed proteinuria, a grade 4 toxicity, and required removal from the study. The study authors concluded that bevacizumab appeared active and was well tolerated in this patient population [26]. Because of its efficacy as a single agent, bevacizumab has also been examined extensively and in combination with standard cytotoxic chemotherapy. Four phase III randomized studies have evaluated its efficacy in patients with advanced epithelial ovarian (EOC), fallopian tube (FTC), and primary peritoneal cancer (PPC). See Tables 6.1 and 6.2.

GOG 218 was a randomized, double-blind phase III study which enrolled 1873 women with newly diagnosed advanced stage EOC [27]. All patients underwent primary debulking surgery followed by standard chemotherapy with six cycles of paclitaxel and carboplatin (CP). Patients were randomized to three groups: the control group received CP with a concurrent placebo followed by placebo maintenance; the bevacizumab-initiation group received CP concurrent with bevacizumab followed by placebo maintenance; and the bevacizumab-throughout group received CP with concurrent bevacizumab and maintenance bevacizumab. Median progression-free survival (PFS) in each group was 10.3, 11.2, and 14.1 months, respectively. The patients in the bevacizumab-throughout group were noted to have a statistical improvement in PFS of 4 months compared to controls, though no differences were noted in overall survival (OS). Side effects were tolerable. Rates of gastrointestinal perforation and fistula formation in the two bevacizumab groups were almost twice those in the control group (1.2 % vs 2.8 % vs 2.6 %) which is consistent with rates seen in metastatic non-gynecologic cancers (2.4 %). The rate of hypertension requiring medical therapy was higher in the groups receiving bevacizumab (16.5 % bevacizumab-initiation, 22.9 % bevacizumab-throughout) than in controls (7.2 %).

ICON 7, another phase III randomized trial, noted similar findings. Perren et al. [28] enrolled 1528 patients with high-risk early stage or advanced EOC, FTC, or PPC. Patients were randomized to either CP or CP with concurrent bevacizumab plus maintenance bevacizumab. PFS was significantly improved for patients receiving bevacizumab (17.4 vs 19.8 months). Controversy exists as to whether a 2-month improvement in PFS constitutes a clinical benefit, particularly since OS did not differ (44.6 vs 45.5 months, respectively).

The OCEANS trial evaluated 484 patients with platinum-sensitive recurrent EOC, FTC, and PPC [29]. This randomized, double-blind, placebo-controlled trial assigned patients to gemcitabine/carboplatin chemotherapy with or without bevacizumab. A statistically significant improvement in response rate (RR) was observed in the bevacizumab group 61.2 % vs the placebo group 48.3 % ($p<0.0001$). PFS was also significantly improved with bevacizumab use (8.6 vs 12.3 months, respectively). However, no difference in OS was observed.

The AURELIA trial was an open-label randomized phase III study which evaluated the effectiveness of chemotherapy (investigator selected liposomal doxorubicin vs paclitaxel vs topotecan) with and without bevacizumab in 361 patients with platinum-resistant EOC [30].

**Table 6.1** Frontline phase III trials for bevacizumab in ovarian cancer

| Trial | Regimen | Patient population | No of patients | PFS months | OS months | >Grade 2 GI events, *n* (%) | >Grade 2 HTN events, *n* (%) |
|---|---|---|---|---|---|---|---|
| GOG 218 [26] | I: CP+Placebo<br>II: CP+Bev<br>III: CP+Bev followed by maintenance Bev | Primary stage III/IV EOC randomized after CRS | 1873 | I: 10.3<br>II: 11.2<br>III: 14.1 | I: 39.3<br>II: 38.7<br>III: 39.7 | I: 7 (1.2)<br>II: 17 (2.8)<br>III: 16 (2.6) | I: 43 (7.2)<br>II: 100 (16.5)<br>III: 139 (22.9) |
| ICON 7 [27] | I: CP<br>II: CP+Bev followed by 12 cycles of maintenance Bev or disease progression | Primary high-risk early stage or advanced EOC/PPC/FTC | 1528 | I: 17.4<br>II: 19.8 | I: 44.6<br>II: 45.5 | I: 3 (<1)<br>II: 10 (1) | I: 2 (<1)<br>II: 46 (6) |

*Bev* bevacizumab, *CP* carboplatin and paclitaxel, *GI* gastrointestinal, *HTN* hypertension, *ICON 7* international collaborative ovarian neoplasm 7, *OS* overall survival, *PFS* progression-free survival, *EOC* epithelial ovarian cancer, *PPC* primary peritoneal cancer, *FTC* fallopian tube cancer, *CRS* cytoreductive surgery

**Table 6.2** Phase III trials for bevacizumab in the recurrent setting

| Trial | Regimen | Patient population | No of patients | PFS, months | Median OS, months | >Grade 2 GI events, *n* (%) | >Grade 2 HTN |
|---|---|---|---|---|---|---|---|
| OCEANS [28] | I: CG + Placebo<br>II: CG + Bev | Platinum-sensitive EOC, FTC, or PPC | 484 | I: 8.6<br>II: 12.3 | I: 35.2<br>II: 33.3 | I: 0 (0)<br>II: 0 (0) | I: 1 (0.4)<br>II: 44 (17.8) |
| Aurelia [29] | I: Standard chemo alone<br>II: Standard chemo + Bev<br>Standard chemo/investigators choice:<br>• Paclitaxel 80 mg/m$^2$ days 1, 8, 15, and 22 q4w<br>• Topotecan 4 mg/m$^2$ days 1, 8, and 15 q4w (or 1.25 mg/m$^2$, days 1–5 q3w)<br>• PLD 40 mg/m$^2$ day 1 q4w | Platinum-resistant ovarian cancer | 361 | I: 3.4<br>II: 6.7 | I: 13.3<br>II: 16.6 | I: 1 (0.6)<br>II: 3 (1.7) | I: 10 (5.5)<br>II: 36 (20.1) |

*OCEANS* ovarian cancer study comparing efficacy and safety of chemotherapy and anti-angiogenic therapy in platinum-sensitive recurrent disease, *Bev* bevacizumab, *CG* carboplatin and gemcitabine, *GI* gastrointestinal, *HTN* hypertension, *OS* overall survival, *PFS* progression-free survival, *EOC* epithelial ovarian cancer, *PPC* primary peritoneal cancer, *FTC* fallopian tube cancer, *CRS* cytoreductive surgery

Median PFS was statistically improved with the addition of bevacizumab compared to chemotherapy alone (6.7 vs 3.4 months). Improvements with bevacizumab were noted with every chemotherapy agent used. As with the other trials there was no difference in OS noted. Gastrointestinal perforation occurred in 2.2 % of patients receiving bevacizumab, and hypertension and proteinuria were also more common.

## Bevacizumab for Other Gynecologic Malignancies

Bevacizumab has been used extensively for the treatment of ovarian cancer, however several studies have also shown benefit in endometrial and cervical cancer. A phase II trial was conducted to determine the activity and tolerability of single-agent bevacizumab in recurrent or persistent endometrial cancer. Of 52 eligible patients, 7 (13.5 %) experienced clinical responses (one complete response and six partial responses). Median PFS was noted to be 4.2 months and OS was 10.5 months [31]. The authors concluded that bevacizumab is active and well-tolerated.

For patients with cervical cancer, GOG 240 examined the addition of bevacizumab to combination chemotherapy in patients with recurrent, persistent, or metastatic disease [32]. In this phase III study, 452 patients were randomized to chemotherapy (cisplatin + paclitaxel or paclitaxel + topotecan) with or without bevacizumab. With combination of the data from the two different chemotherapy arms, addition of bevacizumab was associated with a statistically significant increase in OS (13.3 vs 17.0 month, $p=0.004$) as well as higher RR (26 % vs 48 %, $p=0.008$). As expected, bevacizumab was also associated with increased hypertension, thromboembolism, and gastrointestinal fistula.

## Aflibercept

Aside from bevacizumab, other agents targeting VEGF have been investigated. Aflibercept, also known as VEGF-Trap™, is a manufactured decoy protein that binds with high affinity to VEGF-A and inhibits VEGF1 and 2 binding [33]. In contrast to bevacizumab, which only binds to VEGF-A and forms multimeric complexes, aflibercept monomerically binds, or "traps," the different isoforms of VEGF-A, VEGF-B, and PlGF [34, 35]. Aflibercept has a higher affinity for VEGF-A than bevacizumab. Preclinical trials for aflibercept showed promise and yielded an inhibition of tumor growth, angiogenesis, and a reduction of ascites formation [36]. Hu et al. conducted a preclinical study to assess the efficacy of aflibercept combined with paclitaxel in a mouse model of human ovarian cancer. The study demonstrated tumor burden was reduced by approximately 98 % versus controls [37].

A phase I/II trial assessed the utility of aflibercept with conventional docetaxel in 46 patients with recurrent EOC, FTC, and PPC [38]. No dose-limiting toxicities were noted. The overall RR was 54 % (11 with complete response and 14 with partial response). The most common adverse event specifically associated with aflibercept was grade 1–2 hypertension observed in five patients (11 %). Median PFS and OS were 6.4 and 26.6 months, respectively. Overall, findings showed the combination induced significant antitumor activity. Another phase II trial evaluating aflibercept in the treatment of recurrent or persistent endometrial cancer concluded it met pretrial activity parameters but was associated with significant toxicity. Median PFS and OS were 2.9 and 14.6 months respectively. The most frequent grade 3/4 toxicities was cardiovascular (23 %/5 %), with two treatment-related deaths secondary GI perforation and arterial rupture reported [39].

## Agents Targeting VEGF Receptors

Cediranib and pazopanib are receptor tyrosine kinase inhibitors (TKIs) that bind to and inhibit all three vascular endothelial growth factor receptors (VEGFR-1, -2, -3), thereby blocking VEGF signaling, angiogenesis, and tumor cell growth [40]. In a phase I trial, cediranib showed a 44 % overall RR in patients with recurrent EOC when combined with olaparib, a polyadenosine diphosphate-ribose polymerase (PARP) inhibitor [41]. In a phase II randomized trial for 90 patients with recurrent platinum-sensitive EOC, the combination of olaparib and cediranib showed an improved PFS when compared to olaparib and placebo (17.7 vs 9.0 months, respectively, $p=0.005$) [42]. Unfortunately, grade 3/4 side effects were common with combination therapy and included fatigue, diarrhea, and hypertension, prompting the authors to conclude that though the combination improved PFS and warranted further phase III study, future trials should include quality of life assessments.

A phase II trial evaluating the use of pazopanib in patients with recurrent ovarian cancer showed 11 of 36 patients (31 %) had CA125 improvements with median time to response of 29 days and median response duration of 113 days [43]. Overall RR was 18 % in patients with measurable disease at baseline. The most common adverse events leading to discontinuation of study drug were grade 3 ALT (8 %) and AST (8 %) elevation. Only one grade 4 toxicity (peripheral edema) was reported.

## PI3K/AKT/mTOR Pathway

The PI3K/AKT/mTOR pathway plays a critical role in the regulation of the cell cycle including cell proliferation, metabolism, and survival, as well as protein translation and angiogenesis [44]. PIK3CA amplification (the gene that encodes the p110α catalytic subunit of PI3K, is found in 40 % of EOCs [45], and mutation of PIK3CA is noted in 12 % of ovarian cancers [46] and up to 50 % of type 1 and 30 % of type II endometrial cancers [47, 48]. These changes can lead to increase in kinase activity, causing oncogenesis through activation of AKT, which in turn upregulates mammalian target of rapamycin (mTOR) activity [49]. Ultimately, these pathway changes result in increased cell survival, growth, and chemotherapy resistance [50, 51]. In regards to cervical cancer, high-risk HPV-related E6 has been shown to be associated with downstream mTOR signaling.

When the kinase activity of mTOR is activated, it results in the synthesis of cell cycle proteins such as hypoxia inducible factor-1a (HIF-1a) and cyclin D. HIF-1a then stimulates VEGF leading to increased tumor survival and angiogenesis in oxygen poor environments [52]. The inhibition of the mTOR pathway stops the transmission of proliferative signals resulting in cell cycle arrest and tumor growth inhibition [53]. The prototypic mTOR inhibitor is rapamycin. However, rapamycin has a poor pharmacologic profile including poor water solubility, thus other mTOR inhibitors have been developed for clinical use including everolimus and temsirolimus [54]. Aberrant activity of the mTOR complex appears to be present in many tumor types, including gynecologic cancers [55]. PTEN, phosphatase and tensin homolog, is a tumor suppressor gene that plays a significant role in the pathogenesis of endometrial cancer. PTEN acts as a regulator of the PI3K/AKT pathway and loss of PTEN expression leads to increased PI3K/AKT/mTOR activation [56].

### Temsirolimus

Temsirolimus is a water-soluble ester of rapamycin and has shown variable success in gynecologic cancers. A phase II study evaluated the activity of temsirolimus in patients with recurrent or metastatic endometrial cancer [57]. In the chemotherapy naive cohort, four patients (14 %) had a partial response and 20 (69 %) had stable disease with median duration of 5.1 and 9.7 months, respectively. In the chemotherapy-treated group, one patient (4 %) had a partial response and 12 (48 %) had stable disease with median duration of 4.3 and 3.7 months, respectively. The authors concluded mTOR inhibition with temsirolimus has encouraging single-agent activity in endometrial cancer. Response was higher in chemotherapy-naive patients than in chemotherapy-treated patients and was noted to be independent of PTEN status. Despite its promise, caution is necessary. The GOG-248 trial evaluated temsirolimus alone or in combination with megestrol acetate and tamoxifen in patients with advanced, persistent, or recurrent endometrial cancer [58]. The combination arm was closed early due to high incidence of venous thrombosis in 31 % (7/22) of patients. Also noted was one sudden death and one myocardial infarction. Partial response was noted in 21 % (3/21) of patients. The authors concluded the combination of temsirolimus with megestrol acetate/tamoxifen results in an unacceptable rate of venous thrombosis and its activity is not sufficient to offset its risk of thrombotic events.

Alvarez et al. reported the result of a phase II GOG clinical trial evaluating the combination of temsirolimus and bevacizumab in 53 patients with recurrent or persistent endometrial carcinoma [59]. Twelve patients (41 %) had clinical responses (one complete and 11 partial responses) and 23 (46.9 %) survived progression-free for at least six months. Median PFS and OS were 5.6 and 16.9 months, respectively. Reported toxicities among the 49 eligible patients included two gastrointestinal-vaginal fistulas, two intestinal perforations, and one grade 4 thromboembolic event. Three deaths were also possibly treatment-related. The PFS and OS were found to be 5.6 and 16.9 months, respectively. The combination was deemed active, but not without significant toxicity.

In ovarian cancer, temsirolimus was evaluated by Behbakht et al. in a GOG phase II trial of patients with persistent or recurrent EOC and PPC [60]. Fifty-four patients were eligible for evaluation: 9.3 % experienced a partial response and 24.1 % had PFS ≥ 6 months. The authors concluded temsirolimus appeared to have only modest activity in persistent/recurrent EOC/PPC, and the PFS was deemed too low to warrant inclusion in future phase III studies in unselected patients.

In cervical cancer, two studies have been reported using temsirolums. A phase I study of weekly temsirolimus and topotecan was conducted in patients with advanced and/or recurrent gynecologic malignancies [61]. Two patients with squamous cell cancer of the cervix were included, and one of these experienced stable disease with median time to progression of 3 months. Unfortunately, the combination regimen was not tolerated in patients with prior radiation to the pelvis due to dose-limiting myelotoxicity. On a more promising note, Tinker et al. reported results of a phase II study of temsirolimus in patients with metastatic or recurrent, unresectable locally advanced cervical cancer [62]. One patient (3.0 %) had a partial response lasting 7.2 months, and nine patients (57.6 %) had stable disease with a median duration of 6.5 months (range 2.4–12.0 months). The median progression-free survival was 3.52 months. The single agent was better tolerated, with no toxicities > grade 3 observed.

### Everolimus

Everolimus is an orally bioavailable inhibitor of the mTOR pathway. In a phase II study by Slomovitz, everolimus was administered prior to chemotherapy in patients with recurrent endometrial cancer [63]. Twelve of 28 patients (43 %) remained stable at 8 weeks and six of 28 patients (21 %) had clinical responses at 20 weeks of therapy. This study has ignited further investigation of this drug in combination with other agents [64, 65]. A randomized phase II trial of everolimus and letrozole or tamoxifen/medroxyprogesterone acetate is under development by the GOG for patients with advanced, persistent, or recurrent endometrial carcinoma.

A phase II randomized double-blinded trial of everolimus plus bevacizumab versus placebo plus bevazicumab in patients with recurrent or persistent EOC, PTC, or PPC has been conducted by the GOG. The trial was closed in 2014 and results are expected to be forthcoming.

## EGFR—Epidermal Growth Factor Receptor Pathway

The epidermal growth factor receptor (EGFR) pathway consists of four tyrosine kinase cell surface receptors: EGFR, HER2/neu, Her3, and Her4. EGFR initiates signal transduction pathways including the ras/raf/MEK and PI3K paths that affect cellular proliferation, motility and invasion, apoptosis, and angiogenesis. EGFR is overexpressed in 60–80 % of endometrial cancers, 73 % of cervical carcinomas, 30–90 % of EOCs, and 68 % of vulvar malignancies and is associated with advanced stage and poor prognosis [66–74]. The FDA has approved two tyrosine kinase inhibitors, gefitinib and erlotinib, and two monoclonal antibodies (mAbs), panitumumab and cetuximab, targeting EGFR (see Tables 6.3, 6.4 and 6.5).

**Table 6.3** Trials of targeted therapies for patients with recurrent or metastatic endometrial cancer

| Drug | Target | Clinical phase | No of patients | Response | PFS | Reference |
|---|---|---|---|---|---|---|
| Everolimus | mTOR | II | 28 | PR: 0 %<br>SD: 43 % | 6 months PFS: NR<br>Median PFS: NR | [63] |
| Temsirolimus | mTOR | II | 29 | PR: 14 %<br>SD: 69 % | 6 months PFS: NR<br>Median PFS: 7.3 | [57] |
| Temsirolimus | mTOR | II | 25 | PR: 4 %<br>SD: 48 % | 6 months PFS: NR<br>Median PFS: 3.3 | [57] |
| Deferolimus | mTOR | II | 27 | PR: 7 %<br>SD: 26 % | 6 months PFS: NR<br>Median PFS: NR | [75] |
| Ridaforolimus | mTOR | II | 33 | PR: 8 %<br>SD: 58 % | 6 months PFS: NR<br>Median PFS: NR | [76] |
| Ridaforolimuns | mTOR | II | 114 | PR: 0 %<br>SD: 35 % | 6 months PFS: NR<br>Median PFS:<br>– Ridaforolimus: 3.6 months<br>– Progestins 1.9 months | [77] |
| Trastuzumab | HER2 | II | 23 | PR: 0 %<br>SD: 9 % | 6 months PFS: NR<br>Median PFS: 1.8 months | [78] |
| Erlotinib | EGFR | II | 32 | PR: 13 %<br>SD: 47 % | 6 months PFS: 9.3<br>Median PFS: NR | [79] |
| Gefitinib | EGFR | II | 16 | PR: 4 %<br>SD: 27 % | 6 months PFS: NR<br>Median PFS: NR | [80] |
| Bevacizumab | VEGF | II | 52 | PR: 14 %<br>SD: 50 % | 6 months PFS: 40 %<br>Median PFS: 4.2 months | [31] |
| Thalidomide | VEGF | II | 24 | PR: 13 %<br>SD: 8 % | 6 months PFS: 8 %<br>Median PFS: 1.7 | [81] |
| Sunitinib | VEGFR | II | 16 | PR: 13 %<br>SD: 13 % | 6 months PFS: 19 %<br>Median PFS: NR | [82] |
| Sunitinib | VEGFR | II | 20 | PR: 15 %<br>SD: 25 % | 6 months PFS: 20 %<br>Median PFS: NR | [83] |
| Sorafenib | VEGFR | II | 39 | PR: 5 %<br>SD: 49 % | 6 months PFS: 13 %<br>Median PFS: 3.4 months | [84] |

*NR* not reported, *PFS* progression-free survival, *PR* partial response, *SD* stable disease, *VEGF* vascular endothelial growth factor

## Erlotinib

Erlotinib is a reversible small-molecule TKI of EGFR. Erlotinib has been evaluated in several phase II clinical trials in EOC but only showed marginal activity [87, 105]. A phase II trial evaluated carboplatin in combination with erlotinib for patients with recurrent EOC [90]. Among 54 patients, there were 14 partial responses (57 %) in the platinum-sensitive arm, and only one partial response (7 %) in the platinum-resistant arm. Erlotinib was also evaluated as a single agent in patients with recurrent or metastatic endometrial cancer with only a 12.5 % partial RR noted. Forty-seven percent had stable disease for a median duration of 3.7 months [79].

## Cetuximab

Cetuximab is a monoclonal antibody which binds to EGFR, and has been FDA-approved for metastatic colorectal and head and neck cancer [106, 107]. A phase II trial evaluated the expression of EGFR and the use of cetuximab in combination with carboplatin in platinum-sensitive ovarian cancer patients [86]. Twenty-six of the 28 evaluable patients had EGFR-positive tumors: nine showed an objective response (three complete response, six partial response) and eight had stable disease. Another phase II trial of cetuximab in combination with carboplatin and paclitaxel in patients with advanced EOC or PPC achieved a 38 % PFS at 18 months, though it was not considered

**Table 6.4** Clinical trials targeting EGFR in patients with ovarian cancer

| Drug | Clinical phase | No. of patients | Treatment | Population | Response, $n$ (%) | Conclusions |
|---|---|---|---|---|---|---|
| Cetuximab [85] | II | 25 | Monotherapy<br>Initial dose 400 mg/m$^2$, then 250 mg/m$^2$ weekly for two 3-week cycles | Recurrent | PR: 1 (4)<br>SD: 9 (36)<br>PFS: 2.1 m<br>SR: 54.8 % | Single-agent cetuximab showed minimal activity in patients with recurrent ovarian cancer. Patients with elevated levels of 12 serologic markers at baseline were more likely to have earlier disease progression |
| Cetuximab [86] | II | 28 | Combination<br>Cetuximab 400 mg/m$^2$ initially, followed by weekly infusion of 250 mg/m$^2$, and Carboplatin (AUC 6) every 3 weeks | Recurrent<br>Platinum-sensitive | CR: 3 (10.7)<br>PR: 6 (21.4)<br>SD: 8 (28.6)<br>PFS: 9.4 m | Modest activity in screened patients with EGFR-positive, relapsed platinum-sensitive ovarian or primary peritoneal carcinoma. Cetuximab was associated with an acneiform rash in a majority of patients |
| Erlotinib [87] | II | 34 | Monotherapy<br>150 mg/day for up to 48 weeks, or until disease progression, or dose-limiting toxicity | Recurrent<br>EGFR Positive | PR: 2 (6)<br>SD: 15 (44)<br>PFS: 8 m<br>SR: 35.3 | Patients with rash survived longer than those without ($p=0.009$), correlating with rash grade. The most frequent AEs were rash (68 %) and diarrhea (38 %) |
| Erlotinib [88] | II | I: 28<br>II: 23<br>III: 5 | Combination<br>Paclitaxel (175 mg/m$^2$) and Carboplatin (AUC 6) every 3 weeks for up to six cycles, and Erlotinib 150 mg/day | Primary<br>I: After optimal CRS<br>II: After suboptimal CRS<br>III: Before CRS | CR (I): 8 (29)<br>CR (II): 3 (13) | Erlotinib plus carboplatin-paclitaxel did not improve pCR rates compared with historical experience with carboplatin-paclitaxel alone |
| Erlotinib [89] | Ib | 23 | Combination<br>Docetaxel (75 mg/m$^2$) and Carboplatin (AUC 5) every 3 weeks for up to six cycles, and Erlotinib 75 mg/day | Primary | CR: 5 (21.7)<br>PR: 7 (30.4) | Docetaxel/carboplatin had no measurable effect on erlotinib pharmacokinetics. Common AE were neutropenia, diarrhea, nausea, and rash |
| Erlotinib [90] | II | I: 30<br>II: 14 | Combination<br>Carboplatin (AUC 5) every 3 weeks, and Erlotinib 150 mg/day | Recurrent<br>I: Platinum-sensitive<br>II: Platinum-resistant | CR (I): 3 (10)<br>PR (I): 14 (47)<br>PR (II): 1 (7) | The combination of erlotinib and carboplatin was active in patients with platinum-sensitive disease, but not in platinum-resistant disease |
| Gefitinib [91] | II | 27 | Monotherapy<br>Gefitinib 500 mg/day | Recurrent | PR: 1 (3.7)<br>PFS > 6 m: 14.8 | Gefitinib was well tolerated but had minimal activity in unscreened patients with recurrent ovarian or primary peritoneal carcinoma. First to document activating mutations in catalytic domain of EGFR in 3.5 % (two of 57) of ovarian cancers |

| | | | | | | |
|---|---|---|---|---|---|---|
| Gefitinib [92] | II | 24 | Monotherapy<br>Gefitinib 500 mg/day | Recurrent | OR: 0 (0) | Demonstrated that gefitinib inhibited the phosphorylation of EGFR in >50 % EOC patients |
| Gefitinib [93] | II | 56 | Combination<br>Tamoxifen 40 mg/day and Gefitinib 500 mg/day until progression or unacceptable toxicity | Recurrent | OR: 0 (0)<br>SD: 16 (28.6)<br>PFS: 58 days<br>OS: 253 days | Gefitinib plus tamoxifen did not appear to be efficacious in the treatment of patients with refractory/resistant ovarian cancer The most frequent drug-related AEs were diarrhea and acne-like skin rash |
| Gefitinib [94] | II | I: 26<br>II: 42 | Combination<br>Paclitaxel (175 mg/m2) and Carboplatin (AUC 5) every 3 weeks for 6–8 cycles, and Gefitinib 500 mg/day | Recurrent<br>I: Platinum-sensitive<br>II: Platinum-resistant | I: OR: 16 (61.9)<br>PFS: 9.2 m<br>OS: 25.7 m<br>II: OR: 8 (19.2)<br>PFS: 6.1 m<br>OS: 16.9 m | Gefitinib, in combination with CP, provides a good clinical response but with an increase in hematologic disorders. Grade 3/4 toxicities neutropenia (59 %), diarrhea (25 %), leukopenia (22 %), anemia (13 %), and acne (13 %). Two secondary myelodysplastic syndromes (MDS) and one secondary acute leukemia occurred during treatment |

*CR* complete response, *PR* partial response, *SD* stable disease, *OR* (objective response CR + PR), *PFS* progression-free survival, *SR* 1 year survival rate, *OS* overall survival, *AUC* area under the curve, *CRS* cytoreductive surgery, *no.* number, *pCR* pathologic complete response, *AE* adverse events, *CP* carboplatin and paclitaxel

**Table 6.5** Clinical trials of targeted agents in cervical cancer

| Targeted agent | Target | Regimen | Phase | No of patients | Response | Toxicity | Reference |
|---|---|---|---|---|---|---|---|
| Bevacizumab | VEGF | Bevacizumab (15 mg/kg iv every 21 days) with or without four chemotherapy regimens | III | 450 | OS 17 months in bevacizumab arms versus 13 months in the chemotherapy arms | Treatment with B was associated with more grade 3–4 bleeding (5 % vs 1 %) thrombosis/embolism (9 % vs 2 %), and GI fistula (3 % vs 0 %) | [95] |
| Bevacizumab | VEGF | Bevacizumab (10 mg/kg iv every 2 weeks for three cycles) in combination with definitive radiotherapy and cisplatin chemotherapy | II | 60 | No data | 15 (31 %) protocol-specified treatment-related AEs within 90 days of treatment start; the most common were hematologic (12/15; 80 %). No treatment-related SAEs | [96] |
| Bevacizumab | VEGF | Bevacizumab (15 mg/kg iv every 21 days) with topotecan and cisplatin | II | 27 | ORR: 33.3 % | Grade 3–4 hematologic toxicity was common (thrombocytopenia 82 % leukopenia 74 %, anemia 63 %, neutropenia 56 %). Most patients (78 %) required unanticipated hospital admissions for supportive care and/or management of toxicities | [97] |
| Sunitinib | VEGF | Sunitinib 50 mg daily | II | 19 | No objective responses. Median TTP: 3.5 months | High rate of fistula development (26 %) | [98] |
| Gefitinib | EGFR | Gefitinib 500 mg daily | II | 30 | No objective responses, six (20 %) patients experienced stable disease with a median duration of 111.5 days. Median TTP was 37 days and median OS was 107 days | Most common drug-related AEs were diarrhea, acne, vomiting, and nausea No grade 4 events | [99] |
| Erlotinib | EGFR | Erlotinib 150 mg daily | II | 28 | No objective responses with four (16 %) achieving stable disease; only one patient had a PFS ≥ 6 months (4 %) | Grade 3-related toxicities included diarrhea, nausea, emesis, dehydration, and anorexia. One patient experienced grade 4 renal toxicity | [100] |
| Cetuximab | EGFR | Cetuximab 400 mg/m$^2$ i.v. initial dose followed by 250 mg/m2 weekly | II | 38 | No objective responses with five patients (14.3 %) survived without progression for at least 6 months. Median PFS and OS times were 1.97 and 6.7 months, respectively | Grade 3 adverse events at least possibly related to cetuximab included dermatologic events, GI, anemia, constitutional symptoms, infection, vascular events, pain, and pulmonary, neurologic, vomiting and metabolic events. No grade 4 events | [101] |

| | | | | | | | |
|---|---|---|---|---|---|---|---|
| Temsirolimus | mTOR | Temsirolimus (25 mg i.v. weekly in 4-week cycles) | II | 38 | One patient experienced a partial response (3.0 %). 57.6 % stable disease. Median PFS: 3.52 months | No toxicity grade 3/4 observed. Adverse effects were mild-moderate in most cases and similar to other temsirolimus studies | [102] |
| Hydralazine | HDAC | Hydralazine and valproate (HV) added to cisplatin topotecan (hydralazine at 182 mg for rapid, or 83 mg for slow acetylators, and valproate at 30 mg/kg, continued until disease progression) | III | 36 | Four PRs to CT+HV and one in CT+PLA. 29 and 32 % stable disease, respectively. Median PFS: 6 months for CT+PLA, 10 months for CT+HV | Low incidence of grades 3 and 4 toxicity in both arms. G2/3 thrombocytopenia, edema, drowsiness and tremor were statistically higher in CT+HVarm | [103] |
| rAd-p53 | Proteasome | rAd-p53 combined with chemotherapy (PCG arm) vs chemotherapy alone (CG arm) | II | 40 | ORR 95 % in PCG arm versus 75 % for the CG arm. 1-year OS: 90 and 65 %, respectively | Fever was found in 90 % of PCG patients (mild to medium grade). No serious adverse events relative to rAd-p53 were observed | [104] |

*ORR* overall response rate, *OS* overall survival, *TTP* time to progression, *PFS* progression free survival; *iv* intravenously, *R* randomized, *GI* gastrointestinal a meaningful prolongation of PFS over the expected activity of chemotherapy alone [108]. A phase II trial assessed the combination of cisplatin, topotecan, and cetuximab in patients with advanced cervical cancer [109]. Six (32 %) patients achieved a partial response. Most of the patients receiving this therapy experienced grade 3 or 4 myelosuppression, and unfortunately, three patients died from treatment-related toxicity resulting in early termination of the trial.

## PARP Inhibitors

PARP is a nuclear enzyme that catalyzes the polyADP ribosylation of proteins involved in DNA single-strand break repairs [110]. Inhibition of PARP was shown to be highly selective for cancers that have homologous recombination (HR) deficiencies, such as those containing mutations in one or two genes [111]. PARP inhibitors cause accumulation of single-strand breaks (SSBs) in DNA which in turn lead to double-strand breaks as the replication fork progresses. In the absence of intact double-stranded DNA repair mechanisms (i.e., mutations in BRCA1 and 2), PARP inhibition eventually results in cell death [112]. A great deal of focus has been placed on the use of PARP inhibitors in patients with BRCA mutation-associated ovarian and breast cancers. However, PARP inhibitors may also demonstrate synthetic lethality in cancers deficient in other proteins that mitigate DNA repair [113–117].

Olaparib has been extensively studied in patients with ovarian cancer. Fong et al. evaluated 60 patients with refractory solid tumors in a phase I trial using olapraib [118]. The study noted that only BRCA mutation carriers had a significant objective tumor response. Twelve of the 19 (63 %) derived clinical benefit from treatment, defined as radiologic or tumor-marker responses or meaningful disease stabilization. Out of 19 patients, nine had a partial response (47 %); eight of those patients suffered from ovarian cancer. In a phase II trial evaluating two cohorts of women with confirmed BRCA1 or 2 mutations and recurrent EOC, women were randomized to either olaparib at 400 or 100 mg twice daily [119]. The RR was 33 and 14 %, respectively. The most common toxicities included nausea, anemia, and fatigue. Ledermann et al. [120] presented data on a randomized phase II trial of olaparib maintenance therapy in patients with platinum-sensitive relapsed serous ovarian cancer. Among patients with a BRCA mutation, median PFS was significantly longer in the olaparib group than in the placebo group (11.2 vs 4.3 months, $p<0.0001$). However, OS (58 %) did not differ between the groups. The most common grade 3 or 4 toxicities in the olaparib group were fatigue and anemia.

As stated above, PARP inhibitors are also being investigated in non-germline mutation ovarian cancers. Gelmon et al. conducted a phase II trial of olaparib in high-grade serous/undifferentiated ovarian cancer or triple-negative breast cancer patients irregardless of BRCA mutation status [121]. The RR in BRCA mutants was 41 % with median PFS of 221 days. BRCA mutation-negative patients had an RR of 24 % and PFS of 192 days. This trial highlighted the clinical utility of PARP inhibitors in BRCA wild-type patients. Several other studies investigating PARP inhibitors in conjunction with conventional chemotherapy agents in recurrent or refractory cervical cancer patients are also enrolling [122].

On December 19, 2014, the FDA granted accelerated approval to olaparib (Lynparza™) with a genetic test called BRACAnalysis CDx, a companion diagnostic tool that will detect the presence of germline BRCA mutations. The FDA's decision was based primarily on early clinical trial results where 137 women with germline BRCA mutation associated ovarian cancer treated with olaparib demonstrated an objective RR of 34 % for an average of 7.9 months [123].

## Multi-pathway Targeted Agents

Sorafenib functions as a small-molecule inhibitor that blocks angiogenesis-related receptors including KIT, VEGF, PDGFR as well as Raf [124], which has been studied in ovarian cancer patients with mixed success. A phase II GOG trial assessed its activity and tolerability in patients with recurrent EOC and PPC [125]. Of the 71 eligible patients, 59 patients (83 %) had measurable disease, and 12 (17 %) had detectable disease. There were 32 incidences of grade 3 or 4 toxicities. Fourteen patients (24 %) survived progression-free for at least 6 months. Two patients (3.4 %) had partial responses, 20 had stable disease. The authors concluded sorafenib has modest antitumor activity in patients with recurrent EOC, but at the expense of substantial toxicity.

A phase I study evaluating the use of bevacizumab with sorafenib in patients with advanced solid tumors [126] noted a 43 % partial RR seen among the 13 ovarian cancer patients. Toxicities were common and led to dose reductions in 74 % of patients. Two patients with EOC developed fistulae in areas of rapid tumor regression.

Herzog et al. published findings of a randomized phase II trial assessing maintenance therapy with sorafenib in frontline EOC and PPC patients [127]. Patients were randomized to either sorafenib 400 mg BID or placebo. Greater than 90 % of the 246 patients had ovarian cancer. The most common toxicity was hand–foot skin reaction (39 % vs 0.8 %, respectively). Unfortunately, there was no difference in regards to PFS. The authors concluded that sorafenib could not be recommended as maintenance therapy.

A recent phase II randomized trial, evaluating sorafenib alone or in combination with carboplatin/paclitaxel in women with recurrent platinum-sensitive EOC, FTC, or PPC, showed that sorafenib, both alone and in combination with carboplatin/paclitaxel, has activity [128]. RR was 15 % for patients on sorafenib vs. 61 % for patients on sorafenib plus chemotherapy; stable disease was seen in 35 and 62 %, respectively. Median PFS was 5.6 months for sorafenib vs. 16.8 months for sorafenib plus chemo, but there was no significant difference in OS ($p=0.974$).

## Immunotherapy

Manipulation of the immune system to restore or generate de novo responses to treat malignancy is the primary goal of anticancer immunotherapy. Antitumor immune responses of tumor-reactive T cells and antibodies can be detected in peripheral blood, tumors, and lymphatic channels of patients with advanced EOC [129, 130], indicating the tumor's innate immunogenicity. Unfortunately, tumor-associated immune suppressive mechanisms are many, and include the presence of regulatory T cells (Tregs), and inhibitory signaling from molecules such as CTLA-4.

Most published preclinical trials have demonstrated the requirement of T lymphocytes for the eradication of solid tumors [131]. Cytotoxic T lymphocytes (CTLs) or CD8+ T cells represent the primary effector cells involved in immune-mediated destruction of cancer cells. CTLs recognize, engage, and destroy target cells through the interaction of the antigen-specific receptor (TCR) on the CTL and peptides that are presented by the target cell to the CTL [132, 133]. These antigens are presented in the context of histocompatibility antigens also referred to as human leukocyte antigens (HLA). All somatic cells in the human body express HLA molecules on their surfaces. HLA molecules present on the cell surface serve as an expression of internal proteins cells that have been enzymatically digested into small peptides. These molecules essentially give the immune system an external view of the internal contents of the cell. This information enables CTLs to recognize aberrant changes in the cellular proteins (tumor-associated antigens, TAAs) that are indicative of malignant transformation. The recognition of cancer cells as dangerous results in their targeted destruction by the CTL. The identification of specific peptides that mark the tumor cells as "abnormal" allows for immune targeting of cancer cells. Currently, several TAAs associated with gynecologic cancer have been described and include E6/7, HER2/neu, p53, CA125, STn, FR-α, mesothelin, NY-ESO-1, VEGF, and cdr-2 [134–137] (see Table 6.6).

The most progress in immunotherapy for gynecologic cancers has been made in EOC. Correlation between the presence of CTLs or CD8+ tumor infiltrating lymphocytes (TILs) and prolonged PFS and OS has been shown in patients with advanced-stage EOC [152]. The presence of CD8+ TILs correlates with increased

**Table 6.6** Tumor-associated antigens in gynecologic cancer

| Antigen category | Tumor-associated antigen | Cancer type |
|---|---|---|
| Cancer/testis | NY-ESO-1 [138] | Ovarian |
| Posttranslation modification | MUC1 [139] | Ovarian |
| Posttranslation modification | Cathepsin D [140] | Ovarian |
| Differentiation | EpCAM [141] | Ovarian |
| Differentiation | Mesothelin [142] | Ovarian |
| Amplified | HER2/neu [143] | Breast |
| Amplified | HSP 90 [144] | Ovarian |
| Amplified | HoxB7 [145] | Ovarian |
| Amplified | Folate receptor-α [146] | Ovarian |
| Amplified | Sialyl Tn [147] | |
| Amplified | WT-1 [148] | Ovarian and endometrial |
| Mutational | p53 [149] | Squamous cell |
| Viral | HPV E6 [150] | Cervical |
| Viral | HPV E7 [151] | Cervical |

survival and is a superior marker for prognosis [153]. Zhang et al. documented 5-year OS of 38.0% among patients whose tumors contained TILs and 4.5% among patients whose tumors contained no TILs [152].

Tregs, formerly called suppressor T cells, are a subpopulation of T cells that help to modulate the immune system, prevent the development of autoimmune disorders, inhibit nonspecific T-cell activation, and suppress endogenous tumor-associated antigen (TAA)-specific T-cell immunity [154]. The presence of Tregs, classified as CD4+/CD25+/FoxP3+ T cells, correlates with decreased survival in EOC [155]. Barnett et al. assessed the extent of Treg infiltration in a series of 232 primary serous ovarian cancer specimens. In this series, the extent of infiltration was associated with higher grade and advanced stage [154].

Several broad categories of immune-based strategies have been utilized in patients with gynecologic malignancies: therapeutic vaccination with peptides or pulsed dendritic cells (DCs), adoptive T-cell transfer, monoclonal antibody therapy, and immune checkpoint modulation.

## Peptide Vaccines

The initial identification of specific peptides that mark the tumor cells as "abnormal" and the subsequent re-introduction of these peptides is the basic methodology behind cancer-targeted peptide vaccines. Investigations with various peptide targets are reviewed.

### Her2Neu

Ovarian surface epithelium is weakly positive for HER2 and positive HER2 immunostaining may be found in benign/borderline ovarian tumors as well as in their malignant counterparts [156]. McCaughan et al. described HER2 amplification and expression in all major epithelial ovarian cancer subtypes. HER2 gene amplification was noted in mucinous carcinomas (25%), mixed-type carcinomas (11.9%), clear cell carcinomas (4%), serous papillary carcinomas (3%), and endometrioid carcinomas (2.1%) [157]. In EOC, HER2 expression has been found to be an independent risk factor for decreased survival [158]. Additionally, patients with negative HER2 have been noted to have better chemotherapy responses, and improved survival [159].

A phase I study by Disis et al. evaluated the feasibility of a HER-2/neu vaccine for the treatment of advanced-stage HER2/neu expressing cancers. T-cell expansion was seen in 7/8 (88%) of patients. Most adverse events were grade 1–2. Partial clinical responses were observed in 43%. The study concluded HER2 vaccination was both feasible and well tolerated [160–162]. Further investigation of the HER2 vaccine in gynecologic cancers is needed to establish a clear survival benefit.

### NY-ESO-1

NY-ESO-1 is a cancer-testis antigen which is strongly immunogenic and highly expressed in ovarian cancer. Odunsi et al. evaluated the efficacy of vaccination with NY-ESO in EOC patients, and noted median PFS of 21 months and median OS of 48 months. CD8(+) T cells derived from vaccinated patients were shown to specifically lyse NY-ESO-1-expressing tumor targets [163]. A phase I trial performed by the same group evaluated the potentiation of NY-ESO vaccine based on the theory that DNA methyltransferase inhibitors may augment vaccine efficacy [164]. In this trial, 12 patients with relapsed EOC were evaluated using a dose-escalation of decitabine, as an addition to NY-ESO-1 vaccine and liposomal doxorubicin chemotherapy. The regimen was safe, with limited and clinically manageable toxicities. Disease stabilization or partial clinical response occurred in 6/10 evaluable patients.

### P53

P53 is a tumor suppressor protein encoded on chromosome 17. It also functions as a self-antigen expressed in low levels on normal cells. Induction of p53-specific CTLs with the ability to eliminate p53-presenting tumors without inducing immunopathologic damage to normal tissue has been observed in several studies [165, 166]. In a phase II trial, p53-SLP vaccine was given to patients with ovarian cancer. Cyclophosphamide was also administered in order to decrease Tregs with the goal of improving vaccine immunogenicity [167]. Combination therapy with cyclophosphamide and the p53-SLP vaccine induced higher p53-specific responses compared with p53-SLP monotherapy and produced a clinical response in 20 % (2/10) of patients.

The GOG conducted a phase II trial evaluating p53 peptide vaccine via subcutaneous (SQ) injection or intravenous (IV) pulsed DCs in patients with ovarian cancer at high risk of recurrence [137]. The study involved 22 patients with tumors overexpressing the p53 protein. Nine of 13 patients (69 %) who received SQ injections and five of six patients (83 %) who received IV peptide-pulsed dendritic cells developed an immunologic response. The median OS was 40.8 and 29.6 months, respectively; the median PFS was 4.2 and 8.7 months, respectively. The study concluded either vaccination approach could generate comparable specific immune responses against the p53 peptide with minimal toxicity.

### Adoptive T-Cell Therapy

Adoptive T-cell therapy for cancer consists of removing immune cells from the patient, manipulating them ex vivo to enhance their activity, and then re-infusing them with the goal of improving the immune system's antitumor response [168]. The primary benefit of using CD8+ T cells for adoptive therapy is their ability to specifically target tumor cells through the recognition of differentially expressed tumor proteins presented on the cell surface. A phase I trial by Kershaw et al. evaluated autologous T cells modified to express a chimeric receptor specific for the tumor-associated antigen folate receptor (FR) in patients with metastatic ovarian cancer [169]. FR-specific T cells could consistently be produced from all 14 patients in the study however, there was no evidence of antitumor responses in any patient as determined by computed tomography scan or serum CA125. Poor trafficking of T cells to tumor, as shown by the observed lack of tumor localization of radiolabeled cells, was described as partially responsible for the absence of patient responses.

Natural killer (NK) cells have also been investigated as adoptive therapy. NK cells are part of the normal innate immune response that may function to perform tumor surveillance [170]. A phase II trial conducted by Geller et al. [170] treated 14 women with ovarian cancer with ex vivo activated haplo-identical related NK cells. These cells were transferred after administration of lymphodepleting chemotherapy. Significant toxicities were noted, and at a median of 36 days following transfer, four patients were noted to have a partial response while 12 had stable disease.

### Dendritic Cell Vaccination

DCs function as professional antigen-presenting cells, processing and presenting antigenic material on their surface to T cells [171]. DCs can enhance tumor antigen-specific CTL responses by presenting tumor antigens to CD4 and CD8 T lymphocytes present in lymph nodes adjacent to primary tumors. Activated T cells then eliminate tumor cells and activate B cells to generate tumor antigen-specific antibodies.

Several clinical trials have shown benefit including a randomized phase I/II trial of autologous DCs pulsed with Her-2/neu, hTERT, and PADRE peptides administered with or without cyclophosphamide for 11 patients with advanced ovarian cancer in remission [172]. Of nine patients receiving the full course of vaccinations, three recurred at 6, 17, and 6 months, and six remained disease-free at 36 months of follow up. No grade 3/4 vaccine-related toxicities were noted. The 3-year OS was 90 % with patients receiving cyclophosphamide demonstrating a non-significant survival advantage. Brossart et al. [173] tested HER-2/neu or MUC1-peptide pulsed autologous DC vaccinations in 10 patients with advanced breast or ovarian cancers. Peptide-specific CTL responses were generated in 50 % of the patients, but unfortunately, these were not correlated with clinical responses.

### Monoclonal Antibodies

CA125 is a surface glycoprotein tumor antigen and is elevated in 79 % of all patients with ovarian cancer. CA125–oregovomab complexes can prime dendritic cells, leading to downstream activation of T cells [174]. Oregovomab is a monoclonal antibody that binds to CA125 with high affinity and can produce both cellular and humoral immune responses in ovarian cancer patients [175]. It was initially developed as a technetium 99c-labeled antibody for the immunoscintigraphic detection of recurrent ovarian cancer by virtue of tumor expression of CA125 [176]. However, some patients receiving this imaging agent experienced an unexpected survival advantage, prompting investigations into the antibody's therapeutic potential [177]. Immunologic effects of oregovomab were initially tested in EOC patients in 1998 [178].

In 2004, Gordon et al. evaluated the immune response and clinical outcomes in patients with recurrent EOC when treated with oregovomab and chemotherapy [179]. Oregovomab produced no serious adverse effects and was well tolerated. Significant increases in T-cell responses were measured in 79 % of patients (15 of 19). Immune responses appeared within 12 weeks and were generally maintained or augmented in patients continuing combined treatment. Median OS was 70.4 weeks (4.6–141.6 weeks), and the median PFS was 11 weeks (2.6–114.6 weeks). Patients who mounted a T-cell response to CA125 and/or autologous tumor showed significantly improved survival compared to patients who did not. A phase III trial which recruited 375 stage III and IV EOC patients showed that while bioactivity was demonstrable and the drug was well tolerated, patients receiving oregovomab had similar clinical outcomes vs. placebo [180].

Trastuzumab is a monoclonal antibody targeting HER2 and is commonly used as adjuvant therapy in HER2-expressing breast cancer patients. It has been evaluated as a therapeutic agent in gynecologic malignancies as well. GOG 160, a phase II trial, evaluated trastuzumab in patients with recurrent or refractory EOC or PPC. An overall RR of 7.3 % in the 41 eligible patients with HER2 overexpression was noted. Trastuzumab was relatively well tolerated and several patients demonstrating either response or disease stabilization received treatment for greater than 12 months. Only 11.4 % of tumors exhibited 2+ or 3+ expression and there was no relationship found between HER2 expression and clinical responses or survival [162].

### Immune Checkpoint Modulation

Manipulation of the immune checkpoint inhibitors that serve as checks and balances in the regulation of the immune system [181] has been investigated as an avenue for immune therapy. Most recent advances focus on removing these inhibitors in order to facilitate host antitumor responses. Researchers have sought to identify cytokines that induce the maturation, activation, and migration of inflammatory cells and have used these factors to activate the immune system against tumor cells. Cytokines profoundly affect inflammatory cells, and they activate immune responses by multiple mechanisms.

Several studies evaluating the use of cytokines in patients with gynecologic cancer have yielded mixed results. A phase II trial evaluating IL-12 in patients with EOC-reported therapy was tolerable but there no complete responders and 50 % of patients had stable disease [182]. Vlad et al. evaluated intraperitoneal IL-2 in patients with platinum refractory or resistant EOC [183]. Among 24 patients, six (four complete and two partial) responses were noted with an overall RR of 25 %. The regimen was well tolerated; patients with more circulating IFNα secreting CD8 cells at early time points had better chances for survival.

Cytotoxic T-lymphocyte-associated protein 4 (CTLA-4) is a protein receptor found on the surface of T cells that downregulates the antitumor immune system [184]. Ipilimumab is a monoclonal antibody targeting CTLA-4. This therapy has been extensively studied in patients with melanoma [185–189]. In a phase I/II trial for 11 patients with stage IV ovarian cancers which had previously either received chemotherapy or GVAX (a vaccine product comprised of autologous, irradiated tumor cells engineered to secrete the immune stimulatory cytokine, granulocyte macrophage colony-stimulating factor), ipilimumab was well tolerated with the exception of grade 3 inflammatory toxicities in two patients [189, 190]. Significant antitumor effects were seen in one patient who showed a dramatic fall of serum CA125 levels (43 % reduction) and a substantial regression of hepatic metastasis, complete resolution of mesenteric lymph nodes and omental cake. Ipilimumab is currently being studied in the setting of recurrent/advanced cervical cancer as well.

### Therapeutic Immunotherapies Targeting Cervical Cancer

In cervical cancer, therapeutic strategies targeting HPV have been examined. Efficacy for preventative HPV vaccination in large clinical trials is plentiful, but data in support of therapeutic vaccination are still modest. Cellular immune responses against HPV E6/E7-expressing cells are able to eliminate dysplasic or neoplastic cells driven by HPV infection [191]. Clinical trials have focused on augmentation of the anti-HPV immune response. In 2006, Santin et al. evaluated HPV 16/18 E7 pulsed dendritic cell vaccination in cervical cancer patient with recurrent refractory disease [192]. Autologous DC pulsed with HPV16/18 E7 proteins induced systemic B- and T-cell responses in patients unresponsive to standard treatment modalities. The vaccine was well tolerated in all patients and no local or systemic side effects were seen. ADXS11-001 is an immunotherapy based on a live-attenuated *Listeria monocytogenes* that secretes fusion protein LM-LLO-E7 targeting HPV-associated tumors [193]. Phase I and II trials have been conducted using ADXS11-001. Maciag et al. [194] enrolled 15 patients in a phase I dose-escalation study in women with advanced cervical cancer following failure of traditional therapy and noted dose-limiting toxicity to be reached at 1 × the data, a phase II GOG study is currently in progress for patients with advanced, metastatic, or recurrent cervical cancer that has failed prior systemic chemotherapy. An additional randomized phase II trial in India administering ADXS11-001 with or without cisplatin is also being conducted in 110 patients with recurrent cervical cancer [195].

## Conclusions

Advanced gynecologic malignancies have traditionally been treated with a combination of surgery, chemotherapy, and radiation. These therapies have proven success, though often at the expense of severe toxicities, and in many cases resulting in only temporary responses. In recent years, advances in molecular biology and immunology have allowed more specific targeting of various pathways and factors in tumor immunity that may eventually lead to improved treatment efficacy with fewer side effects. While some progress has been made, results to date are mixed, and much work will be necessary to bring the goals of targeted therapies to fruition.

## References

1. Umene K, Banno K, Kisu I, Yanokura M, Nogami Y, Tsuji K, et al. Aurora kinase inhibitors: potential molecular-targeted drugs for gynecologic malignant tumors (Review). Biomed Rep. 2013;1(3):335–40.
2. Birbrair A, Zhang T, Wang ZM, Messi ML, Olson JD, Mintz A, Delbono O. Type-2 pericytes participate

in normal and tumoral angiogenesis. Am J Phyiol Cell Physiol. 2014;307(1):C25–38.

3. Ide AG, Baker NH, Warren SL. Vascularization of the Brown Pearce rabbit epithelioma transplant as seen in the transparent ear chamber. Am J Roentgenol. 1939;42:891–9.
4. Folkman J, Merler E, Abernathy C, Williams G. Isolation of a tumor factor responsible for angiogenesis. J Exp Med. 1971;133:275–88.
5. Achen MG, Stacker SA. The vascular endothelial growth factor family; proteins which guide the development of the vasculature. Int J Exp Pathol. 1998;79(5):255–65.
6. Folkman J. What is the evidence that tumors are angiogenesis dependent? J Natl Cancer Inst. 1990; 82(1):4–6.
7. Cao Y. Antiangiogenic cancer therapy. Semin Cancer Biol. 2004;14(2):139–45.
8. Ferrara N, Henzel WJ. Pituitary follicular cells secrete a novel heparin-binding growth factor specific for vascular endothelial cells. Biochem Biophys Res Commun. 1989;161:851–8.
9. Ferrara N, Carver Moore K, Chen H, Dowd M, Lu L, O'Shea KS, et al. Heterozygous embryonic lethality induced by targeted inactivation of the VEGF gene. Nature. 1996;380(6573):439–42.
10. Moreira IS, Fernandes PA, Ramos MJ. Vascular endothelial growth factor (VEGF) inhibition--a critical review. Anticancer Agents Med Chem. 2007;7(2):223–45.
11. Ce´be-Suarez S, Zehnder-Fja¨llman A, Ballmer-Hofer K. The role of VEGF receptors in angiogenesis; complex partnerships. Cell Mol Life Sci. 2006;63(5):601–15.
12. Shibuya M, Claesson-Welsh L. Signal transduction by VEGF receptors in regulation of angiogenesis and lymphangiogenesis. Exp Cell Res. 2006;312(5):549–60.
13. Ellis LM, Hicklin DJ. VEGF-targeted therapy: mechanisms of anti-tumour activity. Nat Rev Cancer. 2008;8(8):579–91.
14. Zeng H, Dvorak HF, Mukhopadhyay D. Vascular permeability factor (VPF)/vascular endothelial growth factor (VEGF) peceptor-1 down-modulates VPF/VEGF receptor-2-mediated endothelial cell proliferation, but not migration, through phosphatidylinositol 3-kinase-dependent pathways. J Biol Chem. 2001;276(29):26969–79.
15. Ferrara N, Gerber HP, LeCouter J. The biology of VEGF and its receptors. Nat Med. 2003;9(6):669–76.
16. Merritt WM, Sood AK. Markers of angiogenesis in ovarian cancer. Dis Markers. 2007;23(5-6):419–31.
17. Neufeld G, Cohen T, Gengrinovitch S, Poltorak Z. Vascular endothelial growth factor (VEGF) and its receptors. FASEB J. 1999;13(1):9–22.
18. Garzetti GG, Ciavattini A, Lucarini G, Pugnaloni A, De Nictolis M, Amati S, et al. Vascular endothelial growth factor expression as a prognostic index in serous ovarian cystoadenocarcinomas: relationship with MIB1 immunostaining. Gynecol Oncol. 1999;73(3):396–401.
19. Giatromanolaki A, Sivridis E, Brekken R, Thorpe PE, Anastasiadis P, Gatter KC, et al. The angiogenic "vascular endothelial growth factor/flk-1(KDR) receptor" pathway in patients with endometrial carcinoma: prognostic and therapeutic implications. Cancer. 2001;92(10):2569–77.
20. Guidi AJ, Abu-Jawdeh G, Berse B, Jackman RW, Tognazzi K, Dvorak HF, et al. Vascular permeability factor (vascular endothelial growth factor) expression and angiogenesis in cervical neoplasia. J Natl Cancer Inst. 1995;87(16):1237–45.
21. Obermair A, Kohlberger P, Bancher-Todesca D, Tempfer C, Sliutz G, Leodolter S, et al. Influence of microvessel density and vascular permeability factor/vascular endothelial growth factor expression on prognosis in vulvar cancer. Gynecol Oncol. 1996;63(2):204–9.
22. Shen GH, Ghazizadeh M, Kawanami O, Shimizu H, Jin E, Araki T, et al. Prognostic significance of vascular endothelial growth factor expression in human ovarian carcinoma. Br J Cancer. 2000;83(2): 196–203.
23. Alvarez AA, Krigman HR, Whitaker RS, Dodge RK, Rodriguez GC. The prognostic significance of angiogenesis in epithelial ovarian carcinoma. Clin Cancer Res. 1999;5(3):587–91.
24. Genentech BioOncology™. Avastin® (bevacizumab), product insert. Code revision date: June 2006. ©2006 Genentech, Inc. http://www.gene.com/gene/products/information/oncology/avastin/insert.jsp
25. Ferrara N, Hillian K, Gerber H, Novotny W. Discovery and development of bevacizumab, an anti-VEGF antibody for treating cancer. Nat Rev Drug Discov. 2004;3:391–400.
26. Burger RA, Sill MW, Monk BJ, Greer BE, Sorosky JL. Phase II trial of bevacizumab in persistent or recurrent epithelial ovarian cancer or primary peritoneal cancer: a gynecologic oncology group study. J Clin Oncol. 2007;25(33):5165–71.
27. Burger RA, Brady MF, Bookman MA, Fleming GF, Monk BJ, Huang H, et al. Incorporation of bevacizumab in the primary treatment of ovarian cancer. N Engl J Med. 2011;365(26):2473–83.
28. Perren TJ, Swart AM, Pfisterer J, Ledermann JA, Pujade-Lauraine E, Kristensen G, et al. A phase 3 trial of bevacizumab in ovarian cancer. N Engl J Med. 2011;365(26):2484–96.
29. Aghajanian C, Blank SV, Goff BA, Judson PL, Teneriello MG, Husain A. OCEANS: a randomized, double-blind, placebo-controlled phase III trial of chemotherapy with or without bevacizumab in patients with platinum-sensitive recurrent epithelial ovarian, primary peritoneal, or fallopian tube cancer. J Clin Oncol. 2012;30(17):2039–45.
30. Pujade-Lauraine E, Hilpert F, Weber B, Reuss A, Poveda A, Kristensen G, et al. Bevacizumab

combined with chemotherapy for platinum-resistant recurrent ovarian cancer: the AURELIA open-label randomized phase III trial. J Clin Oncol. 2014;32(13): 1302–8.
31. Aghajanian C, Sill MW, Darcy KM, Greer B, McMeekin DS, Rose PG, et al. Phase II trial of bevacizumab in recurrent or persistent endometrial cancer: a gynecologic oncology group study. J Clin Oncol. 2011;29(16):2259–65.
32. Tewari KS, Sill MW, Long HJ, Penson RT, Huang H, Ramondetta LM, et al. Improved survival with bevacizumab in advanced cervical cancer. N Engl J Med. 2014;370:734–43.
33. Tew WP, Gordon M, Murren J, Dupont J, Pezzulli S, Aghajanian C, et al. Phase 1 study of aflibercept administered subcutaneously to patients with advanced solid tumors. Clin Cancer Res. 2010;16(1): 358–66.
34. Grothey A, Galanis E. Targeting angiogenesis: progress with anti-VegF treatment with large molecules. Nat Rev Clin Oncol. 2009;6:507–18.
35. Rudge JS, Holash J, Hylton D, Russell M, Jiang S, Leidich R. VEGF Trap complex formation measures production rates of VEGF, providing a biomarker for predicting efficacious angiogenic blockade. Proc Natl Acad Sci U S A. 2007;104(47):18363–70.
36. Byrne AT, Ross L, Holash J, Nakanishi M, Hu L, Hofmann JI. Vascular endothelial growth factor-trap decreases tumor burden, inhibits ascites, and causes dramatic vascular remodeling in an ovarian cancer model. Clin Cancer Res. 2003;9(15):5721–8.
37. Hu L, Hofmann J, Holash J, Yancopoulos GD, Sood AK, Jaffe RB. Vascular endothelial growth factor trap combined with paclitaxel strikingly inhibits tumor and ascites, prolonging survival in a human ovarian cancer model. Clin Cancer Res. 2005; 11:6966–71.
38. Coleman RL, Duska LR, Ramirez PT, et al. Phase II multi-institutional study of docetaxel plus aflibercept in recurrent ovarian, primary peritoneal and fallopian tube cancer. J Clin Oncol. 2011;29:5017.
39. Coleman RL, Sill MW, Lankes HA, Fader AN, Finkler NJ, Hoffman JS, et al. A phase II evaluation of aflibercept in the treatment of recurrent or persistent endometrial cancer: a Gynecologic oncology group study. Gynecol Oncol. 2013;130(1):252–3.
40. Wedge SR, Kendrew J, Hennequin LF, Valentine PJ, Barry ST, Brave SR, et al. AZD2171: a highly potent, orally bioavailable, vascular endothelial growth factor receptor-2 tyrosine kinase inhibitor for the treatment of cancer. Cancer Res. 2005;65(10): 4389–400.
41. Liu JF, Tolaney SM, Birrer M, Fleming GF, Buss MK, Dahlberg SE, et al. A Phase 1 trial of the poly(ADP-ribose) polymerase inhibitor olaparib (AZD2281) in combination with the anti-angiogenic cediranib (AZD2171) in recurrent epithelial ovarian or triple-negative breast cancer. Eur J Cancer. 2013;49(14):2972–8.
42. Liu JF, Barry WT, Birrer M, Lee JM, Buckanovich RJ. Combination cediranib and olaparib versus olaparib alone for women with recurrent platinum-sensitive ovarian cancer: a randomized phase 2 study. Lancet Oncol. 2014;15(11):1207–14.
43. Friedlander M, Hancock KC, Rischin D, Messing MJ, Stringer CA, Matthys GM, et al. A phase II, open-label study evaluating pazopanib in patients with recurrent ovarian cancer. Gynecol Oncol. 2010;119(1):32–7.
44. Vivanco I, Sawyers CL. The phosphatidylinositol 3-Kinase AKT pathway in human cancer. Nat Rev Cancer. 2002;2(7):489–501.
45. Shayesteh L, Lu Y, Kuo WL, Baldocchi R, Godfrey T, Collins C, et al. PIK3CA is implicated as an oncogene in ovarian cancer. Nat Genet. 1999;21(1): 99–102.
46. Levine DA, Bogomolniy F, Yee CJ, Lash A, Barakat RR, Borgen PI, Boyd J. Frequent mutation of the PIK3CA gene in ovarian and breast cancers. Clin Cancer Res. 2005;11(8):2875–8.
47. Rudd ML, Price JC, Fogoros S, Godwin AK, Sgroi DC, Merino MJ, Bell DW. A unique spectrum of somatic PIK3CA mutations within primary endometrial cancinomas. Clin Cancer Res. 2011;17(6): 1331–40.
48. Cheung LW, Hennessy BT, Li J, Yu S, Myers AP, Djordjevic B. High frequency of PIK3R1 and PIK3R2 mutations in endometrial cancer elucidates a novel mechanism for regulation of PTEN protein stability. Cancer Discov. 2011;1(2):170–85.
49. Sudo T. Molecular-targeted therapies for ovarian cancer: prospects for the future. Int J Clin Oncol. 2012;17(5):424–9.
50. Hennessy BT, Smith DL, Ram PT, Lu Y, Mills GB. Exploiting the PI3K/AKT pathway for cancer drug discovery. Nat Rev Drug Discov. 2005;4(12):988–1004.
51. Meric-Bernstam F, Gonzalez-Angulo AM. Targeting the mTOR signaling network for cancer therapy. J Clin Oncol. 2009;27(13):2278–87.
52. Hudson CC, Liu M, Chiang GG, Otterness DM, Loomis DC, Kaper F. Regulation of hypoxia-inducible factor 1 expression and function by the mammalian target of rapamycin. Mol Cell Biol. 2000;22(20):7004–14.
53. Mundt A, Yashar C, Mell L. Biological agents and immune therapy. Gynecologic cancer: radiation medicine rounds. New York, NY: Demos Medical Publishing; 2012. p. 401–25.
54. Husseinzadeh N, Husseinzadeh H. mTOR inhibitors and their clinic application in cervical endometrial and ovarian cancers: a critical review. Gynecol Oncol. 2014;133(2):375–81.
55. Wullschleger R, Loewith R, Hall MN. TOR signaling in growth and metabolism. Cell. 2006;124(3): 471–84.
56. Slomovitz BM, Wu W, Broaddus RR, Soliman PT, Wolf J, Sun CC. mTOR inhibition is a rational target

for the treatment of endometrial cancer. Proc Am Soc Clin Oncol. 2004;22:5076.
57. Oza AM, Elit L, Tsao MS, Kamel-Reid S, Biagi J, Provencher DM. Phase II study of temsirolimus in women with recurrent or metastatic endometrial cancer: a trial of the NCIC Clinical Trials Group. J Clin Oncol. 2011;29(24):3278–85.
58. Fleming GF, Filliaci VL, Hanjani P, Burks JJ, Davidson SA, Leslie KK, et al. Hormone therapy plus temsirolimus for endometrial cancer (EC): Gynecologic Oncology Group trial #248. J Clin Oncol. 2011;29:335.
59. Alvarez EA, Brady WE, Walker JL, Rotmensch J, Zhou XC, Kendrick JE, et al. Phase II trial of combination bevacizumab and temsirolimus in the treatment of recurrent or persistent endometrial carcinoma: a Gynecologic Oncology Group study. Gynecol Oncol. 2013;129(1):22–7.
60. Behbakht K, Sill MW, Darcy KM, Rubin SC, Mannel RS, Waggoner S, et al. Phase II trial of the mTOR inhibitor, temsirolimus and evaluation of circulating tumor cells and tumor biomarkers in persistent and recurrent epithelial ovarian and primary peritoneal malignancies: a Gynecologic Oncology Group study. Gynecol Oncol. 2011;123(1):19–26.
61. Temkin SM, Yamada SD, Fleming GF. A phase I study of weekly temsirolimus and topotecan in the treatment of advanced and/or recurrent gynecologic malignancies. Gynecol Oncol. 2010;11(3):473–6.
62. Tinker AV, Ellard S, Welch S, Moens F, Allo G, Tsao MS, et al. Phase II study of temsirolimus (CCI-779) in women with recurrent, unresectable, locally advanced or metastatic carcinoma of the cervix. A trial of the NCIC Clinical Trials Group (NCIC CTG IND 199). Gynecol Oncol. 2013;130(2):269–74.
63. Slomovitz BM, Lu KH, Johnston T, Coleman RL, Munsell M, Broaddus RR, et al. A phase 2 study of the oral mammalian target of rapamycin inhibitor, everolimus, in patients with recurrent endometrial carcinoma. Cancer. 2010;23:5415–9.
64. Milani A, Geuna E, Mittica G, Valabrega G. Overcoming endocrine resistance in metastatic breast cancer: current evidence and future directions. World J Clin Oncol. 2014;5(5):990–1001.
65. Coussy F, Teixeira L, Giacchetti S, Cuvier C, Hocini H, Espié M. New targeted therapies in breast cancer. Gynecol Obstet Fertil. 2014;42(11):787–94.
66. Bansal N, Yendluri V, Wenham RM. The molecular biology of endometrial cancers and the implications for pathogenesis, classification, and targeted therapies. Cancer Control. 2009;16(1):8–13.
67. Growdon WB, Boisvert SL, Akhavanfard S, Oliva E, Dias-Santagata DC, et al. Decreased survival in EGFR gene amplified vulvar carcinoma. Gynecol Oncol. 2008;111(2):289–97.
68. Kersemaekers AM, Fleuren GJ, Kenter GG, Van den Broek LJ, Uljee SM, Hermans J, et al. Oncogene alterations in carcinomas of the uterine cervix: overexpression of the epidermal growth factor receptor is associated with poor prognosis. Clin Cancer Res. 1999;5(3):577–86.
69. Kim JW, Kim YT, Kim DK, Song CH, Lee JW. Expression of epidermal growth factor receptor in carcinoma of the cervix. Gynecol Oncol. 1996; 60(2):283–7.
70. Oonk MH, de Bock GH, van der Veen DJ, Ten Hoor KA, de Hullu JA, Hollema H, et al. EGFR expression is associated with groin node metastases in vulvar cancer, but does not improve their prediction. Gynecol Oncol. 2007;104(1):109–13.
71. Zagouri F, Bozas G, Kafantari E, Tsiatas M, Nikitas N, Dimopoulos MA, Papadimitriou CA. Endometrial cancer: what is new in adjuvant and molecularly targeted therapy? Obstet Gynecol Int. 2010;2010: 749579.
72. Moscatello DK, Holgado-Madruga M, Godwin AK, Ramirez G, Gunn G, Zoltick PW, Gunn G, et al. Frequent expression of a mutant epidermal growth factor receptor in multiple human tumors. Cancer Res. 1995;55(23):5536–9.
73. Bartlett JM, Langdon SP, Simpson BJ, Stewart M, Katsaros D, Sismondi P, et al. The prognostic value of epidermal growth factor receptor mRNA expression in primary ovarian cancer. Br J Cancer. 1996;73(3):301–6.
74. Fischer-Colbrie J, Witt A, Heinzl H, Speiser P, Czerwenka K, Sevelda P, et al. EGFR and steroid receptors in ovarian carcinoma: comparison with prognostic parameters and outcome of patients. Anticancer Res. 1997;17(18):613–9.
75. Colombo N, McMeekin S, Schwartz P, Kostka J, Sessa C, Gehrig P, et al. A phase II trial of the mTOR inhibitor AP23573 as a single agent in advanced endometrial cancer. J Clin Oncol. 2007;25:5516.
76. Mackay H, Welch S, Tsao MS, Biagi JJ, Elit L, Ghatage P, et al. Phase II study of oral ridaforolimus in patients with metastatic and/or locally advanced recurrent endometrial cancer: NCIC CTG IND 192. J Clin Oncol. 2011;29:5013.
77. Oza AM, Poveda A, Clamp AR, Pignata S, Scambia G, Del Campo JM, et al. A randomized phase II (RP2) trial of ridaforolimus (R) compared with progestin (P) or chemotherapy (C) in female adult patients with advanced endometrial carcinoma. J Clin Oncol. 2011;29:509.
78. Fleming GF, Sill MW, Darcy KM, McMeekin DS, Thigpen JT, Alder LM, et al. Phase II trial of trastuzumab in women with advanced or recurrent, HER2-positive endometrial carcinoma: a Gynecologic Oncology Group study. Gynecol Oncol. 2010;116:15–20.
79. Oza AM, Eisenhauer EA, Elit L, Cutz JC, Sakurada A, Tsao MSA, et al. A phase II study of erlotinib in recurrent or metastatic endometrial cancer, NCIC IND-148. J Clin Oncol. 2008;26(26):4319–25.
80. Leslie KK, Sill MW, Darcy KM, Baron AT, Wilken JA, Godwin AK, et al. Efficacy and safety of gefitinib and potential prognostic value of soluble EGFR, EGFR mutations, and tumor markers in a Gynecologic Oncology Group phase II trial of persistent or recurrent endometrial cancer. J Clin Oncol. 2009;27:e16542.

81. McMeekin DS, Sill MW, Benbrook D, Darcy KM, Stearns-Kurosawa DJ, Eaton L, et al. A phase II trial of thalidomide in patients with refractory endometrial cancer and correlation with angiogenesis biomarkers: a Gynecologic Oncology Group study. Gynecol Oncol. 2007;105(2):508–16.
82. Welch S, Mackay HJ, Hirte H, Fleming GF, Morgan R, Wang L, et al. A phase II study of sunitinib in recurrent or metastatic endometrial carcinoma: a trial of the PMH Phase II Consortium. J Clin Oncol. 2009;28:15s.
83. Correa R, Mackay H, Hirte HW, Morgan R, Welch S, Fleming GF, et al. A phase II study of sunitinib in recurrent or metastatic endometrial carcinoma: a trial of the Princess Margaret Hospital, the University of Chicago, and California Cancer Phase II Consortia. J Clin Oncol. 2010;28.
84. Nimeiri HS, Oza AM, Morgan RJ, Huo D, Elit L, Knost J. Sorafenib (SOR) in patients (pts) with advanced/recurrent uterine carcinoma (UCA) or carcinosarcoma (CS): a phase II trial of the University of Chicago, PMH, and California Phase II Consortia. J Clin Oncol. 2008;26:15S.
85. Schilder RJ, Pathak HB, Lokshin AE, Holloway RW, Alvarez RD, Aghajanian C, et al. Phase II trial of single agent cetuximab in patients with persistent or recurrent epithelial ovarian or primary peritoneal carcinoma with the potential for dose escalation to rash. Gynecol Oncol. 2009;113(1):21–7.
86. Secord AA, Blessing JA, Armstrong DK, Rodgers WH, Miner Z, Barnes MN, et al. Phase II trial of cetuximab and carboplatin in relapsed platinum-sensitive ovarian cancer and evaluation of epidermal growth factor receptor expression: a Gynecologic Oncology Group study. Gynecol Oncol. 2008; 108(3):493–9.
87. Gordon AN, Finkler N, Edwards RP, Garcia AA, Crozier M, Irwin DH, et al. Efficacy and safety of erlotinib HCL, an epidermal growth factor receptor (HER1/EGFR) tyrosine kinase inhibitor, in patients with advanced ovarian carcinoma: results from a phase II multicenter study. Int J Gynecol Cancer. 2005;15(5):785–92.
88. Blank SV, Christos P, Curtin JP, Runowicz CD, Goldman N, Sparano JA, et al. Erlotinib added to carboplatin and paclitaxel as first-line treatment of ovarian cancer, phase II study based on surgical reassessment. Gynecol Oncol. 2010;119(3):451–6.
89. Vasey PA, Gore M, Wilson R, Rustin G, Gabra H, Guastalla JP, et al. A phase Ib trial of docetaxel, carboplatin and erlotinib in ovarian, fallopian tube and primary peritoneal cancers. Br J Cancer. 2008; 98(11):1774–80.
90. Hirte H, Oza A, Swenerton K, Ellard SL, Grimshaw R, Fisher B, Seymour L. A phase II study of erlotinib (OSI-774) given in combination with carboplatin in patients with recurrent epithelial ovarian cancer (NCIC CTG IND.149). Gynecol Oncol. 2010; 118(3):308–12.
91. Schilder RJ, Sill MW, Chen X, Darcy KM, Decesara SL, Lewandowski G, et al. Phase II study of gefitinib in patients with relapsed or persistent ovarian or primary peritoneal carcinoma and evaluation of epidermal growth factor receptor mutations and immunohistochemical expression: a Gynecologic Oncology Group Study. Clin Cancer Res. 2005; 11(15):5539–48.
92. Posadas EM, Liel MS, Kwitkowski V, Minasian L, Godwin AK, Hussain MM, et al. A phase II and pharmacodynamic study of gefitinib in patients with refractory or recurrent epithelial ovarian cancer. Cancer. 2007;109(7):1323–30.
93. Wagner U, du Bois A, Pfisterer J, Huober J, Loibl S, Luck HJ, et al. Gefitinib in combination with tamoxifen in patients with ovarian cancer refractory or resistant to platinum-taxane based therapy – a phase II trial of the AGO Ovarian Cancer Study Group (AGO-OVAR 2.6). Gynecol Oncol. 2007;105(1): 132–7.
94. Pautier P, Joly F, Kerbrat P, Bougnoux P, Fumoleau P, Petit T, et al. Phase II study of gefitinib in combination with paclitaxel (P) and carboplatin (C) as secondline therapy for ovarian, tubal or peritoneal adenocarcinoma (1839IL/0074). Gynecol Oncol. 2010;116(2):157–62.
95. Tewari KS, Sill M, Long HJ, Ramondetta LM, Landrum LM, Oaknin A, et al. Incorporation of bevacizumab in the treatment of recurrent and metastatic cervical cancer: a phase III randomized trial of the Gynecologic Oncology Group. J Clin Oncol. 2013;31(18):3.
96. Schefter TE, Winter K, Kwon JS, Stuhr K, Balaraj K, Yaremko BP, et al. A phase II study of bevacizumab in combination with definitive radiotherapy and cisplatin chemotherapy in untreated patients with locally advanced cervical carcinoma: preliminary results of RTOG 0417. Int J Radiat Oncol Biol Phys. 2012;83(4):1179–84.
97. Zighelboim I, Wright JD, Gao F, Case AS, Massad LS, Mutch DG, et al. Multicenter phase II trial of topotecan, cisplatin and bevacizumab for recurrent or persistent cervical cancer. Gynecol Oncol. 2013; 130(1):64–8.
98. Mackay HJ, Tinker A, Winquist E, Thomas G, Swenerton K, Oza A, et al. A phase II study of sunitinib in patients with locally advanced or metastatic cervical carcinoma, NCIC CTG Trial IND.184. Gynecol Oncol. 2010;116(2):163–7.
99. Goncalves A, Fabbro M, Lhommé C, Gladieff L, Extra JM, Floquet A, et al. A phase II trial to evaluate gefitinib as second- or third-line treatment in patients with recurring locoregionally advanced or metastatic cervical cancer. Gynecol Oncol. 2008;108(1):42–6.
100. Schilder RJ, Sill MW, Lee YC, Mannel R. A phase II trial of erlotinib in recurrent squamous cell carcinoma of the cervix: a Gynecologic Oncology Group Study. Int J Gynecol Cancer. 2009;19(5):929–33.

101. Santin AD, Sill MW, McMeekin DS, Leitao Jr MM, Brown J, Sutton GP, et al. Phase II trial of cetuximab in the treatment of persistent or recurrent squamous or non-squamous cell carcinoma of the cervix: a Gynecologic Oncology Group study. Gynecol Oncol. 2011;122(3):495–500.
102. Tinker AV, Ellard S, Welch S, Tinker AV, Ellard S, Welch S, et al. Phase II study of temsirolimus (CCI-779) in women with recurrent, unresectable, locally advanced or metastatic carcinoma of the cervix. A trial of the NCIC Clinical Trials Group (NCIC CTG IND 199). Gynecol Oncol. 2013;130(2):269–74.
103. Coronel J, Cetina L, Pacheco I, Trejo-Becerril C, González-Fierro A, de la Cruz-Hernandez E, et al. A double-blind, placebo-controlled, randomized phase III trial of chemotherapy plus epigenetic therapy with hydralazine valproate for advanced cervical cancer. Preliminary results. Med Oncol. 2011;28 Suppl 1:S540–6.
104. Zhou J, Liu F, Xiao J. Recombinant adenovirus-p53 combined with chemo- therapy in treatment of locally advanced cervical cancer (a phase II study). J Clin Oncol. 2013;31.
105. Nimeiri HS, Oza AM, Morgan RJ, Friberg G, Kasza K, et al. Efficacy and safety of bevacizumab plus erlotinib for patients with recurrent ovarian, primary peritoneal, and fallopian tube cancer. A trial of the Chicago, PMH, and California phase II consortia. Gynecol Oncol. 2008;110(1):49–55.
106. Bonner JA, Harari PM, Giralt J, Azarnia N, Shin DM, Cohen RB, et al. Radiotherapy plus cetuximab for squamous-cell carcinoma of the head and neck. N Engl J Med. 2006;354(6):567–78.
107. Jonker DJ, O'Callaghan CJ, Karapetis CS, Zalcberg JR, Tu D, Au HJ, et al. Cetuximab for the treatment of colorectal cancer. N Engl J Med. 2007;357:2040–8.
108. Konner J, Schilder RJ, DeRosa FA, Gerst SR, Tew WP, Sabbatini PJ, et al. A phase II study of cetuximab/paclitaxel/carboplatin for the initial treatment of advanced-stage ovarian, primary peritoneal, or fallopian tube cancer. Gynecol Oncol. 2008;110(2):140–5.
109. Kurtz JE, Hardy-Bessard AC, Deslandres M, Lavau-Denes S, Largillier R, et al. Cetuximab, topotecan and cisplatin for the treatment of advanced cervical cancer: a phase II GINECO trial. Gynecol Oncol. 2009;113(1):16–20.
110. Beck C, Robert I, Reina-San-Martin B, Schreiber V, Dantzer F. Poly(ADP-ribose) polymerases in double-strand break repair: focus on PARP1, PARP2 and PARP3. Exp Cell Res. 2014;329(1):18–25.
111. Farmer H, McCabe N, Lord CJ, Tutt AN, Johnson DA, Richardson TB, et al. Targeting the DNA repair defect in BRCA mutant cells as a therapeutic strategy. Nature. 2005;434(7035):917–21.
112. Boulton S, Kyle S, Durkacz BW. Interactive effects of inhibitors of poly(ADP-ribose) polymerase and DNA-dependent protein kinase on cellular responses to DNA damage. Carcinogenesis. 1999;20(2):199–203.
113. Saffhill R, Ockey CH. Strand breaks arising from the repair of the 5-bromodeoxyuridine-substituted template and methyl methanesulphonate-induced lesions can explain the formation of sister chromatid exchanges. Chromosoma. 1985;92(3):218–24.
114. Duan W, Gao L, Zhao W, Leon M, Sadee W, Webb A, et al. Assessment of FANCD2 nuclear foci formation in paraffin-embedded tumors: a potential patient-enrichment strategy for treatment with DNA inter-strand crosslinking agents. Transl Res. 2013;161(3):156–64.
115. McCabe N, Turner NC, Lord CJ, Kluzek K, Bialkowska A, Swift S, et al. Deficiency in the repair of DNA damage by homologous recombination and sensitivity to poly(ADP-ribose) polymerase inhibition. Cancer Res. 2006;66(16):8109–15.
116. Turner N, Tutt A, Ashworth A. Hallmarks of 'BRCAness' in sporadic cancers. Nat Rev Cancer. 2004;4(10):814–9.
117. Donawho CK, Luo Y, Luo Y, Penning TD, Bauch JL, Bouska JJ, et al. ABT-888, an orally active poly(ADP-ribose) polymerase inhibitor that potentiates DNA-damaging agents in preclinical tumor models. Clin Cancer Res. 2007;13(9):2728–37.
118. Fong PC, Boss DS, Yap TA, Tutt A, Wu P, Mergui-Roelvink M, et al. Inhibition of poly(ADP-ribose) polymerase in tumors from BRCA mutation carriers. N Engl J Med. 2009;361(2):123–34.
119. Audeh MW, Carmichael J, Penson RT, Friedlander M, Powell B, Bell-McGuinn KM, et al. Oral poly(ADP-ribose) polymerase inhibitor olaparib in patients with BRCA1 or BRCA2 mutations and recurrent ovarian cancer: a proof-of-concept trial. Lancet. 2010;376(9737):245–51.
120. Ledermann J, Harter P, Gourley C, Friedlander M, Vergote I, Rustin G. Olaparib maintenance therapy in patients with platinum-sensitive relapsed serous ovarian cancer: a preplanned retrospective analysis of outcomes by BRCA status in a randomised phase 2 trial. Lancet Oncol. 2014;8:852–61.
121. Gelmon KA, Tischkowitz M, Mackay H, Swenerton K, Robidoux A, Tonkin K, et al. Olaparib in patients with recurrent high-grade serous or poorly differentiated ovarian carcinoma or triple-negative breast cancer: a phase 2, multicentre, open-label, non-randomised study. Lancet Oncol. 2011;12(9):852–61.
122. Reinbolt RE, Hays JL. The role of PARP inhibitors in the treatment of gynecologic malignancies. Front Oncol. 2013;3:237.
123. FDA News Release "FDA approved Lynparza to treat advanced ovarian cancer" for immediate release December 19, 2014. http://www.fda.gov/newsevents/newsroom/pressannouncements/ucm427554.htm
124. Wilhelm SM, Adnane L, Newell P, Villanueva A, Llovet JM, Lynch M. Preclinical overview of sorafenib, a multikinase inhibitor that targets both Raf and VEGF and PDGF receptor tyrosine kinase signaling. Mol Cancer Ther. 2008;7(10):3129–40.

125. Matei D, Sill MW, Lankes HA, DeGeest K, Bristow RE, Mutch D, et al. Activity of sorafenib in recurrent ovarian cancer and primary peritoneal carcinomatosis: a gynecologic oncology group trial. J Clin Oncol. 2011;29(1):69–75.
126. Azad NS, Posadas EM, Kwitkowski VE, Steinberg SM, Jain L, Annunziata CM, et al. Combination targeted therapy with sorafenib and bevacizumab results in enhanced toxicity and antitumor activity. J Clin Oncol. 2008;26(22):3709–14.
127. Herzog TJ, Scambia G, Kim BG, Lhommé C, Markowska J, Ray-Coquard I, et al. A randomized phase II trial of maintenance therapy with Sorafenib in front-line ovarian carcinoma. Gynecol Oncol. 2013;130(1):25–30.
128. Schwandt A, von Gruenigen VE, Wenham RM, Frasure H, Eaton S, Fusco N, et al. Randomized phase II trial of sorafenib alone or in combination with carboplatin/paclitaxel in women with recurrent platinum sensitive epithelial ovarian, peritoneal, or fallopian tube cancer. Invest New Drugs. 2014;32(4):729–38.
129. Zsiros E, Tanyi J, Balint K, Kandalaft LE. Immunotherapy for ovarian cancer: recent advances and perspectives. Curr Opin Oncol. 2014;26(5):492–500.
130. Schlienger K, Chu CS, Woo EY, Rivers PM, Toll AJ, Hudson B, et al. TRANCE- and CD40 ligand-matured dendritic cells reveal MHC class I-restricted T cells specific for autologous tumor in late-stage ovarian cancer patients. Clin Cancer Res. 2003;9(4):1517–27.
131. Shiao S, Ganesan A, Rugo H, Coussen L. Immune microenvironments in solid tumors: new targets for therapy. Genes Dev. 2011;25(24):2559–72.
132. Bright RK. Book review: peptide based cancer vaccines. Leukemia. 2002;16:970–1.
133. Mantia-Smaldone GM, Corr B, Chu CS. Immunotherapy in ovarian cancer. Hum Vaccin Immunother. 2012;8(9):1179–91.
134. Disis ML, Goodell V, Schiffman K, Knutson KL. Humoral epitope-spreading following immunization with a HER-2/neu peptide based vaccine in cancer patients. J Clin Immunol. 2004;24(5):571–8.
135. Disis ML, Gooley TA, Rinn K, Davis D, Piepkorn M, Cheever MA, et al. Generation of T-cell immunity to the HER-2/neu protein after active immunization with HER-2/neu peptide-based vaccines. J Clin Oncol. 2002;20(11):2624–32.
136. Odunsi K, Qian F, Matsuzaki J, Mhawech-Fauceglia P, Andrews C, Hoffman EW, et al. Vaccination with an NY-ESO-1 peptide of HLA class I/II specificities induces integrated humoral and T cell responses in ovarian cancer. Proc Natl Acad Sci U S A. 2007;104(3):12837–42.
137. Rahma OE, Ashtar E, Czystowska M, Szajnik ME, Wieckowski E, Bernstein S, et al. A gynecologic oncology group phase II trial of two p53 peptide vaccine approaches: subcutaneous injection and intravenous pulsed dendritic cells in high recurrence risk ovarian cancer patients. Cancer Immunol Immunother. 2012;61(3):373–84.
138. Stockert E, Jäger E, Chen YT, Scanlan MJ, Gout I, Karbach J, et al. A survey of the humoral immune response of cancer patients to a panel of human tumor antigens. J Exp Med. 1998;187(8):1349–54.
139. Richards ER, Devine PL, Quin RJ, Fontenot JD, Ward BG, McGuckin MA. Antibodies reactive with the protein core of MUC1 mucin are present in ovarian cancer patients and healthy women. Cancer Immunol Immunother. 1998;46(5):245–52.
140. Chinni SR, Falchetto R, Gercel-Taylor C, Shabanowitz J, Hunt DF, Taylor DD. Humoral immune responses to cathepsin D and glucose-regulated protein 78 in ovarian cancer patients. Clin Cancer Res. 1997;3(9):1557–64.
141. Kim JH, Herlyn D, Wong KK, Park DC, Schorge JO, Lu KH, et al. Identification of epithelial cell adhesion molecule autoantibody in patients with ovarian cancer. Clin Cancer Res. 2003;9(13):4782–91.
142. Ho M, Hassan R, Zhang J, Wang QC, Onda M, Bera T, et al. Humoral immune response to mesothelin in mesothelioma and ovarian cancer patients. Clin Cancer Res. 2005;11(10):3814–20.
143. Chapman C, Murray A, Chakrabarti J, Thorpe A, Woolston C, Sahin U, et al. Autoantibodies in breast cancer: their use as an aid to early diagnosis. Ann Oncol. 2007;18(5):868–73.
144. Luo LY, Herrera I, Soosaipillai A, Diamandis EP. Identification of heat shock protein 90 and other proteins as tumour antigens by serological screening of an ovarian carcinoma expression library. Br J Cancer. 2002;87(3):339–43.
145. Naora H, Yang YQ, Montz FJ, Seidman JD, Kurman RJ, Roden RB. A serologically identified tumor antigen encoded by a homeobox gene promotes growth of ovarian epithelial cells. Proc Natl Acad Sci U S A. 2001;98:4060–5.
146. Kalli KR, Oberg AL, Keeney GL, Christianson TJ, Low PS, Knutson KL, Hartmann LC. Folate receptor alpha as a tumor target in epithelial ovarian cancer. Gynecol Oncol. 2008;108(3):619–26.
147. Kobayashi H, Terao T, Kawashima Y. Serum sialyl Tn as an independent predictor of poor prognosis in patients with epithelial ovarian cancer. J Clin Oncol. 1992;10(1):95–101.
148. Coosemans A, Vergote I, Van Gool SW. Wilms' tumor gene 1 immunotherapy in pelvic gynecological malignancies. Expert Rev Clin Immunol. 2014;10(6):705–11.
149. Scanlan MJ, Chen YT, Williamson B, Gure AO, Stockert E, Gordan JD, et al. Characterization of human colon cancer antigens recognized by autologous antibodies. Int J Cancer. 1998;76(5):652–8.
150. Bleul C, Muller M, Frank R, Gausepohl H, Koldovsky U, Mgaya HN, et al. Human papillomavirus

type 18 E6 and E7 antibodies in human sera: increased anti- E7 prevalence in cervical cancer patients. J Clin Microbiol. 1991;29(8):1579–88.
151. Muller M, Viscidi RP, Sun Y, Guerrero E, Hill PM, Shah F, et al. Antibodies to HPV-16 E6 and E7 proteins as markers for HPV-16-associated invasive cervical cancer. Virology. 1992;187(2):508–14.
152. Zhang L, Conejo-Garcia JR, Katsaros D, Gimotty PA, Massobrio M, Regnani G, et al. Intratumoral T cells, recurrence, and survival in epithelial ovarian cancer. N Engl J Med. 2003;348:203–13.
153. Hwang WT, Adams SF, Tahirovic E, et al. Progrostic significance of tumor infiltrating T cells in ovarian cancer: a meta-analysis. Gynecol Oncol. 2012; 124(2):192–8.
154. Sakaguchi S, Wing K, Onishi Y, Prieto-Martin P, Yamaquchi T. Regulatory T cells: how do they suppress immune responses? Int Immunol. 2009;21(10):1105–11.
155. Curiel TJ, Coukos G, Zou L, Alvarez X, Cheng P, Mottram P, et al. Specific recruitment of regulatory T cells in ovarian carcinoma fosters immune privilege and predicts reduced survival. Nat Med. 2004; 10(9):942–9.
156. Wang DP, Konishi I, Koshiyama M, Nanbu Y, Iwai T, Nonogaki H, et al. Immunohistochemical localization of c-erbB-2 protein and epidermal growth factor receptor in normal surface epithelium, surface inclusion cysts, and common epithelial tumours of the ovary. Virchows Arch A Pathol Anat Histopathol. 1992;421(5):393–400.
157. McCaughan H, Um I, Langdon SP, Harrison DJ, Faratian D. HER2 expression in ovarian carcinoma: caution and complexity in biomarker analysis. J Clin Pathol. 2012;65(7):670–1.
158. Lassus H, Leminen A, Vayrynen A, Cheng G, Gustafsson JA, Isola J, et al. ERBB2 amplification is superior to protein expression status in predicting patient outcome in serous ovarian carcinoma. Gynecol Oncol. 2004;92(1):31–9.
159. Felip E, Del Campo JM, Rubio D, Vidal MT, Colomer R, Bermejo B. Overexpression of c-erbB-2 in epithelial ovarian cancer. Prognostic value and relationship with response to chemotherapy. Cancer. 1995;75(8):2147–52.
160. Disis ML, Goodell V, Schiffman K, Knutson KL. Humoral epitope-spreading following immunization with a HER-2/neu peptide based vaccine in cancer patients. J Clin Immunol. 2004;24(5):571–8.
161. Disis ML, Dang Y, Coveler AL, Marzbani E, Kou ZC, Childs JS, et al. HER-2/neu vaccine-primed autologous T-cell infusions for the treatment of advanced stage HER-2/neu expressing cancers. Cancer Immunol Immunother. 2014;63(2):101–9.
162. Bookman MA, Darcy KM, Clarke-Pearson D, Boothby RA, Horowitz IR. Evaluation of monoclonal humanized anti-HER2 antibody, trastuzumab, in patients with recurrent or refractory ovarian or primary peritoneal carcinoma with overexpression of HER2: a phase II trial of the Gynecologic Oncology Group. J Clin Oncol. 2003;21(2):283–90.
163. Odunsi K, Matsuzaki J, Karbach J, Neumann A, Mhawech-Fauceglia P, Miller A, et al. Efficacy of vaccination with recombinant vaccinia and fowlpox vectors expressing NY-ESO-1 antigen in ovarian cancer and melanoma patients. Proc Natl Acad Sci U S A. 2012;109(15):5797–802.
164. Odunsi K, Matsuzaki J, James SR, Mhawech-Fauceglia P, Tsuji T, Miller A, et al. Epigenetic potentiation of NY-ESO-1 vaccine therapy in human ovarian cancer. Cancer Immunol Res. 2014;2(1):37–49.
165. Vierboom MPM, Nijman HW, Offringa R, van der Voort EL, van Hall T, van den Broek L, et al. Tumor eradication by wild-type p53-specific cytotoxic T lymphocytes. J Exp Med. 1997;186(5):695–704.
166. Zwaveling S, Vierboom MPM, Ferreira Mota SC, Hendriks JA, Ooms ME, Sutmuller RP, et al. Antitumor efficacy of wild-type p53-specific CD4+ T-helper cells. Cancer Res. 2002;62(21):6187–93.
167. Vermeij R, Leffers N, Hoogeboom BN, Hamming IL, Wolf R, Reyners AK, et al. Potentiation of a p53-SLP vaccine by cyclophosphamide in ovarian cancer: a single-arm phase II study. Int J Cancer. 2012;131(5):E670–80.
168. Rosenberg SA, Restifo NP, Yang JC, Morgan RA, Dudley ME. Adoptive cell transfer: a clinical path to effective cancer immunotherapy. Nat Rev Cancer. 2008;8(4):299–308.
169. Kershaw MH, Westwood JA, Parker LL, Wang G, Eshhar Z, Mavroukakis SA, et al. A phase I study on adoptive immunotherapy using gene-modified T cells for ovarian cancer. Clin Cancer Res. 2006;12(20):6106–15.
170. Geller MA, Cooley S, Judson PL, Ghebre R, Carson LF, Argenta PA, et al. A phase II study of allogeneic natural killer cell therapy to treat patients with recurrent ovarian and breast cancer. Cytotherapy. 2011;13(1):98–107.
171. Steinman RM, Banchereau J. Taking dendritic cells into medicine. Nature. 2007;449(7161):419–26.
172. Chu CS, Boyer J, Schullery DS, Gimotty PA, Gamerman V, Bender J, et al. Phase I/II randomized trial of dendritic cell vaccination with or with- out cyclophosphamide for consolidation therapy of advanced ovarian cancer in first or second remission. Cancer Immunol Immunother. 2012;61(5):629–41.
173. Brossart P, Wirths S, Stuhler G, Reichardt VL, Kanz L, Brugger W. Induction of cytotoxic T-lymphocyte responses in vivo after vaccinations with peptide-pulsed dendritic cells. Blood. 2000;96(9):3102–8.
174. Oregovomab: anti-CA-125 monoclonal antibody B43.13—AltaRex, B43.13, MAb B43.13, monoclonal antibody B43.13. Drugs R D 2006;7(6):379–83.
175. Liu B, Nash J, Runowicz C, Swede H, Stevens R, Li Z. Ovarian cancer immunotherapy: opportunities, progresses and challenges. J Hematol Oncol. 2010;3:7.
176. Mobus VJ, Baum RP, Bolle M, Kreienberg R, Noujaim AA, Schultes BC, et al. Immune responses

to murine monoclonal antibody-B43.13 correlate with prolonged survival of women with recurrent ovarian cancer. Am J Obstet Gynecol. 2003;189(1):28–36.
177. Tse C, Collins A, Oehler M, Zippelius A, Heinzelmann-Schwarz V. Antibody-based immunotherapy for ovarian cancer: where are we at? Ann Oncol. 2014;25(2):322–31.
178. Schultes BC, Baum RP, Niesen A, Noujaim AA, Madiyalakan R. Anti-idiotype induction therapy, anti-CA125 antibodies (Ab3) mediated tumor killing in patients treated with Ovarex mAb B43.13 (Ab1). Cancer Immunol Immunother. 1998;46(4):201–12.
179. Gordon AN, Schultes BC, Gallion H, Edwards R, Whiteside TL, Cermak JM, et al. CA125- and tumor-specific T-cell responses correlate with prolonged survival in oregovomab-treated recurrent ovarian cancer patients. Gynecol Oncol. 2004; 94(2):340–51.
180. Berek J, Taylor P, McGuire W, Smith LM, Schultes B, Nicodemus CF. Oregovomab maintenance monoimmunotherapy does not improve outcomes in advanced ovarian cancer. J Clin Oncol. 2009;27(3): 418–25.
181. Hodi FS, Butler M, Oble DA, Seiden MV, Haluska FG, Kruse A, et al. Immunologic and clinical effects of antibody blockade of cytotoxic T lymphocyte-associated antigen 4 in previously vaccinated cancer patients. Proc Natl Acad Sci U S A. 2008;105(8):3005–10.
182. Hurteau JA, Blessing JA, DeCesare SL, Creasman WT. Evaluation of recombinant human interleukin-12 in patients with recurrent or refractory ovarian cancer: a gynecologic oncology group study. Gynecol Oncol. 2001;82(1):7–10.
183. Vlad AM, Budiu RA, Lenzner DE, Wang Y, Thaller JA, Colonello K. A phase II trial of intraperitoneal interleukin-2 in patients with platinum-resistant or platinum-refractory ovarian cancer. Cancer Immunol Immunother. 2010;59(2):293–301.
184. Pardoll D. The blockade of immune checkpoints in cancer immunotherapy. Nat Rev Cancer. 2012; 12(4):252–64.
185. Topalian SL, Weiner GJ, Pardoll DM. Cancer immunotherapy comes of age. J Clin Oncol. 2011;29(36):4828–48.
186. Phan GQ, Yang JC, Sherry RM, Hwu P, Topalian SL, Schwartzentruber DJ, et al. Cancer regression and autoimmunity induced by cytotoxic T lymphocyte-associated antigen 4 blockade in patients with metastatic melanoma. Proc Natl Acad Sci U S A. 2003; 100(14):8372–7.
187. Ribas A, Camacho LH, Lopez-Berestein G, Pavlov D, Bulanhaqui CA, Millham R, et al. Antitumor activity in melanoma and anti-self-responses in a phase I trial with the anti-cytotoxic T lymphocyte-associated antigen 4 monoclonal antibody CP-675,206. J Clin Oncol. 2005; 23(35):8968–77.
188. Attia P, Phan GQ, Maker AV, Robinson MR, Quezado MM, Yang JC, et al. Autoimmunity correlates with tumor regression in patients with metastatic melanoma treated with anti-cytotoxic T-lymphocyte antigen-4. J Clin Oncol. 2005;23(25): 6043–53.
189. Hodi FS, Mihm MC, Soiffer RJ, Haluska FG, Bulter M, Seiden MV, et al. Biologic activity of cytotoxic T lymphocyte-associated antigen 4 antibody blockade in previously vaccinated metastatic melanoma and ovarian carcinoma patients. Proc Natl Acad Sci U S A. 2003;100(8):4712–7.
190. Hodi FS, Butler M, Oble DA, Seiden MV, Haluska FG, Kruse A, et al. Immunologic and clinical effects of antibody blockade of cytotoxic T lymphocyte-associated antigen 4 in previously vaccinated cancer patients. Proc Natl Acad Sci U S A. 2008;105(8): 3005–10.
191. Wallecha A, French C, Petit R, Singh R, Amin A, Rothman J. Lm-LLO-based immunotherapies and HPV-associated disease. J Oncol. 2012;2012: 542851.
192. Santin A, Bellone S, Palmieri M, Ravaggi A, Romani C, Tassi R, et al. HPV16/18 E7-pulsed dendritic cell vaccination in cervical cancer patients with recurrent disease refractory to standard treatment modalities. Gynecol Oncol. 2006;100(3): 469–78.
193. Kim SH, Castro F, Gonzalez D, Maciag PC, Paterson Y, Gravekamp C. Mage-b vaccine delivered by recombinant Listeria monocytogenes is highly effective against breast cancer metastases. Br J Cancer. 2008;99(5):741–9.
194. Maciag PC, Radulovic S, Rothman J. The first clinical use of a live-attenuated Listeria monocytogenes vaccine: a Phase I safety study of Lm-LLO-E7 in patients with advanced carcinoma of the cervix. Vaccine. 2009;27(30):3975–83.
195. Petit R, Mehta A, Jain M, Gupta S, Nagarkar R, Kumar V, et al. ADXS11-001 immunotherapy targeting HPV-E7: final results from a Phase II study in Indian women with recurrent cervical cancer. J Immunother Cancer. 2014;2 Suppl 3:92.

# Part IV

# Fertility Preservation in the Setting of Malignant Disease

# Preservation of Fertility in Gynecological Malignancies

7

Janos L. Tanyi

**Abstract**

Survival rate of reproductive aged women with gynecologic cancer has steadily been improving. As cancer therapy and cancers themselves may carry the risk of infertility and many of these young female cancer patients did not complete their family planning yet at the time of cancer diagnosis, fertility preservation has an emerging importance. Oncofertility is a rising concept requiring the contributions of both gynecologic oncology and reproductive medicine. All patients should be adequately informed at the time of diagnosis about the risk of infertility and the available methods for fertility preservation so they will have maximal chance to make an optimal decision without any significant impact and delay in oncologic outcome. The current treatment options for gynecologic malignancies include a wide variety of cytotoxic chemotherapy, different radiation treatments, multiple surgeries and anti-estrogen therapy, or any combination of these. Although these therapies can significantly reduce mortality, it can cause long-term toxicity, such as induction of an early menopause and fertility impairment even when the ovaries and the uterus left in place. At the present time, there are several potential options available including both standard and experimental assisted technologies. Embryo and sperm banking are the standard methods but many experts also count oocyte cryopreservation as a standard technique. Ovarian tissue harvesting, cryopreservation, and transplantation are safe but still believed as experimental as their utilization is still limited and their true value needs to be determined. Several pioneering procedures are being actively investigated, including uterus transplantation and in vitro follicle maturation, which may magnify

J.L. Tanyi, MD, PhD (✉)
Division of Gynecologic Oncology, Department of Obstetrics and Gynecology, University of Pennsylvania Health System,
3400 Civic Center Boulevard, 3rd Floor West Pavilion, Philadelphia, PA 19104, USA
e-mail: janos.tanyi@uphs.upenn.edu



A. Giordano, M. Macaluso (eds.), *Gynecological Cancers*, Current Clinical Oncology,
DOI 10.1007/978-3-319-32907-9_7

the number of fertility preservation options for young cancer patients in the future. It is with great importance to start to discuss fertility preservation options even in the gynecologic oncologist's office and initiate the referral to fertility specialists immediately. The application of structured psychosocial supportive care also helps these patients through of this demanding time. In this chapter, the current data and concepts regarding fertility preservation of female patients with gynecological malignancies are reviewed.

**Keywords**
Fertility preservation • Gynecological malignancies • Oncofertility • Trachelectomy • Embryo cryopreservation • Oocyte cryopreservation • Oophoropexy • Gonadal shielding • Gonadal suppression

## Introduction

A cancer diagnosis and the subsequent sometimes radical treatments in young female patients can cause limited fertility or even infertility. Approximately 10 % of all female cancer survivors are younger than 40 years of age [1]. For example, although infrequent, about 6–7 % of women with breast cancer are diagnosed <40 years in Western countries [2]. Overall, the number of young cancer survivors increases as more effective treatments are available. Currently, the 5-year survival rate for the 15- to 39-year age group has a wide distribution ranging from 23 % for stomach cancer to 99 % for thyroid cancer, with an overall average of 80 % [3]. Because of an increase in delay of first pregnancy due to cultural, professional, educational, and personal reasons, many of these young cancer survivors have not completed their families when diagnosed [4]. As such, most young cancer survivors end up living with the negative effects of cancer for a long time and the restricted fertility can be among these long-term effects. About 70 % of young cancer patients have the desire for childbearing therefore preserving fertility should be an essential part of their comprehensive treatment plan [5, 6]. It is well known that the probability of young cancer patients having children is reduced in contrast to the general population and furthermore, women are more affected than men [7]. Fertility preservation referred to as oncofertility is often the only option for cancer patients with a high risk of infertility to have offspring in the future [8]. The standard treatment of many gynecological cancers is removal of the uterus and adnexa even if this approach permanently harms the reproductive capacity of young women. This practice has slowly changed toward less radical surgeries in young women with early-stage gynecological cancer desiring future fertility. Not all patients diagnosed with gynecological cancer have the opportunity to discuss fertility preservation options before the start of treatment [9]. Oncofertility is a new, emerging concept and should be an integral part of everyday oncology practice. The future role of oncofertility is to help these patients in optimal decision making without significant delay and impact in their oncologic outcome. The main purpose of this review is to summarize the current data and methodology about oncofertility focusing from the gynecologic oncologic perspective.

## The Concept of Oncofertility

Oncofertility is a new area of specialized care that has brought great attention in the past decade. Historically, oncofertility has been relatively overlooked because the priority for its major beneficiaries—young patients with cancer—was longer survival. In the past, there were only few options available but with recent developments there is more reason for optimism nowadays.

Unfortunately, there is sparse knowledge about the real sensitivity of germ cells to the wide range of agents used for treating cancer and hematological or autoimmune diseases, and dietary factors or environmental hazards and tobacco [10, 11]. Thus it is difficult to predict which patient will benefit from the fertility preservation. The question arises whether oncofertility should be accepted as a new field or should stay within the domain of reproductive endocrinology and infertility. The concept of oncofertility was first proposed in 2006 in order to improve fertility outcomes of young adults who were diagnosed with cancer of any kind and are scheduled to undergo therapy for cancer [10]. In the same year, an Oncofertility Consortium, funded by National Institute of Health (NIH), was established. Oncofertility might be defined as "the application of surgical, medical, or laboratory procedures to preserve the potential for genetic parenthood in adults or children with cancer diagnosis who are at risk of sterility before the end of the natural reproductive lifespan." This endeavor should address both medical and social needs in circumstances where fertility is threatened by gonadotoxic agents used therapeutically. In 2006, Lee et al. with The American Society of Clinical Oncology (ASCO) published guidelines addressing the concept of oncofertilityand the necessity for early pretreatment counseling for young patients who will undergo cancer treatment [12]. Generally, sperm and embryo banking are the standard methods used for patients whose fertility under risk while oocyte banking and ovarian tissue cryopreservation are often considered experimental. On the contrary, the American Society of Reproductive Medicine (ASRM) currently states that oocyte cryopreservation is no longer considered to be experimental [1].

## The Impact of Cancer Therapies on the Reproductive Capability

In order to be independently fertile, a woman must have the following: a functioning neuroendocrine system that provides that capability to maintain a pregnancy; a healthy pool of ovarian follicles; and a receptive uterus that will support embryo implantation and fetal development to term [13]. It is well known that all women are born with approximately two million primordial follicles, but the number of follicles decreases to 500,000 at the onset of menarche by age 12 years. By the late thirties, this number falls to under 25,000, and when menopause occurs, it reaches around 1000 [14]. Cancer treatments decrease the number of primordial follicles which dictates a woman's reproductive lifespan. Since younger patients have a larger starting pool of follicles, they can tolerate larger doses of irradiation and chemotherapy compared with older patients before manifesting menopausal or infertility symptoms [14, 15].

## Radiation-Associated Damage

It is very difficult to predict how radiation will affect fertility. It is known that the reproductive consequences of radiotherapy are highly dependent on the dose, site, duration of exposure, frequency of treatments, and whether or not it is administered in isolation or in combination with chemotherapy [16]. Radiation therapy is used to treat multiple gynecological malignancies, causing ovarian damage and infertility by atrophy of the ovary and reduced primordial follicle reserve. The accepted dose at which half of the follicles are irreversibly lost in humans (LD50) is 4 Gy [17]. There are two ways that ionizing radiation damages the ovaries. First is the direct damage to DNA by photons, x-rays, gamma rays, and neutrons. The second is the indirect effects of radiation on other adjacent substances in the cell such as water leading to the formation of free radicals that cause DNA damage [18]. Many factors influence the degree of ovarian damage caused by ionizing radiation such as the patient's age, dose, type of radiation used and the length of radiation as well as use of concomitant chemotherapy [19]. Multiple forms of radiation treatment are administered in gynecologic oncology including external-beam radiation therapy, interstitial or intracavitary brachytherapy, and proton therapy. Radiation therapy is associated with increased risk of developing acute ovarian failure, particularly if both ovaries are within the radiation field.

Radiotherapy can damage follicles, targeting them for either repair or elimination [13, 20]. It is well known that actively dividing cells are more susceptible to radiation-induced damage and death, but oocytes in the young adult are arrested in prophase of meiosis I, so they are more resistant to radiation than cells in mitosis [13]. Primordial follicles, which are considered to be quiescent, show more resistance to radiation than growing follicles [13, 20]. Wallace et al. published the dose necessary to destroy 50 % of immature human oocytes (LD50) is less than 2 Gy [21]. Other studies published that the effective sterilizing dose of radiation was inversely correlated with age [18, 22]. At birth it is 20.3 Gy but it decreases to 16.5 Gy at age 20 [18]. Ovaries of younger women are more resistant to permanent damage from irradiation due to the higher number of primordial follicles [18]. In addition to causing ovarian damage, radiotherapy also has adverse effect on the uterus, causing decreased uterine blood flow, impaired uterine growth, and decreased uterine volume. These uterine changes not only impact fertility, but also increase the incidence of complications during pregnancy, such as premature labor, and low birth weight or even early fetal loss [23, 24]. Radiation, particularly targeting the head and neck area, can severely affect the function of the hypothalamus and pituitary axis [25, 26]. Rose et al. published cases of hypothalamic dysfunction after chemotherapy even in the absence of cranial irradiation [27].

## Chemotherapy-Associated Damage

Chemotherapy is administered to treat almost all malignancies and it also has a major effect on fertility. Regardless of the difficulty in foreseeing how chemotherapy will impact the reproductive axis, several main points can be stated. Chemotherapies have different mechanisms of action and different gonadotoxic capabilities. Overall, chemotherapeutic agents target dividing cells. However, most human follicles, though primordial, are arrested in meiotic division. Nonetheless, they can still be injured by chemotherapeutic drugs. The increase in follicle depletion during chemotherapy comes from the increased follicle sensitivity to the cytotoxic effects combined the given number of follicles that continue to undergo atresia during reproductive cycle until menopause [28]. The mechanism of action by which chemotherapy damages follicles is still unclear. Meirow et al. published a hypothesis that follicular apoptosis and follicular "burn out," are the possible mechanisms behind this phenomenon [29]. They hypothesized that there is an increased activation of follicles from the resting pool, causing an accelerated atresia, and premature burn-out of the primordial follicle reserve [29]. Furthermore, cortical fibrosis may develop when chemotherapy leads to hyalinization of cortical blood vessels called endarteritis obliterans, which results in cortical ischemia harming the growth and survival of primordial follicles [29]. Histological evidence of ovarian specimens revealed that chemotherapeutic drugs diminish the primordial follicle pool, promote ovarian atrophy, limit ovarian blood vasculature, decreased ovarian weight, and create stromal fibrosis [30, 31]. The number of studies evaluating the impact of chemotherapeutic drugs on ovaries is limited (Table 7.1) [32–41]. Following Docetaxel administration, poor follicle health was mainly due to effects on granulosa cells, demonstrating that the effects of Docetaxel on oocytes was possibly secondary to granulosa cell damage [37]. Docetaxel damages mainly growing follicles without direct effect on the primordial follicle reserve [37]. In mice, ovarian stroma cells exhibit an earlier DNA damage response than granulosa cells in response to drug accumulation of doxorubicin, however the granulosa cells are more sensitive, responding with greater levels of DNA damage [38]. Doxorubicin crosses the blood–follicle barrier and accumulates in oocytes and granulosa cells [36]. The mechanism of doxorubicin-induced apoptosis involves chromosomal disintegration, activation of the mitochondria followed by activation of PERK and caspase-12 and inactivation of PARP [36]. Intensive research is underway to evaluate preventive agents to decrease chemotherapy-induced follicle death. For example, sphingosine-1-phosphate (S1P), a ceramide-induced death

**Table 7.1** Impact of chemotherapy on the ovary and the human follicle reserve

| Agent | Impact on reproductive organs | References |
|---|---|---|
| Docetaxel alone | Granulosa cell damage, induction of somatic cell apoptosis | Lopes et al. [32] |
| Cyclophosphamide alone | Apoptosis in primordial follicles, oocytes, granulosa cells. Damaged granulosa cell nuclei in human. Follicle loss and apoptotic DNA fragmentation in the ovary | Oktem et al. [33]<br>Raz et al. [34]<br>Meng et al. [35]<br>Li et al. [36] |
| Doxorubicin alone | Apoptosis of primordial, pre-antral follicles, oocytes, granulosa cells, stroma, and blood vessels. Stroma cell-enriched populations exhibited an earlier DNA damage response than granulosa cells. Chromosomal disintegration, activation of the mitochondria | Roti Roti et al. [37]<br>Bar-Joseph et al. [38]<br>Li et al. [36] |
| Cyclophosphamide combined with vincristine and carmustine | Deterioration of the quality of the pre-antral follicles. Abnormalities in granulosa cell nuclei<br>Cortical fibrosis and blood vessels damage | Meirow et al. [39] |
| Non-sterilizing doses of alkylating and non-alkylating chemotherapy | Damage to cortical blood vessel and proliferation of small vessels. The cortex showed focal areas of fibrosis with disappearance of follicles. Decreased estrogen production. Decreased number of primordial follicles | Oktem et al. [40] |

pathway inhibitor, significantly reduced cyclophosphamide and doxorubicin-induced apoptotic follicle death in human ovarian xenografts [42]. The most damaging agents are the alkylating agents (notably cyclophosphamide, ifosfamide, nitrosoureas, chlorambucil, melphalan, busulfan, and procarbazine). One of the most studied is cyclophosphamide, which is used to treat many solid tumors as well as hematologic malignancies [43]. It is a member of the nitrogen mustard family and attacks an alkyl group to the guanine base of DNA and known to damage oocytes and granulosa cells in a dose-dependent manner [44]. Interestingly, cyclophosphamide is not cell cycle-specific therefore damage occurs at different stages of the cell cycle, including resting primordial follicles [44]. When cyclophosphamide was used in combination with other agents, deterioration in follicular quality was observed, manifested mainly as an increase in abnormal granulosa cell nuclei and in oocyte vacuolization [39]. Many other classes of chemotherapeutic drug groups include platinum derivatives (carboplatin, cisplatin, and oxalyplatin), antibiotics, antimetabolites, plant alkaloids, and taxanes are used for treatment. Carboplatin and cisplatin have also been shown to be gonadotoxic with an estimated odds ratio (OR) of 1.77 for ovarian failure [30]. The effects of latest targeted therapies, such as monoclonal antibody targeting neovascularization bevacizumab, are not known yet.

## Preservation of Female Fertility

Previously, gamete and embryo storage was the most frequently used and studied method of fertility preservation, however new options are available as research breakthroughs are translated into clinical practice (Table 7.2). According to The American Society of Clinical Oncology (ASCO) and The American Society of Reproductive Endocrinology (ASRM), sperm and embryo cryopreservation are still the recognized standard procedures for fertility preservation purposes for young women and men [12]. Other available options which still recognized as experimental but offered in health care facilities with special expertise and services in place will be also discussed in this chapter. As there are many fertility preservation options available today, individual patient-related characteristics will determine the best approach. These characteristics include a patient's age, pretreatment ovarian reserve, location of malignancy, the type and duration of adjuvant or neoadjuvant treatment.

**Table 7.2** Current options for fertility preservation in women

| Type | Method | Time requirements | Delay in cancer treatment |
|---|---|---|---|
| Surgical | Ovarian transposition | Immediate, outpatient procedure | No |
| | Trachelectomy | Immediate, inpatient procedure | No |
| | Ovarian tissue preservation | Immediate, outpatient procedure | Yes |
| | Ovarian tissue autologous transplant | Immediate, outpatient procedure | N/A |
| | Gonadal shielding | Concurrent with radiotherapy | No |
| | Uterus transplantation | After anticancer treatment | No |
| Non-surgical | Gonadal suppression with GnRH | Concurrent with chemotherapy | No |
| | Embryo cryopreservation | 10–14 days from menses | Yes |
| | Oocyte cryopreservation | 10–14 days from menses | Yes |
| | Development of ovarian follicle in vitro ovarian follicle culture | Experimental, different timing | N/A |
| Other | Progesterone treatment in early-stage endometrial cancer | 3–12 months | No |
| | Fertility sparing surgery in early-stage ovarian cancer | Immediate, in- or outpatient procedure | No |
| | Surrogacy | N/A | N/A |
| | Oocyte donation | N/A | No |

## Surgical Methods

### Ovarian Transposition (Oophoropexy)

Pelvic irradiation is a common treatment for cancer, specifically for cancers involving the lower genital tract. Pelvic irradiation can cause ovarian follicle depletion and cortical fibrosis as well as uterine damage resulting in pregnancy loss and premature labor. Alleviating these effects of radiation is of main importance in preserving fertility, and the two most frequently used techniques are ovarian transposition and gonadal shielding. Oophoropexy, also known as ovarian transposition (OT), is a relatively simple procedure of elevating and suspending the ovaries out from the pelvis and the future radiation field. Historically, ovaries are transposed behind uterus in Hodgkin's disease with extra pelvic shielding, however in cervical cancer ovaries should be transposed higher in lateral abdominal walls lateral to psoas muscles. The surgery should be performed before radiation therapy and can be done as an outpatient procedure or at the time of hysterectomy or other pelvic surgery. It is suggested that the ovaries should be moved out of any pelvic radiation field at least to the level above the pelvic brim [45]. Ovarian vessel pedicle length is limiting factor for upper distance of OT. In one study the lowest limit of transposed ovaries spared from RT was reported to be 1.5 cm above iliac crest. Locations lower than this point leaded to ovarian failure in higher rates [46]. Potential complications are pain because of ovarian torsion or cyst formation necessitating surgical interventions. It is suggested to mark the ovaries with surgical clips to determine the location when planning the radiotherapy field. Some experts suggest to repositioning the ovaries in a subsequent surgery to perform in vitro fertilization but spontaneous pregnancies have occurred and published without repositioning the ovaries back to their original location [47]. Functional ovaries with good blood supply do not need to be repositioned unless the patient is unable to conceive [47]. The rates of ovarian preservation with oophoropexy were reported as high as 90 % [48]. It is important to suspend the ovaries above the pelvic rim because under the pelvic rim the method has very low protective value and it reduces radiation exposure to the ovaries to only 5–10 % [49]. The most important factors causing failures are scatter radiation, radiation dose, vascular compromise, patient age, and whether the ovaries are shielded during the radiation procedure [50]. Published success rates are reported between 16 and 90 % and the most frequent complications were chronic pelvic pain, metastasis to the transposed ovaries and to surgical wounds [50, 51].

## Radical Trachelectomy

Contrary to radical hysterectomy, the gold standard for the radical trachelectomy (RT) is the vaginal approach (Dargent operation). RT is an available option for young women (<40 years) desiring to preserve fertility but the indications are strict (Table 7.3) [52]. RT is generally recommended for patients with tumor size less than or equal of 2 cm primarily located on the ectocervix (without endocervical lesion or extension). Metastatic workup should be negative including all pelvic lymph nodes and distant sites. The suggested stages are stage Ia1 with lymphovascular space involvement (LVSI) or stage Ia2 or Ib1 without LVSI. Currently, no histologic subtype is listed as a contraindication, although some view glandular lesions as higher risk and less support for neuroendocrine tumors. The procedure can be done vaginally or abdominally (by laparotomy, laparoscopy, or robotic-assisted route) but the vaginal approach with laparoscopic pelvic lymph node dissection gained greater popularity due to benefits of minimally invasive surgery. Technically, during RT half of the lower parametrium and paracolpos is excised and approximately two-thirds of cervix is removed. The uterine artery is saved and Doppler ultrasonograpy study should be done in order to evaluate a good uterine artery blood flow [53]. Morbidity associated with trachelectomy is low but includes infection, pelvic pain, and malodorous vaginal discharge. As intact cervix is requirement for a term pregnancy, the rate of preterm delivery increased after RT and a well-known morbidity of this surgery. The cancer recurrence and mortality rates were reported up to 5 % and 3.2 %, respectively [52, 54]. Mangler et al. reported a comprehensive follow-up study of 96 women after RT. Of these women 70 % tried to get pregnant and 80 % of these achieved pregnancy successfully. The rate of early pregnancy loss was 16 %. One-third of all who got pregnant suffered of preterm contractions and 43 % had premature rupture of membranes. The measured average cervical length of pregnant women after RT was 13 mm. Interestingly only the percentage

**Table 7.3** Fertility sparing in early endometrial, cervical and ovarian carcinomas

| Tumor type | Stage and histology | Consideration |
|---|---|---|
| Epithelial ovarian carcinomas | FIGO IA, clear cell cancer | Consider fertility sparing surgery: unilateral salpingo-oophorectomy |
| | FIGO IC, GI+II, serous, mucinous, endometrioid | Consider fertility sparing surgery: unilateral salpingo-oophorectomy |
| | FIGO IC, clear cell cancer | No fertility sparing surgery |
| | FIGO IA+IC, GIII | No fertility sparing surgery |
| Ovarian sex cord stromal tumors | FIGO stage I | Consider fertility sparing surgery: unilateral salpingo-oophorectomy |
| Ovarian germ cell tumors | FIGO stage I | Consider fertility sparing surgery: unilateral salpingo-oophorectomy |
| Endometrial carcinoma | Presumed stage IA, grade 1 with no myometrial invasion, nor extrauterine disease and no lymph node involvement | Consider progesterone treatment |
| Cervical carcinoma | Stage Ia1 with LVSI<br>Stage Ia2 or Ib1 without LVSI<br>Tumor size <2 cm<br>No evidence of lymph node metastases<br>No distant metastasis<br>No unfavorable histology (neuroendocrine) | Consider fertility sparing surgery: radical trachelectomy with lymphadenectomy |

*FIGO* The International Federation of Gynecology and Obstetrics, *LVSI* lymphovascular space involvement of premature rupture of membrane was increased compared to control group in the same gestational age, while the newborns' Apgar scores, cord pH values, weight and body length and duration of stay in the hospital were similar [55].

## Ovarian Tissue Preservation Followed by Autotransplantation

Although still considered to be experimental, ovarian tissue banking, where ovarian tissue is surgically removed and cryopreserved, is an alternative to other conventional methods [56]. The ovarian tissue can be later reimplanted, either at orthotopic (pelvis) or heterotopic sites (forearm, abdomen), after completion of the anticancer treatment in order to protect and restore reproductive function in female cancer patients [57]. Cryopreservation of ovarian tissue is a promising option for fertility preservation because it can be done without the need for ovarian stimulation and a sperm donor. It also can be the only suitable method to preserve fertility for prepubertal girls [56, 58], and also a favored option for single women, for women who cannot delay cancer treatment for stimulation, and women with hormone-sensitive malignancies [59]. The procedure is surgical removal and cryopreservation of small pieces of the ovarian cortex and each of these small cortex pieces can contain hundreds of primordial follicles [59]. The biggest challenge in this approach is to develop procedures to support the maturation of these primordial follicles to produce mature, fertilizable oocytes because most follicles that survive cryopreservation are the small primordial follicles [60]. The follicle viability and developmental potential is preserved following cryopreservation, thawing, and reimplantation [60] because the primordial follicles are much more tolerant of cryopreservation than mature oocytes due to their size, decreased metabolism, and absence of a metaphase spindle and the protective zona pellucida and cortical granules [61–64]. An alternative method is in vitro follicle maturation (IVM) procedure where the immature follicle cells within the cortical tissue are retrieved and matured in vitro. IVM followed by vitrification (fast freezing procedure in which crystal formation and cellular damage is prevented) of oocytes has resulted in four published successful live births to date [65, 66].

## Autologous Transplantation of Cryopreserved Ovarian Tissue

Autologous transplantation of cryopreserved ovarian tissue is gaining more and more popularity and is the only tissue banking approach that targets primarily women with premature ovarian failure (POF). One study reported 46 ovarian transplantations and 29 live births from 46 women, 16 of those live births were from women with autologous ovarian transplantation who received prior chemotherapy [67]. The first reported live births in humans was from patients previously treated for Hodgkin's lymphoma, in which cryopreserved thawed tissue was reimplanted into an intraperitoneal location adjacent to the atrophic ovaries [68]. In this procedure, cryopreserved and thawed cortical strips are transplanted back into the patient, to either an orthotopic or heterotopic site. Another report of a successful live birth following ovarian homolog autografting of cryopreserved tissue to the remaining ovary in a 28-year-old patient was published. This patient had the history of several years of ovarian failure following cancer treatment but she resumed spontaneous menstrual periods only 2 months after the transplantation [69]. Although, the relatively small piece of ovarian tissue has a limited endocrine function longer term. Heterotopic transplantation offers the advantages of accessibility for implantation and removal of the tissue if necessary and less need for anesthesia. Although there are successful animal models where fresh monkey ovarian tissue was transplanted to heterotopic sites, creating multiple oocytes and after fertilization resulted live birth, the human results are not as advanced yet [70]. In the human, several reports of heterotopic transplantation to the abdominal wall and forearm [71, 72] have confirmed that transplanted cortical strips lead to follicle development and resumption of menstrual cycling and resulted in the production of a four-cell embryo [71]. The major limitation of the autologous transplantation is the potential for ischemia before it can develop appropriate blood supply. This ischemia may result in the rejection of the tissue graft or follicle atresia [73]. Unfortunately, about 20 % of the grafts failed by 6 months [74, 75]. Multiple methods to prevent ischemia have been published including using angiogenesis-promoting factors, such as VEGF, or selecting a site of implantation known to be responsive to angiogenesis [74]. Theoretical concerns regarding ovarian transplantation is the risk of reintroducing malignant cells to the patient after completing cancer treatment however, this risk varies with cancer type and stage, along with the number of malignant cells transferred [75, 76]. In animal models, when these human ovaries were transplanted to immunosuppressed mice tumor development was detected in the peritoneal cavity [77]. Another controversial alternative is the uterus transplantation. Up to the present time only two reports of uterus transplantation were published, one from cadaver and other from live donor [78, 79]. Over the last two decades there was tremendous effort invested into uterine transplantation and after the first few transplantations there have been no successful clinical pregnancy achieved [79–81]. The very first human live birth after uterus transplantation was just reported in 2014 [82]. This report is a proof-of-concept for uterus transplantation and in the future it can be a treatment option for uterine factor infertility [82]. This report presents that in 2013, a 35-year-old woman with congenital absence of the uterus (Rokitansky syndrome) underwent transplantation of the uterus donated by a living, 61-year-old, two-parous woman. The recipient and the donor had essentially uneventful postoperative recoveries and she had her first menstruation occurred 43 days after transplantation and she continued to menstruate regularly. The recipient and her partner had 11 embryos cryopreserved and 12 months after transplantation, the recipient underwent her first single embryo transfer, which resulted in a living pregnancy. She was kept on continuous immunosuppression (tacrolimus, azathioprine, and corticosteroids) during the entire pregnancy but there were three episodes of mild rejection which all were reversed by corticosteroid treatment. Fetal growth parameters and blood flows of the uterine arteries and umbilical cord were normal throughout pregnancy. At the 32nd week of the pregnancy caesarean section was performed because of abnormal fetal heart rate and pre-eclampsia and a healthy preterm male infant was born with 1175 g weight and with APGAR scores 9, 9, and 10 [82]. Indeed, it was a great success and the future of uterus transplantation is promising although many details are still unsolved such as the use of high doses of immune-suppressants which increases the risk of recurrence.

## Gonadal Shielding

Gonadal shielding is a method that uses lead or bismuth plates to externally cover the gonads in order to reduce their exposure to radiation. In the past, ovaries are transposed behind uterus in Hodgkin's disease with extra pelvic shielding, however this historic method had limited protection. The combination of gonadal shielding with ovarian transposition during radiation therapy can even further diminish the dose of radiation delivered to the reproductive organs. Expertise of the radiation oncologist is required to ensure that the shielding is appropriately placed and does not increase the dose delivered to reproductive organs [83].

## Non-surgical Methods

### Gonadal Suppression

Oral contraceptives were the first hormonal method to be used for gonadal suppression but they do not completely inhibit the follicular growth [84, 85]. Stronger ovarian suppression can be achieved with gonadotropin-releasing hormone analogs (GnRH) and this is the most commonly used method of hormonal suppression today [86]. Ovarian suppression with GnRH agonists (GnRHa) is noninvasive and is mostly used in the case of non-gynecological malignancies. The exact mechanism by which GnRHa protects the ovary during chemotherapy is still under debate. Some hypothesize that GnRHa causes ovarian suppression and non-cycling cells are then generally more resistant to chemotherapeutic agents than the rapidly proliferating cells. It has also been proposed that GnRHa provides ovarian protection by reducing the ovarian blood flow. Uterine blood flow has been shown to be reduced after administration of GnRHa and it effectively decreases the quantity of chemotherapy drugs reaching the ovary [87]. Another theory is that the protective effect of GnRH manifested by inhibiting the hypothalamic–pituitary–ovarian (HPO) axis and inducing a prepubertal state. Physiologically in humans, GnRH is secreted in a pulsatile fashion, stimulating gonadotropin release that initiates the ovulatory cycle and ovarian steroidogenesis. When GnRH agonists are administered, the surge in GnRH overwhelms the pituitary GnRH receptors, results in a subsequent downregulation of the pituitary GnRH receptors and decrease in gonadotropin release. The continuous inhibition of the pituitary–ovarian axis will decrease the estrogen level down to a pre-pubertal level [88]. Although these theories are all persuading there are conflicting results from different studies which require further clarifications. One study found no effect of GnRH agonists of restoration of menses after chemotherapy [64, 89, 90], while another recent study showed the ovarian failure rate was significantly decreased in women undergoing chemotherapy for non-gynecologic malignancy with the use of GnRH agonists [91]. All of these studies used menstrual cycles as the representation of ovarian function, although ultrasonographic evaluation of antral follicles would have been a better indicator. A randomized study of 18 women with Hodgkin's disease where GnRH was administered prior to and during chemotherapy concluded that it was an ineffective method to conserve fertility [92]. On the contrary, another study showed the co-administration of GnRHa with chemotherapy in women for 6 months led to the return of regular menses and ovulation in 96.9 % of women versus only 63 % of women treated with chemotherapy alone [93]. In a meta-analysis, Megan et al. concluded that concurrent administration of GnRH analogs increases the chances of maintaining ovarian function and childbearing potential by 65–68 % over chemotherapy alone [94]. Although gonadal suppression with GnRH analogs in patients undergoing chemotherapy is controversial, the risks and benefits of success rates and known side effects of hypoestrogenism and osteoporosis should be discussed with the patient. The American Society of Clinical Oncology (ASCO) urges women to participate in clinical trial to collect more knowledge about the protective effect of GnRH analogs on gonadal function during chemotherapy as the available literature still presents insufficient evidence [12].

## Embryo Cryopreservation

The mainstay of fertility preservation is the low temperature banking of reproductive cells or embryos. Previously this has been done using a slow freezing technique but more recently vitrification is the preferred methodology. The novel advance of the field started with a discovery in the 1950s when glycerol cryoprotective properties were identified. By the 1960s, human semen was being cryopreserved, and multiple sperm banks were established the following years [95]. Today, embryo cryopreservation is the most established and widespread technique for fertility preservation in women. The method has been available since 1983 and the first live birth as a result of embryo freezing was published in 1984 [96, 97].

The process of embryo cryopreservation for fertility preservation is identical to the IVF process used in infertile women. First involves induction of superovulation with FSH and hCG injections, serial blood tests, and ultrasounds to monitor follicle development. Multifollicular growth is stimulated by these exogenous gonadotropins and the oocytes are retrieved about 14–21 days later as an outpatient procedure under ultrasonographic guidance. The retrieved oocytes are fertilized with sperm and the good quality embryos are selected in 3–4 days later and frozen down for later use. Today, as advanced reproductive technologies are available such us in vitro fertilization with embryo transfer (IVF-ET), these embryos can be used later when all cancer treatments are completed. Several studies evaluated the outcome of embryo cryopreservation and found that generally the number of oocytes was lower in cancer patients but the live birth rates were the same [98, 99]. Limitation of this technique is that embryo cryopreservation is not appropriate for children, young adults without a partner, and those patients who do not desire to use donor sperm. Furthermore, this method requires couple of weeks delay in the onset of cancer therapy as hormonal stimulation and oocyte retrieval should be completed first [100]. In established IVF cycles, hormonal stimulation is started in luteal phase of menstrual cycle with GnRH agonists and completed with exogenous gonadotropins in early follicular phase. As patients can be anywhere in their cycles, sometimes delay is inevitable. Another pitfall of ovarian stimulation is that in patients with hormone-sensitive malignancies, such as breast, endometrial or ovarian cancers, there is the further concern regarding the presence of ER and PR receptors on the tumor cells and the safety of ovarian stimulation because of the high estradiol levels [101]. For these women, the use of aromatase inhibitors can be an option to minimize supra physiologic estrogen exposure [102, 103]. Studies proved that application of Letrozole along with gonadotropins did not worsen oocyte yield or fertilization rates [104]. Women who do not want to delay their cancer treatment or they do not have an actual male partner there is another technique than embryo cryopreservation is available called oocyte vitrification.

## Oocyte Cryopreservation/ Vitrification

The cryopreservation and banking of human semen was spread very quickly in the 1960s and 1970s and the first case of oocyte banking was reported shortly thereafter, but this cell type turned out to be more problematic to cryopreserve [105]. Concern about the biological safety of the technology was quickly raised when evidence was published that cooling caused various oocyte defects [106]. The technique of oocyte cryopreservation is the collecting and freezing of unfertilized mature eggs from reproductive aged women. There are two cooling mechanisms known: slow freezing and vitrification. For oocyte freezing, similar to embryo cryopreservation, the oocytes are first exposed to low concentrations of permeating cryoprotectants (glycerol, DMSO, ethylene glycol, propylene glycol), and non-permeating factors such as sucrose, glucose, or fructose. The oocytes are then loaded in small volumes into straws and cooled to about −5 to −7 °C where they equilibrate for several minutes. Following this process the solution is cooled gradually, at a speed of 0.3–0.5 °C/min, to reach temperature between −30 and −65 °C. Long-term storage happens in liquid nitrogen thereafter [107]. Although the first live birth as a result of oocyte freezing was occurred in 1986, the method of oocyte cryopreservation was not well accepted due to technical challenges [105]. Up to 2004, only 150 pregnancies were created from cryopreserved oocytes [108]. Although the first problem of oocyte cryopreservation, the hardening of the zona pellucida was quickly solved when the emerging new technologies such as intracytoplasmic sperm injection was introduced but the survival rates of the oocytes continued to be very low and only over the last couple of years reached to 70–80 % [109, 110]. Freezing of oocytes remains to be a huge need for women without male partners, and despite continuing debate about its efficiency, it is likely to stay available for a long period of time. Over the last couple of years, vitrification started to replace cryopreservation as it is an ultra-rapid cooling that minimizes cell injury and the formation of ice crystals resulting in survival rates >90 % [111]. The process of vitrification is the combination of two steps: a preliminary equilibration step similar to cryopreservation and a subsequent vitrification phase in which cells undergo a high osmotic gradient that completes cells' dehydration followed by the ultra-rapid cooling with liquid nitrogen. The warming of oocytes must be just as rapid in order to prevent recrystallization of water.

The same cryoprotectants are used during both slow freezing and vitrification but the second procedure requires higher concentrations of the protectants [112]. The introduction of vitrification made a significant impact on techniques of oocyte preservation, with an increase to about 900 published live births worldwide, of which an estimated 500 live births from oocyte preservation occurred in the United States [113, 114].

## In Vitro Ovarian Follicle Development, Ovarian Follicle Culture, and Maturation

In vitro follicle culture is the most promising and state-of-the-art technique of assisted reproductive technology. The big advantage of this alternative approach is that the follicle maturation happens in vitro and so excludes the need of ovarian tissue transplant and therefore eliminates the risk of reimplanting cancer cells into the patient. Follicle development and maturation is a multifaceted process that requires complex communication network between the oocyte, the hormonal milieu, and presence of the adjacent, supportive somatic cells. At each stage of follicle growth and maturation, the oocyte is dependent on the follicular granulosa cells and the communication between the oocyte and the surrounding somatic supportive cells. The recreation of this complex network outside of the human body brought new challenges and required extensive research to reach the point where it is today. The in vitro ovarian follicle culture systems are titled as two- and three-dimensional culture systems and as organ culture or single cell system culture. The two-dimensional systems which are not so frequently used nowadays are less optimal for culture because of their inability to maintain the structural arrangements of cells as seen in vivo. In the original two-dimensional culture systems, the follicles were located on a flat surface in the culture dish and lost their three-dimensional arrangement [115]. The major problem of the two-dimensional systems were that these systems were not able to create the architecture between the oocyte, granulosa cells and supportive somatic cells and pertinent communication links between the cellular elements become disrupted, thereby impeding oocyte growth and maturation [10]. The three-dimensional culture systems revolutionized the field when the biomaterial alginate was introduced which makes the cellular microenvironment more similar to in vivo by preserving cellular spatial arrangements, growth, and communication with surrounding cells with the oocyte. This system utilizes alginate, a hydrogel derived from brown algae which cross-links in the presence of divalent cations such as $Ca^{2+}$ but can be degraded for follicle recovery using an alginate-specific enzyme, alginate lyase. One of the major advantages of alginate is that it does not interact biochemically with mammalian cells, therefore permitting the creation of a culture environment where follicles can grow, produce antral cavities and mature oocytes [116–119]. The three-dimensional culture system was tested experimentally using follicles from multiple species including humans [57, 73, 75, 76, 78, 120] and follicles from three-dimensional cultures were successfully fertilized, implanted, and produced healthy pups in mice experiments [121]. Adjuvant treatments, hormones, and enzymes such as insulin, selenium, and transferrin are added in order to regulate growth, help the cell interactions just as in a physically supported environment. In spite of the impressive development, there are still scientific obstacles in this technology which makes it currently unable to grow immature human follicles through terminal meiotic maturation when they can be fertilized and transferred to the female recipient [10]. Early experiments created viable, healthy human follicles that were able to grown in vitro for 30 days and these results hold tremendous promise [122].

The other two approaches are the organ culture and the isolated follicle culture. Organ culture is the removal and culture of strips from the ovarian cortex. These tissue pieces are removed laparoscopically and keep the original structure of the ovarian tissue and maintain the interactions between the follicle and adjacent stromal cells. Human primordial follicles developed through secondary follicle stage and were able to survive as long as 4 weeks with the usage of this organ culture [79, 80, 120]. The main problem with in vitro organ culture is the development of ischemia as there is revascularization in the in vitro culture. Another disadvantage is the inability to observe and follow the follicles during culture by microscopy due to the surrounding tissue and the risk of culturing empty tissue pieces, especially when the patients have decreased ovarian reserve due to age, disease, or previous cancer therapy [76]. The isolated follicle culture involves a process where the individual follicles are removed from the surrounding cortical tissue prior to culture. The follicles are isolated from the ovary through an enzymatic or mechanical approach. This culture system allows for the investigator to follow and monitor each single follicle during the maturation process. This isolated follicle cultures can be done on two-dimensional collagen-coated surfaces or in three-dimensional methods as explained above.

## Special Situations for Fertility Sparing in Gynecologic Oncology

### Hormonal Treatment in Endometrial Hyperplasia or Early Endometrial Carcinoma

Roughly 5 % of women with endometrial cancer (EC) and an even higher percentage with complex atypical endometrial hyperplasia (CAH) are diagnosed under the age of 40 [123]. As the age of the first pregnancy increases, the incidence of EC in women still considering future childbearing will increase. For many of these younger women, hysterectomy as a standard of care is completely unacceptable due to strong desire to maintain fertility. Most of these ECs under age 40 years of age are still in early-stage and low-grade disease (grade 1) which associated with a favorable prognosis and allows the practitioner some time to apply medical management [124–126]. The use of progesterone-based agents proved to be safe but the careful patient selection is critical (Table 7.3). The optimal candidates are those patients who have early-stage, well-differentiated (presumed grade 1 and stage IA) disease without lymph node involvement, myometrial invasion, and extrauterine spread. The first step after the histologic confirmation of the disease, an imaging, usually MRI or ultrasound should be done to rule out myometrial invasion and lymph node metastasis. Patients without myometrial invasion and lymph node involvement are thought to be the best candidates for this treatment which can include theoretically patients with stage II diseases. Most of the gynecologic oncologists do not support progesterone treatment on young women with stage II diseases as the recurrence rate is extremely high [127]. Progestin therapy, most frequently with medroxyprogesterone acetate or megestrol acetate, has been effective in reversing malignant changes in up to 76 % of cases [125, 126]. In a study by Ramirez et al., 81 patients with grade 1 EC were treated and 62 patients (76 %) responded to treatment with a median time to response of 12 weeks (range, 4–60 weeks) [126]. Unfortunately, the recurrence rate was high, 15 patients (24 %) who initially responded to treatment recurred with a median time to recurrence was 19 months (range, 6–44 months [126]. Most of the experts suggest hysterectomy shortly after the childbearing plans are accomplished because of the high recurrence rate. There is a recently more frequently applied alternative of the oral or injectable progesterones, the progestin-based intrauterine devices, although the data are limited. A prospective pilot study reported negative histology on follow-up biopsy in seven of 11 patients at 6 months, and in six of eight patients at 12 months who underwent the progesterone IUD placement secondary to presumed stage IA, grade 1 EC [128]. Westin et al. conducted a phase 2 study with levonorgestrel intrauterine system (LIUS) to treat CAH and grade 1 EC [129]. Although the overall response rate in 1 year was only 58 % but when divided by histology, response rate was 85 % for CAH and 33 % for EEC [129]. Another systematic review showed 74 % of the patients with CAH achieved a pathological complete response (CR) for 6 months or longer with oral progestins [130]. It is very important that if the response should be considered temporary or incomplete, periodic sampling of the endometrium is strongly advised. Penner and colleagues suggested that lack of response to progestin therapy is more common when the first response assessment (after 3 months of treatment) shows lack of response, despite adjacent stromal decidualization [131]. There are many agents tested such as megestrol acetate, hydroxyprogesterone acetate, 17a-hydroxyprogesterone caproate, norethindrone, but usually the medroxyprogesterone acetate (MPA) is the most commonly used. The suggested treatment time is 3–6 months but can be extended up to 12 months. The usually given daily dose is 200–800 mg of MPA or 40–200 mg of Megestrol acetate. Other "progesterone-like drugs" such as gonadotropin-releasing hormone agonists, aromatase inhibitors, and selective estrogen receptor modulators were all reported to be similarly effective. The close follow-up of these women in every 3 months are very important and should be done by gynecologic oncologists.

## Fertility Preservation in Early Ovarian Cancer

The patients with epithelial ovarian cancer (EOC) are usually diagnosed in postmenopausal years and only very few of them are in the reproductive ages. About 7 % of these patients are under 40 and over 60 % of them have stage I disease at the time of diagnosis [132]. Amongst those younger patients who wish to preserve her childbearing potential and who appears to have a curable cancer (i.e., a localized tumor with endometrioid, mucinous, or low-grade serous histology), it is appropriate to save the uterus and the contralateral ovary and perform a fertility saving surgery, only a unilateral salpingo-oophorectomy. Fertility preservation is suggested with stage IA clear cell carcinoma or stage IC, Grade 1 and 2 serous, mucinous or endometrioid carcinomas. No fertility sparing surgery allowed in the case of stage IB or IC clear cell carcinoma or any subtype of ovarian cancer if it is a stage IC grade 3 [133]. If in spite of this fact the patient still wishes to retain fertility with disease extending beyond IA grade 1, 2, she should be warned and extensively consented about the high possibility of recurrences [134]. The remaining ovary and the whole abdominal cavity should be carefully evaluated and any abnormalities should be biopsied during surgery and sent for frozen section. If the frozen section is uncertain whether the tumor is benign, borderline, or malignant, the final histology should be awaited and the staging procedure needs to be done in second setting. If both ovaries contain invasive tumor on frozen section ovarian preservation is usually not allowed. For non-epithelial (sex cord stromal and germ cell tumors) tumors, fertility-sparing surgery with unilateral salpingo-oophorectomy is acceptable for patients with stage IA disease who wish to preserve of their reproductive capabilities. A comprehensive review of 376 patients with ovarian sex cord stromal tumors found no survival differences between patients with stage I–II disease who underwent fertility sparing surgery without hysterectomy and patients who underwent standard surgery [135]. Borderline ovarian tumors are relatively rare and usually occur about 15 years earlier than EOC. Most of the patients with borderline tumors are diagnosed in early stage and because of the generally favorable prognosis fertility preservation such unilateral salpingo-oophorectomy or ovarian cystectomy is the preferred approach by most of the gynecologic oncologists [136].

## Conclusion

Usually cancer treatments have the potential to harm all measures of the female reproductive axis, thus pushing patients into premature menopause or infertility. In the past, a cancer diagnosis was equivalent with losing all future childbearing potential. The growing numbers of children and reproductive-age women surviving cancer have resulted in an increased attention about fertility preservation. Fertility preservation, as nowadays called oncofertility is a newly described concept, an emerging and rapidly expanding field of medical research. Oncofertility is an interdisciplinary field that was created not only to try to reach fertility preservation options for cancer patients but also to increase nationwide awareness of these possibilities. Oncofertility requires a team-based approach where gynecologic oncologists and reproductive endocrinologists need to unite their effort to provide the highest quality care for their young patients. The recently formed oncofertility consortium is a great platform of this endeavor. Gynecologic oncologist has a unique position to be the advocate of their patients and be the first who provides critical information to the patient about the available fertility preservation options. There is a crucial need for new clinical trials to elucidate controversial issues such as application of aromatase inhibitors during ovulation induction of patients with hormone-sensitive cancer or GnRH agonists in ovarian preservation during chemotherapy. There is urgent need to develop more site-specific, targeted oncologic treatments which have significantly less adverse effect on the healthy reproductive organs. The great improvement of the reproductive technology over the past decades widened the horizon for patient to preserve their future ability to be a parent after successful cancer treatment. It is expected that the great development in complex culture systems, in tissue preservation techniques, and organ transplantation will make oocyte preservation, ovarian tissue banking, and ovarian or even uterus transplantation available in the near future.

## References


1. Dursun P, Dogan NU, Ayhan A. Oncofertility for gynecologic and non-gynecologic cancers: fertility sparing in young women of reproductive age. Clin Rev Oncol Hematol. 2014;92:258–67.
2. DeSantis C, Siegel R, Bandi P, Jemal A. Breast cancer statistics, 2011. Cancer J Clin. 2011;61:409–18.
3. Gondos A, Hiripi E, Holleczek B, et al. Survival among adolescents and young adults with cancer in Germany and the United States: an international comparison. Int J Cancer. 2013;133:2207e15.
4. Cooke A, Mills TA, Lavender T. 'Informed and uninformed decision making' – women's reasoning, experiences and perceptions with regard to advanced maternal age and delayed childbearing: a meta-synthesis. Int J Nurs Stud. 2010;47:1317–29.
5. Schover LR. Patient attitudes toward fertility preservation. Pediatr Blood Cancer. 2009;53:281e4.
6. Gardino SL, Russell AE, Woodruff TK. Adoption after cancer: adoption agency attitudes and perspectives on the potential to parent post-cancer. Cancer Treat Res. 2010;156:153e70.
7. Magelssen H, Melve KK, Skjaerven R, et al. Parenthood probability and pregnancy outcome in patients with a cancer diagnosis during adolescence and young adulthood. Hum Reprod. 2008;23:178e86.
8. Kim SS. Fertility preservation in female cancer patients: current developments and future directions. Fertil Steril. 2006;85:1e11.
9. Forman EJ, Anders CK, Behera MA. A nationwide survey of oncologists regarding treatment-related infertility and fertility preservation in female cancer patients. Fertil Steril. 2010;94(5):1652–6.
10. Woodruff TK. The oncofertility consortium—addressing fertility in young people with cancer. Nat Rev Clin Oncol. 2010;7(8):466–75.
11. Soares SR, Melo MA. Cigarette smoking and reproductive function. Curr Opin Obstet Gynecol. 2008;20(3):281–91.
12. Lee SJ, Schover LR, Partridge AH, Patrizio P, Wallace WH, Hagerty K, et al. American Society of Clinical Oncology recommendations on fertility preservation in cancer patients. J Clin Oncol. 2006;24(18):2917–31.
13. Duncan FE, Jozefik JK, Kim AM, Hirshfeld-Cytron J, Woodruff TK. The gynecologist has a unique role in providing oncofertility care to young cancer patients. US Obstet Gynecol. 2011;6(1):24–34.
14. Faddy MJ, Gosden RG, Gougeon A, et al. Accelerated disappearance of ovarian follicles in midlife: implications for forecasting menopause. Hum Reprod. 1992;7:1342–6.
15. Bath LE, Wallace WHB, Critchley HOD. Late effects of the treatment of childhood cancer on the female reproductive system and the potential for fertility preservation. BJOG. 2002;109: 107–14.
16. Critchley HO. Factors of importance for implantation and problems after treatment for childhood cancer. Med Pediatr Oncol. 1999;33:9–14.
17. Wallace WH, Shalet SM, Hendry JH, Morris-Jones PH, Gattamaneni HR. Ovarian failure following abdominal irradiation in childhood: the radiosensitivity of the human oocyte. Br J Radiol. 1989;62(743):995–8.
18. Wallace WH, Thomson AB, Saran F, Kelsey TW. Predicting age of ovarian failure after radiation to a field that includes the ovaries. Int J Radiat Oncol Biol Phys. 2005;62(3):738–44.
19. Meirow D, Nugent D. The effects of radiotherapy and chemotherapy on female reproduction. Hum Reprod Update. 2001;7(6):535–43.
20. Ogilvy-Stuart AL, Shalet SM. Effect of radiation on the human reproductive system. Environ Health Perspect. 1993;101 Suppl 2:109–16.
21. Wallace WHB, Thomson AB, Kelsey TW. The radiosensitivity of the human oocyte. Hum Reprod. 2003;18:117–21.
22. Langan RC, Prieto PA, Sherry RM, Zlott D, Wunderlich J, Csako G, Costello R, White DE, Rosenberg SA, Yang JC. Assessment of ovarian function after preparative chemotherapy and total body radiation for adoptive cell therapy. J Immunother. 2011;34(4):397–402.

23. Critchley HO, Bath LE, Wallace WH. Radiation damage to the uterus – review of the effects of treatment of childhood cancer. Hum Fertil (Camb). 2002;5:61–6.
24. Agha A, Sherlock M, Brennan S, et al. Hypothalamic-pituitary dysfunction after irradiation of nonpituitary brain tumors in adults. J Clin Endocrinol Metab. 2005;90:6355–60.
25. Constine LS, Woolf PD, Cann D, et al. Hypothalamic-pituitary dysfunction after radiation for brain tumors. N Engl J Med. 1993;328:87–94.
26. Rose SR, Schreiber RE, Kearney NS, et al. Hypothalamic dysfunction after chemotherapy. J Pediatr Endocrinol Metab. 2004;17:55–66.
27. Reynaud K, Driancourt MA. Oocyte attrition. Mol Cell Endocrinol. 2000;163(1-2):101–8.
28. Meirow D, Biederman H, Anderson RA, Wallace WH. Toxicity of chemotherapy and radiation on female reproduction. Clin Obstet Gynecol. 2010;53(4):727–39.
29. Meirow D. Reproduction post-chemotherapy in young cancer patients. Mol Cell Endocrinol. 2000;169(1-2):123–31.
30. Nicosia SV, Matus-Ridley M, Meadows AT. Gonadal effects of cancer therapy in girls. Cancer. 1985;55(10):2364–72.
31. Soleimani R, De Sutter P. In situ identification of follicles in ovarian cortex as a tool for quantifying follicle density, viability and developmental potential in strategies to preserve female fertility. Hum Reprod. 2011;26(4):955–6.
32. Lopes F, Smith R, Anderson RA, Spears N. Docetaxel induces moderate ovarian toxicity in mice, primarily affecting granulosa cells of early growing follicles. Mol Hum Reprod. 2014;20(10):948–59.
33. Oktem O, Oktay K. A novel ovarian xenografting model to characterize the impact of chemotherapy agents on human primordial follicle reserve. Cancer Res. 2007;67(21):10159–62.
34. Raz A, Fisch B, Okon E, Feldberg D, Nitke S, Raanani H, Abir R. Possible direct cytotoxicity effects of cyclophosphamide on cultured human follicles: an electron microscopy study. J Assist Reprod Genet. 2002;19(10):500–6.
35. Meng Y, Xu Z, Wu F, Chen W, Xie S, Liu J, Huang X, Zhou Y. Sphingosine-1-phosphate suppresses cyclophosphamide induced follicle apoptosis in human fetal ovarian xenografts in nude mice. Fertil Steril. 2014;102(3):871–7.
36. Li F, Turan V, Lierman S, Cuvelier C, De Sutter P, Oktay K. Sphingosine-1-phosphate prevents chemotherapy-induced human primordial follicle death. Hum Reprod. 2014;29(1):107–13.
37. Roti Roti EC, Leisman SK, Abbott DH, Salih SM. Acute doxorubicin insult in the mouse ovary is cell- and follicle-type dependent. PLoS One. 2012;7(8), e42293.
38. Bar-Joseph H, Ben-Aharon I, Rizel S, Stemmer SM, Tzabari M, Shalgi R. Doxorubicin-induced apoptosis in germinal vesicle (GV) oocytes. Reprod Toxicol. 2010;30(4):566–72.
39. Meirow D, Dor J, Kaufman B, Shrim A, Rabinovici J, Schiff E, Raanani H, Levron J, Fridman E. Cortical fibrosis and blood-vessels damage in human ovaries exposed to chemotherapy. Potential mechanisms of ovarian injury. Hum Reprod. 2007;22(6):1626–33.
40. Oktem O, Oktay K. Quantitative assessment of the impact of chemotherapy on ovarian follicle reserve and stromal function. Cancer. 2007;110(10):2222–9.
41. Abir R, Ben-Haroush A, Felz C, Okon E, Raanani H, Orvieto R, Nitke S, Fisch B. Selection of patients before and after anticancer treatment for ovarian cryopreservation. Hum Reprod. 2008;23(4):869–77.
42. Waxman J. Chemotherapy and the adult gonad: a review. J R Soc Med. 1983;76(2):144–8.
43. Koyama H, Wada T, Nishizawa Y, Iwanaga T, Aoki Y. Cyclophosphamide-induced ovarian failure and its therapeutic significance in patients with breast cancer. Cancer. 1977;39(4):1403–9.
44. Kurt M, Uncu G, Cetintas SK, Kucuk N, Guler S, Ozkan L. Successful spontaneous pregnancy in a patient with rectal carcinoma treated with pelvic radiotherapy and concurrent chemotherapy: the unique role of laparoscopic lateral ovary transposition. Eur J Gynaecol Oncol. 2007;28(5):408–10.
45. Sonoda Y, Abu-Rustum NR, Gemignani ML, Chi DS, Brown CL, Poynor EA, et al. A fertility-sparing alternative to radical hysterectomy: how many patients may be eligible? Gynecol Oncol. 2004;95(3):534–8.
46. Thomas PR, Winstanly D, Peckham MJ, Austin DE, Murray MA, Jacobs HS. Reproductive and endocrine function in patients with Hodgkin's disease: effects of oophoropexy and irradiation. Br J Cancer. 1976;33(2):226–31.
47. Bisharah M, Tulandi T. Laparoscopic preservation of ovarian function: an underused procedure. Am J Obstet Gynecol. 2003;188(2):367–70.
48. Sonmezer M, Oktay K. Fertility preservation in female patients. Hum Reprod Update. 2004;10(3):251–66.
49. Nakagawa K, Kanda Y, Yamashita H, Hosoi Y, Oshima K, Ohtomo K, Ban N, Yamakawa S, Nakagawa S, Chiba S. Preservation of ovarian function by ovarian shielding when undergoing total body irradiation for hematopoietic stem cell transplantation: a report of two successful cases. Bone Marrow Transplant. 2006;37(6):583–7.
50. Oktay K, Sonmezer M. Fertility issues and options in young women with cancer. Recent Results Cancer Res. 2008;178:203–24.
51. Dursun P, LeBlanc E, Nogueira MC. Radical vaginal trachelectomy (Dargent's operation): a critical review of the literature. Eur J Surg Oncol. 2007;33(8):933–41.
52. Klemm P, Tozzi R, Kohler C, Hertel H, Schneider A. Does radical trachelectomy influence uterine blood supply? Gynecol Oncol. 2005;96(2):283–6.
53. Lanowska M, Mangler M, Spek A, Grittner U, Hasenbein K, Chi-antera V, et al. Radical vaginal trachelectomy (RVT) combined with laparoscopic lymphadenectomy: prospective study of 225 patients

with early-stage cervical cancer. Int J Gynecol Cancer. 2011;21(8):1458–64.
54. Mangler M, Speiser D, Nguyen BD, Cremer M, Koehler C, Schneider A, et al. Neonatal outcome in infants of patients with radical vaginal trachelectomy. J Perinat Med. 2012;40(5):503–9.
55. Oktay K, Aydin BA, Karlikaya G. A technique for laparoscopic transplantation of frozen-banked ovarian tissue. Fertil Steril. 2001;75(6):1212–6.
56. Practice Committee of the American Society for Reproductive. Ovarian tissue and oocyte cryopreservation. Fertil Steril. 2004;82(4):993–8.
57. Simon B, Lee SJ, Partridge AH, et al. Preserving fertility after cancer. CA Cancer J Clin. 2005;55: 211–28.
58. Marhhom E, Cohen I. Fertility preservation options for women with malignancies. Obstet Gynecol Surv. 2007;62:58–72.
59. Newton H, Aubard Y, Rutherford A, et al. Low temperature storage and grafting of human ovarian tissue. Hum Reprod. 1996;11:1487–91.
60. Seli E, Tangir J. Fertility preservation options for female patients with malignancies. Curr Opin Obstet Gynecol. 2005;17:299–308.
61. Oktay K, Newton H, Aubard Y, et al. Cryopreservation of immature human oocytes and ovarian tissue: an emerging technology? Fertil Steril. 1998;69:1–7.
62. Maltaris T, Dimmler A, Muller A, et al. Comparison of two freezing protocols in an open freezing system for cryopreservation of rat ovarian tissue. J Obstet Gynaecol Res. 2006;32:273–9.
63. Gook DA, Edgar DH, Borg J, et al. Diagnostic assessment of the developmental potential of human cryopreserved ovarian tissue from multiple patients using xenografting. Hum Reprod. 2005;20:72–8.
64. Chian RC, Gilbert L, Huang JY, Demirtas E, Holzer H, Benjamin A, et al. Live birth after vitrification of in vitro matured human oocytes. Fertil Steril. 2009;91(2):372–6.
65. Chian RC, Uzelac PS, Nargund G. In vitro maturation of human immature oocytes for fertility preservation. Fertil Steril. 2013;99(5):1173–81.
66. Donnez J, Silber S, Andersen CY, Demeestere I, Piver P, Meirow D, et al. Children born after autotransplantation of cryopreserved ovarian tissue. a review of 13 live births. Ann Med. 2011;43(6):437–50.
67. Donnez J, Dolmans MM, Demylle D, et al. Live birth after orthotopic transplantation of cryopreserved ovarian tissue. Lancet. 2004;364:1405–10.
68. Meirow D, Levron J, Eldar-Geva T, et al. Pregnancy after transplantation of cryopreserved ovarian tissue in a patient with ovarian failure after chemotherapy. N Engl J Med. 2005;53:318–21.
69. Lee DM, Yeoman RR, Battaglia DE, et al. Live birth after ovarian tissue transplant. Nature. 2004;428: 137–8.
70. Oktay K, Buyuk E, Veeck L, et al. Embryo development after heterotopic transplantation of cryopreserved ovarian tissue. Lancet. 2004;363:837–40.
71. Wolner-Hanssen P, Hagglund L, Ploman F, et al. Autotransplantation of cryopreserved ovarian tissue to the right forearm 4(1/2) years after autologous stem cell transplantation. Acta Obstet Gynecol Scand. 2005;84:695–8.
72. Silber SJ, Lenahan KM, Levine DJ, et al. Ovarian transplantation between monozygotic twins discordant for premature ovarian failure. N Engl J Med. 2005;353:58–63.
73. Nomi M, Atala A, Coppi PD, et al. Principals of neovascularization for tissue engineering. Mol Aspects Med. 2002;23:463–83.
74. Shaw JM, Bowles J, Koopman P, et al. Fresh and cryopreserved ovarian tissue samples from donors with lymphoma transmit the cancer to graft recipients. Hum Reprod. 1996;11:1668–73.
75. Donnez J, Dolmans MM, Martinez-Madrid B, et al. The role of cryopreservation for women prior to treatment of malignancy. Curr Opin Obstet Gynecol. 2005;17:333–8.
76. Abir R, Nitke S, Ben-Haroush A, et al. In vitro maturation of human primordial ovarian follicles: clinical significance, progress in mammals, and methods for growth evaluation. Histol Histopathol. 2006;21:887–98.
77. Scott JE, Zhang P, Hovatta O. Benefits of 8-bromoguanosine 3′,5′-cyclic monophosphate (8-brcGMP) in human ovarian cortical tissue culture. Reprod Biomed Online. 2004;8:319–24.
78. Scott JE, Carlsson IB, Bavister BD, et al. Human ovarian tissue cultures: extracellular matrix composition, coating density, and tissue dimensions. Reprod Biomed Online. 2004;9:287–93.
79. Wright CS, Hovatta O, Margara R, et al. Effects of follicle-stimulating hormone and serum substitution on the in-vitro growth of human ovarian follicles. Hum Reprod. 1999;14:1555–62.
80. Hovatta O, Silye R, Abir R, et al. Extracellular matrix improves survival of both stored and fresh human primordial and primary ovarian follicles in long-term culture. Hum Reprod. 1997;12:1032–6.
81. Falcone T, Attaran M, Bedaiwy MA, Goldberg JM. Ovarian function preservation in the cancer patient. Fertil Steril. 2004;81(2):243–57.
82. Brännström M, Johannesson L, Bokström H, Kvarnström N, Mölne J, Dahm-Kähler P, Enskog A, Milenkovic M, Ekberg J, Diaz-Garcia C, Gäbel M, Hanafy A, Hagberg H, Olausson M, Nilsson L. Live birth after uterus transplantation. Lancet. 2014;S0140–6736(14):61728–31.
83. Imai A, Furui T. Chemotherapy-induced female infertility and protective action of gonadotropin-releasing hormone analogues. J Obstet Gynaecol. 2007;27(1):20–4.
84. Longhi A, Pignotti E, Versari M, Asta S, Bacci G. Effect of oral contraceptive on ovarian function in young females undergoing neoadjuvant chemotherapy treatment for osteosarcoma. Oncol Rep. 2003;10(1):151–5.
85. Blumenfeld Z, Von Wolff M. GnRH-analogues and oral contraceptives for fertility preservation in women during chemotherapy. Hum Reprod Update. 2008;14(6):543–52.

86. Reinsch RC, Murphy AA, Morales AJ, Yen SS. The effects of RU 486 and leuprolide acetate on uterine artery blood flow in the fibroid uterus: a prospective, randomized study. Am J Obstet Gynecol. 1994;170(6):1623–7.
87. Periti P, Mazzei T, Mini E. Clinical pharmacokinetics of depot leuprorelin. Clin Pharmacokinet. 2002;41(7):485–504.
88. Yavas G, Dogan NU, Yavas C, Benzer N, Yuce D, Celik C. Prospec-tive assessment of quality of life and psychological distress in patients with gynecologic malignancy: a 1-year prospective study. Int J Gynecol Cancer. 2012;22(6):1096–101.
89. Munster PN, Moore AP, Ismail-Khan R, Cox CE, Lacevic M, Gross-King M, et al. Randomized trial using gonadotropin-releasing hormone agonist triptorelin for the preservation of ovarian function during (neo)adjuvant chemotherapy for breast cancer. J Clin Oncol. 2012;30(5):533–8.
90. Navarria I, Usel M, Rapiti E, Neyroud-Caspar I, Pelte MF, Bouchardy C, et al. Young patients with endometrial cancer: how many could be eligible for fertility-sparing treatment? Gynecol Oncol. 2009;114(3):448–51.
91. Waxman JH, Ahmed R, Smith D, Wrigley PF, Gregory W, Shalet S, Crowther D, Rees LH, Besser GM, Malpas JS, et al. Failure to preserve fertility in patients with Hodgkin's disease. Cancer Chemother Pharmacol. 1987;19(2):159–62.
92. Blumenfeld Z, Avivi I, Eckman A, Epelbaum R, Rowe JM, Dann EJ. Gonadotropin-releasing hormone agonist decreases chemotherapy-induced gonadotoxicity and premature ovarian failure in young female patients with Hodgkin lymphoma. Fertil Steril. 2008;89(1):166–73.
93. Clowse ME, Behera MA, Anders CK, Copland S, Coffman CJ, Leppert PC, Bastian LA. Ovarian preservation by GnRH agonists during chemotherapy: a meta-analysis. J Womens Health (Larchmt). 2009;18(3):311–9.
94. Sherman JK. Synopsis of the use of frozen human semen since 1964: state of the art of human semen banking. Fertil Steril. 1973;24(5):397–412.
95. Trounson A, Mohr L. Human pregnancy following cryopreservation, thawing and transfer of an eight-cell embryo. Nature. 1983;305(5936):707–9.
96. Zeilmaker GH, Alberda AT, van Gent I, Rijkmans CM, Drogendijk AC. Two pregnancies following transfer of intact frozen-thawed embryos. Fertil Steril. 1984;42(2):293–6.
97. Quintero RB, Helmer A, Huang JQ, Westphal LM. Ovarian stimulation for fertility preservation in patients with cancer. Fertil Steril. 2010;93(3):865–8.
98. Friedler S, Koc O, Gidoni Y, Raziel A, Ron-El R. Ovarian response to stimulation for fertility preservation in women with malignant disease: a systematic review and meta-analysis. Fertil Steril. 2012;97(1):125–33.
99. Baynosa J, Westphal LM, Madrigrano A, Wapnir I. Timing of breast cancer treatments with oocyte retrieval and embryo cryopreservation. J Am Coll Surg. 2009;209(5):603–7.
100. Stern CJ, Toledo MG, Gook DA Seymour JF. Fertility preservation in female oncology patients. Aust N Z J Obstet Gynaecol. 2006;46(1):15–23.
101. Kim J, Oktay K, Gracia C, Lee S, Morse C, Mersereau JE. Which patients pursue fertility preservation treatments? A multicenter analysis of the predictors of fertility preservation in women with breast cancer. Fertil Steril. 2012;97(3):671–6.
102. Lee S, Oktay K. Does higher starting dose of FSH stimulation with letrozole improve fertility preservation outcomes in women with breast cancer? Fertil Steril. 2012;98(4):961–4.
103. Reddy J, Oktay K. Ovarian stimulation and fertility preservation with the use of aromatase inhibitors in women with breast cancer. Fertil Steril. 2012; 98(6):1363–9.
104. Chen C. Pregnancy after human oocyte cryopreservation. Lancet. 1986;1(8486):884–6.
105. Pickering SJ, Johnson MH. The influence of cooling on the organization of the meiotic spindle of the mouse oocyte. Hum Reprod. 1987;2(3):207–16.
106. Saragusty J, Arav A. Current progress in oocyte and embryo cryopreservation by slow freezing and vitrification. Reproduction. 2011;141(1):1–19.
107. Stachecki JJ, Cohen J. An overview of oocyte cryopreservation. Reprod Biomed Online. 2004;9(2):152–63.
108. Palermo G, Joris H, Devroey P, Van Steirteghem AC. Pregnancies after intracytoplasmic injection of single spermatozoon into an oocyte. Lancet. 1992;340(8810):17–8.
109. Fabbri R, Porcu E, Marsella T, Rocchetta G, Venturoli S, Flamigni C. Human oocyte cryopreservation: new perspectives regarding oocyte survival. Hum Reprod. 2001;16(3):411–6.
110. Kuwayama M. Highly efficient vitrification for cryopreservation of human oocytes and embryos: the cryotop method. Theriogenology. 2007;67(1):73–80.
111. Harp R, Leibach J, Black J, Keldahl C, Karow A. Cryopreservation of murine ovarian tissue. Cryobiology. 1994;31(4):336–43.
112. Revelli A, Molinari E, Salvagno F, Delle Piane L, Dolfin E, Ochetti S. Oocyte cryostorage to preserve fertility in oncological patients. Obstet Gynecol Int. 2012;2012:525896. doi:10.1155/2012/525896. Epub 2012 Jan 15.
113. Noyes N, Porcu E, Borini A. Over 900 oocyte cryopreservation babies born with no apparent increase in congenital anomalies. Reprod Biomed Online. 2009;18(6):769–76.
114. Rudick B, Opper N, Paulson R, Bendikson K, Chung K. The status of oocyte cryopreservation in the United States. Fertil Steril. 2010;94(7):2642–6.
115. Gomes JE, Correia SC, Gouveia-Oliveira A, Cidadao AJ, Plancha CE. Three-dimensional environments preserve extracellular matrix compartments of ovarian follicles and increase FSH-dependent growth. Mol Reprod Dev. 1999;54(2):163–72.

116. West ER, Shea LD, Woodruff TK. Engineering the follicle microenvironment. Semin Reprod Med. 2007;25:287–99.
117. Pangas SA, Saudye H, Shea LD, et al. Novel approach for the three-dimensional culture of granulosa cell-oocyte complexes. Tissue Eng. 2003;9:1013–21.
118. Xu M, West E, Shea LD, et al. Identification of a stage-specific permissive in vitro culture environment for follicle growth and oocyte development. Biol Reprod. 2006;75:916–23.
119. Kreeger PK, Fernandes NN, Woodruff TK, et al. Regulation of mouse follicle development by follicle-stimulating hormone in a three-dimensional in vitro culture system is dependent on follicle stage and dose. Biol Reprod. 2005;73:942–50.
120. Louhio H, Hovatta O, Sjoberg J, et al. The effects of insulin, and insulin-like growth factors I and II on human ovarian follicles in long-term culture. Mol Hum Reprod. 2000;6:694–8.
121. Xu M, Kreeger PK, Shea LD, et al. Tissue-engineered follicles produce live, fertile offspring. Tissue Eng. 2006;12:2739–46.
122. Xu M, Barrett SL, West-Farrell E, Kondapalli LA, Kiesewetter SE, Shea LD, Woodruff TK. In vitro grown human ovarian follicles from cancer patients support oocyte growth. Hum Reprod. 2009;24(10):2531–40.
123. Trimble EL, Harlan LC, Clegg L, et al. Pre-operative imaging, surgery, and adjuvant therapy for women diagnosed with cancer of the corpus uteri in community practice in the US. Gynecol Oncol. 2005;96:741–8.
124. Ushijima K, Yahata H, Yoshikawa H, et al. Multicenter phase II study of fertility-sparing treatment with medroxyprogesterone acetate for endometrial carcinoma and atypical hyperplasia in young women. J Clin Oncol. 2007;25:2798–803.
125. Jadoul P, Donnez J. Conservative treatment may be beneficial for young women with atypical endometrial hyperplasia or endometrial adenocarcinoma. Fertil Steril. 2003;80:1315–24.
126. Ramirez P, Frumovitz M, Bodurka D, et al. Hormonal therapy for the management of grade 1 endometrial adenocarcinoma: a literature review. Gynecol Oncol. 2004;95:133–8.
127. Gallos ID, Yap J, Rajkhowa M, Luesley DM, Coomarasamy A, Gupta JK. Regression, relapse, and live birth rates with fertility-sparing therapy for endometrial cancer and atypical complex endometrial hyperplasia: a systematic review and meta-analysis. Am J Obstet Gynecol. 2012;207(4):266.e1–12.
128. Montz FJ, Bristow RE, Bovicelli A, et al. Intrauterine progesterone treatment of early endometrial cancer. Am J Obstet Gynecol. 2002;186(4):651–7.
129. Westin S, Sun C, Broaddus R, Pal N, Nath V, Urbauer D, Schmeler K, Lu K, Bodurka D, Johnston T. Prospective phase II trial of the Levonorgestrel Intrauterine System (Mirena) to treat complex atypical hyperplasia and grade 1 endometrioid endometrial cancer. Gynecol Oncol. 2012;125 Suppl 1:S9.
130. Baker J, Obermair A, Gebski V, et al. Efficacy of oral or intrauterine device-delivered progestin in patients with complex endometrial hyperplasia with atypia or early endometrial adenocarcinoma: a meta-analysis and systematic review of the literature. Gynecol Oncol. 2012;125:263–70.
131. Penner K, Dorigo O, Aoyama C, et al. Predictors of resolution of complex atypical hyperplasia or grade 1 endometrial adenocarcinoma in premenopausal women treated with progestin therapy. Gynecol Oncol. 2012;124:542–8.
132. Plaxe SC, Braly PS, Freddo JL, McClay E, Kirmani S, Howell SB. Profiles of women age 30–39 and age less than 30 with epithelial ovarian cancer. Obstet Gynecol. 1993;81(5 Pt 1):651–4.
133. Satoh T, Hatae M, Watanabe Y, et al. Outcomes of fertility-sparing surgery for stage I epithelial ovarian cancer: a proposal for patient selection. J Clin Oncol. 2010;28(10):1727–32.
134. Kashima K, Yahata T, Fujita K, Tanaka K. Outcomes of fertility-sparing surgery for women of reproductive age with FIGO stage IC epithelial ovarian cancer. Int J Gynaecol Obstet. 2013;121(1):53–5.
135. Zhang M, Cheung MK, Shin JY, et al. Prognostic factors responsible for survival in sex cord stromal tumors of the ovary—an analysis of 376 women. Gynecol Oncol. 2007;104:396–400.
136. Guvenal T, Dursun P, Hasdemir PS, et al. Effect of surgical staging on 539 patients with borderline ovarian tumors: a Turkish Gynecologic Oncology Group study. Gynecol Oncol. 2013;131(3):546–50.

# Part V

# Racial/Ethnic Disparities in Gynecological Cancer Screening, Treatment and Survival

# Racial/Ethnic Disparities in Gynecological Cancer Screening, Treatment, and Survival

8

Fong W. Liu, Robert E. Bristow, and Ana I. Tergas

**Abstract**

Differences in cancer screening and treatment have been associated with race and ethnic classification. Several disparities have been identified in gynecologic cancer screening and therapy, most often affecting black and Hispanic women. The causes of health disparities are multifactorial and involve systemic, provider, and patient factors, including cultural attitudes, socioeconomic status, education level, and geographic barriers. This chapter documents the disparities in gynecologic cancer screening, treatment, and survival for women with cancers of the cervix, uterus, ovaries, vagina, and vulva. Each disease site has specific areas where minimizing differences in access to care can potentially minimize the disparate health outcomes seen among specific racial and ethnic groups.

**Keywords**

Cervical cancer • Uterine cancer • Ovarian cancer • Vulvar cancer • Vaginal cancer • Health disparities

F.W. Liu, MD, MPH (✉)
Division of Gyncologic Oncology, Department of Obstetrics and Gynecology, Beth Israel Deaconess Medical Center, Harvard Medical School, 330 Brookline Ave, Boston, MA 02215, USA
e-mail: fongl1@uci.edu; rbristow@uci.edu

R.E. Bristow, MD, MBA
Department of Obstetrics and Gynecology, Division of Gynecologic Oncology, University of California at Irvine, 101 The City Drive, Orange, CA 92868, USA

A.I. Tergas, MD, MPH
Division of Gynecologic Oncology, Department of Obstetrics and Gynecology, Columbia University Medical Center, 161 Fort Washington Ave, New York, NY 10011, USA
e-mail: ait2111@cumc.columbia.edu

## Introduction

Over the last two decades reducing disparities in health outcomes has been a priority of the Institute of Medicine and the Department of Health and Human Services. Several factors influence the perpetuation of health inequalities, including health systems characteristics, patient and cultural perspectives, provider factors, and social and historical determinants of care. The focus of this chapter is on identifying health disparities in gynecologic cancer and the areas where intervention will have the greatest impact. The purpose of



A. Giordano, M. Macaluso (eds.), *Gynecological Cancers*, Current Clinical Oncology,
DOI 10.1007/978-3-319-32907-9_8

intervention is to reduce mortality and morbidity from gynecologic malignancy and key point of intervention is increasing access to services on both screening and treatment levels.

Black patients bear the most disparate burden of incidence and mortality for a number of chronic medical problems, including diabetes, heart disease, stroke, and multiple malignancies. While racial differences in incidence and mortality are improving for black women with cervical cancer, disparities in uterine cancer incidence and mortality are particularly striking. The historical impact of segregation and unequal access should not be diminished as an important mechanism by which factors like socioeconomic status (SES), differential health education, familiarity and trust of the health care system are mediated and have a direct influence on health care outcomes. As the research suggests, these social determinants of care have an important effect on the receipt of guideline-adherent care, especially in ovarian cancer, where the coordination of complex surgical and chemotherapeutic interventions at high volume centers significantly improves survival.

Hispanic women in the USA come from a number of different countries and comprise of both white and black racial identifications. While they are the largest minority group in the USA, the disparities in disease incidence and health outcomes are less consistent, which can likely be attributed to the heterogeneity of the racial classification. The studies on gynecologic cancer in Hispanic women are largely limited based on classification of Hispanic women in large population databases. For example, the SEER-Medicare database uses the North American Association of Central Cancer Registries Hispanic Identification Algorithm (NHIA) for cases diagnosed since 1992. The NHIA variable is an algorithm that uses Spanish/Hispanic surname or Spanish origin to classify cases as Hispanic [1]. A method of accurately capturing Hispanic ethnicity and its impact on health outcomes has not been identified; however, as the largest minority group in the USA, increasing literature, not only in medical outcomes and public health but also in sociologic and anthropological studies, regarding this population of women will help better delineate nuances among the various groups that identify as Hispanic.

## Cervical Cancer

### Incidence and Stage at Diagnosis

Cervical cancer is the third most common gynecologic cancer in the USA with an estimated 12,900 cases per year [2]. Racial/ethnic minorities bear a greater burden of cervical cancer than white women in the USA. For instance, the lifetime probability of developing cervical cancer in the USA for black women is 0.84 % (1 in 119) and 1.05 % (1 in 95) for Hispanic women, compared to 0.65 % (1 in 153) for white women [2]. With age-adjusted incidence rates of 10.5 and 11.8 per 100,000, respectively, black and Hispanic women are 34 and 60 % more likely to develop cervical cancer compared to white women [2, 3].

Recent trends in cervical cancer incidence appear favorable with a narrowing of the racial/ethnic incidence gap. Overall incidence continues to decline, albeit at a slower rate during the most recent years, with incidence rates declining faster among black and Hispanic women compared to white women [4]. From 2000 to 2009, the average annual percent decline in cervical cancer age-adjusted incidence rates was 1.9 % for white women, 3.2 % for black women, and 3.8 % for Hispanic women. Looking at these rates more closely, it appears that this trend is most pronounced in young women [5]. From 2007 to 2011, rates in women younger than 50 years of age were stable among white women and decreased by 3.4% per year among black women; in women 50 years or older, rates declined by 2.5 % per year in whites and by 3.8 % per year in blacks [2]. In fact, among women under age 50, incidence rates of cervical cancer for white and black women have recently converged [5].

Hispanic women living in the USA represent a heterogeneous group of women from several different countries of origin and of varying immigration status. Hispanic women have the highest incidence rates of any racial/ethnic group in the USA, particularly among first-generation immigrants [6]. Cervical cancer is more common in economically developing countries, such as Central and South American countries, where women have limited access to routine cervical cancer screening. A study on the geographic variation of cervical cancer incidence found that the highest rates were found among Hispanic women living in the Midwest, likely due to the large numbers of recent immigrants living in this region of the country [7].

## Screening

Women can be screened for cervical cancer either with the Papanicolaou (Pap) test or with an HPV test. The Pap test, which has been widely implemented in developed countries since the 1950s, is an effective method for cervical cancer screening in settings where the health care and civil infrastructure supports multiple rounds of screening and recalls for further diagnostic evaluation. Primary HPV testing for cervical cancer screening has only recently been approved and no data is yet available on its impact on cervical cancer screening rates. Even though currently there is a disparity in cervical cancer incidence between black and white women for all ages, in 2010, the rate of Pap testing within the previous 3 years was similar between both groups (78 %) [8].

For Hispanic women, screening rates have improved in recent decades. The proportion of Hispanic women who obtained cervical cancer screening increased from 64 to 75 % from 1987 to 2010 [9, 10]. Rates of screening for Hispanic women differ by country of origin, with Puerto Rican and Cuban women (≥80 %) having the highest rates of cervical cancer screening compared to Mexican women (71.6 %) [6]. However, among women of all races, screening rates are lowest in older women, women with no health insurance, and recent immigrants [11]. These patterns of screening correlate with the patterns of cervical cancer incidence as discussed above.

In order for screening to be effective, women should obtain adequate follow-up and treatment for any detected abnormalities. A large study of 10,004 women in a US-based cervical cancer screening program demonstrated that less than half of women with two consecutive abnormal Pap smears received appropriate follow-up diagnostic evaluation with colposcopy, and black women were the most likely to receive no follow-up [12]. Thus, varying rates of cervical cancer screening and adherence with follow-up may contribute to disparities in cervical cancer incidence, stage at diagnosis, and mortality.

## HPV Vaccine

Persistent infection with high-risk human papillomavirus (HPV) genotypes is necessary for the development of cervical cancer and its precursors, as well as other anogenital and oropharyngeal cancers in women and men. Genital HPV is the most common sexually transmitted infection in the USA, with an estimated 14 million new cases of infection among individuals aged 15–59 years occurring each year [13, 14]. Approximately half of these new infections occur among young persons aged 15–24 years [13]. In a prospective cohort study, Ho et al. evaluated over 600 female college students and found a cumulative 36-month incidence rate of HPV infection of 43 % [15]. Black female adolescents and women have the highest rates of HPV infection compared to other racial/ethnic groups [16, 17]. However, first generation Mexican immigrants have a higher prevalence of HPV infection than US-born Mexican women [18].

There are currently three US Food and Drug Administration-approved HPV vaccines. The vaccines are highly efficacious, with efficacy rates ranging from 92 to 100 % in various clinical trials [19–23]. Currently, the Advisory Committee on Immunization Practices (ACIP) recommends the routine use of the HPV vaccine in females aged 11 or 12 years, with catch-up vaccination for females aged 13–26 years [24]. The ACIP also recommends routine vaccination with the quadrivalent vaccine for males age 11 through 26 years. All vaccines are given as a three-dose series, and are most effective if given prior to initiation of sexual activity [24].

Despite the recommendation for routine vaccination, vaccination rates are low across all races/ethnicities. In 2012, only 53.8 and 33.4 % of US female adolescents age 13–17 years, respectively, initiated and completed the HPV vaccine series [25]. Initiation and completion rates for US male adolescents are even lower: 20.8 and 6.8 % [25]. Initiation and completion rates are similar among white and black female adolescents (51.1 and 50.1 %, respectively) [15]. Vaccine completion rates are also similar between white and black adolescents (33.7 and 29.0 %, respectively). However, there may be a developing disparity between vaccination rates between black and white female adolescents given that, since 2011, the HPV vaccine initiation rate for non-Hispanic black girls has decreased by 6 %, whereas the initiation rate for non-Hispanic white girls has increased by 3 % [26]. Perhaps somewhat unexpectedly, the HPV vaccine initiation rate for Hispanic adolescents (62.9 %) is higher than both white and black adolescents, and completion rates (35.5 %) are similar [25]. While there is no disparity in HPV vaccination rates by race/ethnicity among female adolescents, there is a difference seen in women. Among women aged 19–26 years, black women (29.1 %) and Hispanic women (18.7 %) had lower coverage compared with whites (42.2 %) in 2012 [27].

Parental attitudes and behavior are crucial to vaccine uptake. Generally there is no difference in HPV vaccine acceptability by race/ethnicity, although racial/ethnic groups face different barriers and facilitators for vaccination [26]. For instance, fear that the vaccine was experimental is a unique concern among black mothers [26]. A focus group study among black mothers of adolescent daughters in the USA found four key factors that impacted HPV vaccination: having a personal experience with cervical pre-cancer or cancer, knowledge of HPV as a cause of cervical cancer, anticipation of sexual initiation of their daughters, and physician recommendation of HPV vaccination [28]. Focus group participants indicated that if physicians did not initiate a discussion about HPV vaccination, this raised doubt about the safety and effectiveness of the vaccine among the mothers [28]. Barriers common to Hispanics include language, safety concerns, not knowing where to obtain the vaccine, lack of health insurance, especially among poor and undocumented immigrants, lower rates of provider recommendation compared with whites, and logistical challenges associated with receipt of all three doses in the series [26].

## Treatment and Survival

Cervical cancer mortality has decreased steadily over the past several decades due to prevention and early detection from widespread implementation of screening in developing countries. In the USA, mortality rates declined more rapidly in black women than for white women (2.6 % per year compared to 1.9 % per year, respectively) [4]. However, despite this progress, black women are still at higher risk of dying from cervical cancer compared to white women, as are Hispanic women (see Table 8.1). The lifetime probability of dying from invasive cervical cancer in the USA is 0.40 (1 in 250) for black women and 0.21 (1 in 479) for white women [3].

Higher death rates among racial/ethnic minority women have been largely attributed to socioeconomic disparities and a lack of access to care [29]; however, differences in treatment also play a key role. Several studies have demonstrated that there are significant disparities in treatment based on race/ethnicity [30–32]. Using data from a state cancer registry, researchers demonstrated that, after adjustment for stage and insurance status, black women were 50 % less likely to receive surgery compared to white women [32].

**Table 8.1** Mortality rates among black, Hispanic, and white women in the USA, 2005–2009

| | Mortality rate[a] | Rate ratio[b] |
|---|---|---|
| White women | 2.2 | – |
| Black women | 4.3 | 1.97* |
| Hispanic women | 3.0 | 1.50* |

*Statistical significant ($P<0.05$)

[a]Rates are per 100,000 and age adjusted to the 2000 US standard population

[b]Rate ratios compare mortality rates for blacks and Hispanics to white women as the reference group

This trend was also seen in a study using SEER data 1985–2009 [31]. Black women were less likely to receive cancer-directed surgery compared to white women (32.4 % vs 46 %), and more likely to receive radiotherapy (36.3 % vs 26.4 %) [31]. In order to demonstrate the importance of equal access to care, researchers conducted a study of women with cervical cancer treated within the US Military Health Care System [33], a system hypothesized to be a model of equal access to care. In this study of 1553 women with invasive cancer in the automated tumor registry from 1988 to 1999, there was no racial disparity in the stage distribution or the percentage of patient receiving surgery or radiation as initial treatment. Furthermore, 5- and 10-year overall survival rates were similar between black and white women.

Disparities in survival rates are seen between black and white women, but not between Hispanic and white women. The overall 5-year relative survival rate for cervical cancer among black women in the USA is 59 %, compared to 69 % among white women [8]. In contrast, 5-year relative survival rate for Hispanic women with cervical cancer in 74 % [6]. This difference in survival rates reflects the distribution of stage at diagnosis. Black women are more likely to be diagnosed with regional- or distant-stage disease compared with white women, despite similar screening rates reported in national surveys (see Table 8.2). In contrast, the stage distribution for Hispanic women is similar to that of white women. While screening rates may be similar among racial/ethnic groups, this racial disparity in stage at diagnosis may be due to differences in the quality of screening and lack of follow-up after abnormal results [12, 34, 35].

**Table 8.2** Stage distribution for invasive cervical cancer among white, black and Hispanic women in the USA, 2005–2009

| | Localized, % | Regional, % | Distant, % | Unstaged, % |
|---|---|---|---|---|
| White | 49 | 35 | 12 | 4 |
| Black | 40 | 41 | 14 | 5 |
| Hispanic | 48 | 37 | 10 | 4 |

## Conclusions

In 1991, the Centers for Disease Control and Prevention (CDC) established the National Breast and Cervical Cancer Early Detection Program (NBCCEDP) to provide breast and cervical cancer screening and diagnostic services to low-income, uninsured women. It has provided screening and diagnostic services to over 4.3 million women in the USA since its inception. Continued efforts in public education and outreach are needed to ensure that minority women, especially black women, receive the follow-up care necessary to help reduce disparities in cervical cancer diagnosis. Appropriations should also be made to raise awareness for parents and young adults regarding the efficacy and safety of HPV vaccines.

## Uterine Cancer

### Incidence and Stage at Diagnosis

Uterine cancer is the most common gynecologic malignancy in American women, with 54,870 new cases and 10,170 deaths estimated in 2015 [2]. Although they have a 30 % decreased incidence compared to white women, black women with endometrial cancer are 2.5 times more likely to die with their disease [36]. Figure 8.1 shows the trend in incidence and mortality of endometrial cancer in the USA over the last decade [37]. Several studies utilizing large databases have shown the disparate incidence of uterine cancer among different races, and highlight the disproportionate number of highly aggressive uterine cancers among black women [38–44].

A little over half of black women present with more favorable, localized uterine cancer as opposed to 71 % of white patients and 68 % of patients overall [2]. While 39 % of Black patients have regional or distant metastases at the time of presentation, only 26 % of whites do [40]. There are conflicting reports on the stage at which Hispanic women are diagnosed with uterine cancer, with some studies demonstrating later stage disease than their non-Hispanic white counterparts

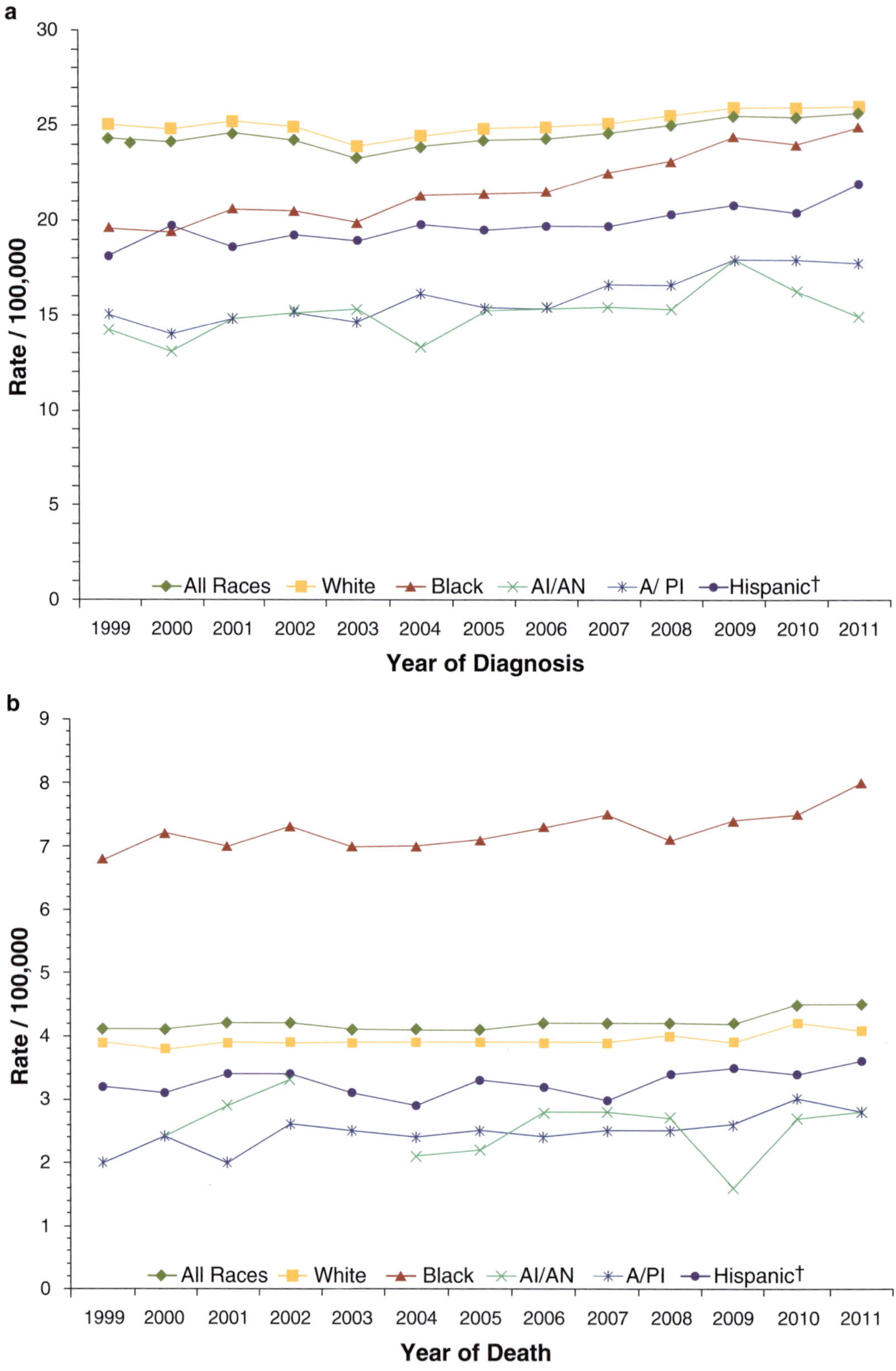


**Fig. 8.1** Uterine cancer incidence (**a**) and mortality (**b**) rates by race and ethnicity in the USA, 1999–2011. Rates are per 100,000 persons and are age-adjusted to the 2000 US standard population (19 age groups—Census P25-1130). Incidence rates cover approximately 90 % of the US population. (*Dagger*) Hispanic origin is not mutually exclusive from race categories (white, black, A/PI = Asian/Pacific Islander, AI/AN = American Indian/Alaska Native). (National Cancer Institute and the Centers for Disease Control and Prevention, 2015)

[45, 46] while others have found similar stages at presentation [47]. The most marked difference between Hispanic women and white women is the younger age at diagnosis, which was fairly consistent across studies [45–48].

## Histologic Subtype: Molecular and Genetic Factors

Black patients are up to three times more likely to present with less favorable subtypes (sarcomas, clear cell carcinomas, serous carcinomas, and carcinosarcomas) and higher-grade tumors [38]. More aggressive cell times are also seen more commonly in Hispanic women compared to white women; however, the disparity is not as drastic [46–48] Little research has been done to determine why these histologic differences exist. With the establishment of The Cancer Genome Atlas and the massive amount of genetic and epigenetic data that it provides, research on the potential molecular basis for such drastic differences in histology between racial groups may now be possible with genome wide association studies (GWAS). Endometrioid endometrial cancer has a distinct genetic profile when compared to type II endometrial cancers. Racial differences in molecular and genetic factors may explain the histologic and survival discrepancy.

Microsatellite instability (MSI) and mutations in the tumor suppressor gene PTEN are more common in type I endometrial cancer, which portends more favorable prognosis [49–51]. PTEN mutations are less common in black compared to white women; however, the evidence on MSI is conflicting [52]. In contrast, mutations in tumor suppressor gene p53 are more common in type II endometrial cancer and are associated with poorer prognosis. Three recent studies have found p53 expression to be more common in the tumors of Black patients [53–55]. These studies did not stratify for type I vs. type II endometrial cancer, and the differences in p53 expression may be due to the fact that Blacks are more likely to have type II tumors. The HER2/neu oncogene has also been associated with treatment resistance and poor survival in breast, ovarian, and endometrial cancers and may be more frequently upregulated in the tumors of Blacks. A study of 27 women with uterine papillary serous carcinoma (UPSC) found heavy HER2/neu receptor expression in 70 % of the Black women but only 24 % of the white women [56]. When adjusted for race and age, heavy HER2/neu expression was associated with earlier death (adjusted HR 28.00) and presumably more aggressive disease.

Other studies have shown no difference in the gene expression profiles of endometrial cancers from Black women. A 2006 study of 39 patients from Memorial Sloan Kettering concluded that molecular factors did not play a role in endometrial cancer's survival disparity, as they found no statistically significant differences in gene expression between groups of white and black women [57]. A recent multi-ethnic GWAS study failed to identify novel single-nucleotide polymorphisms for uterine cancer but confirmed prior associations with genetic markers near the HNF1 homeobox B gene [58]. Another GWAS study found an association with a locus upstream from TET2, previously associated with prostate cancer; however, this was conducted in a population of European ancestry [59].

## Treatment and Survival

The mortality rate associated with endometrial cancer in the USA has largely remained stable over the last decade (Fig. 8.1). Black women have consistently had worse survival compared to white women, with mortality rates 80 % higher despite an overall incidence 30 % by comparison [60]. Even among patients with the less aggressive endometrioid subtype, black women had an associated 5 year survival 40–50 % lower than their white counterparts [38]. The mortality disparity among Hispanic women is markedly less pronounced than that for black women. Among Hispanic women, country of origin appears to mediate survival. In a cohort study of 69,764 women, including 1572 Hispanic women, mortality for US-born and foreign-born Hispanics was higher compared to non-Hispanic Whites after adjustments for demographics, tumor characteristics, and treatment; however, over time, the mortality disparity persisted only for foreign-born Hispanics [46].

Several recent studies confirm that black women are less likely to undergoing definitive surgery, including hysterectomy and lymphadenectomy [41, 61, 62]. Preliminary studies have also shown this difference in treatment for Hispanic women, with fewer receiving hysterectomy and combination treatment with radiation [46, 48]. Encouragingly, the treatment inequities between the black and white patients appear to be improving [42, 63, 64].

Disparities in mortality rates, however, persist in equal treatment environments. In a study reviewing data from four randomized treatment trials for advanced endometrial cancers, black patients had a lower response rate to treatment compared to white women (35 % vs. 43 %); however, despite receiving identical treatment and completing therapy at similar rates, Black patients had an increased risk of death when compared to whites (HR = 1.26, 95 % CI 1.06–1.51) [65]. This may be further evidence that molecular or genetic factors are the source of racial disparities in survival.

Biologic factors do not solely explain the survival disparity seen in endometrial cancer, and socioeconomic factors have also been explored as a contributing factor to worse survival among ethnic groups. Ethnic minorities are more likely than Whites to live in poverty and reside in underserved areas. They are less likely to receive higher education, to possess private health insurance, and to have regular primary health care. Lower SES and lack of health care funding could explain a delay in definitive treatment, as time may be wasted while patients without private insurance await enrollment into government programs or referral to a gynecologic oncologist.

In a study of 39,510 cases of uterine cancer and the impact of insurance status on survival, black women were less likely to have privately funded insurance; however, after adjusting for zip code, education level, clinical factors, and insurance status, the hazard ratio of death for Blacks dropped from 2.35 (95 % CI 2.20–2.51) to 1.28 (95 % CI 1.17–1.40), suggesting that health care access and SES account for some, but not all, of the disparities observed in this population [66]. Another study found that the effect of SES remained important only in women with the less aggressive endometrial histology [61]. In women with aggressive endometrial tumors, race, age, and median family income were not associated with stage at diagnosis. This suggests that, while some cancers are too aggressive to catch in their early stages, there is a large group of patients with less aggressive tumors that could benefit from improved access to care and earlier diagnosis.

Comorbidities, like obesity and diabetes, are more prevalent in black and Hispanic populations; however, several studies have examined the influence of comorbid conditions on survival with mixed results [39, 45, 61, 67, 68]. Comorbid conditions could also contribute to disease-related mortality by preventing women from receiving curative surgical treatment. However, it is difficult to determine whether comorbid conditions are at the root of the discrepancy due to limitations of population databases, which do not always collect data on comorbid conditions or surgical risks. The alternative theory that comorbid factors might influence surgical treatment or surgery-related mortality associated with uterine cancers has not borne out in the literature. Current research does not support that comorbidity increases disease specific mortality from endometrial cancer.

## Conclusions

In uterine malignancies, the effect of racial predispositions toward genetic traits cannot be overlooked and future studies specifically addressing these discrepancies will hopefully identify therapeutic targets or new methods of screening by which racial disparities in uterine cancer incidence and mortality may be reduced. Culturally appropriate education models and health care navigation support systems have been associated with increased screening for breast and cervical cancers among minorities, but no such interventions have been evaluated in endometrial cancer. Increasing awareness among women regarding the symptoms of uterine cancer and the appropriate referral from primary care providers to oncologists remain vital components in reducing the gap in survival.

## Ovarian Cancer

### Incidence and Stage at Diagnosis

The National Cancer Institute has estimated 21,290 cases of and 14,180 deaths from ovarian cancer in 2015 [2]. It is the leading cause of gynecologic cancer related mortality among American women, with approximately 70 % of patients presenting with advanced disease. Optimal ovarian cancer care requires that patients have access to specialty-trained surgeons and tertiary care centers that provide multidisciplinary oncologic care. Studies have shown the positive relationship between surgeon and hospital case volume and clinical outcome for malignancies treated with technically complex surgical procedures [69–72]. Racial classification and insurance status have previously been associated with substandard ovarian cancer care [73–75].

The overall incidence of ovarian cancer has decreased over the last two decades (Fig. 8.2), with rates decreasing by 2.0 % per year from 2001 to 2010 [2]. During this time period incidence rates have fallen more for white and Hispanic women, declining by 2.3 and 2.1 % per year respectively, compared to 1.5 % per year in blacks [76]. Similar to other gynecologic cancers, black women are less likely to be diagnosed with early stage disease after adjusting for clinicopathologic characteristics, age, and sociodemographic factors [77–79] Hispanic women had similar rates of early stage disease when compared to white patients. No significant differences in histology have been clearly demonstrated between racial groups [80].

### Screening

No effective screening method has been established for ovarian cancer given its low overall prevalence and lack of a clinically identifiable pre-invasive state. The multi-institutional Prostate, Lung, Colorectal, and Ovarian Cancer randomized screening trial confirmed that among the general population in the USA, serial transvaginal ultrasound and CA-125 levels did not impact mortality from ovarian cancer [81].

### Genetics

Although screening has not been effective in improving outcomes in the general population, women at high risk of developing ovarian cancer, including those with hereditary breast and ovarian cancer syndrome (HBOC) and hereditary nonpolyposis colorectal cancer/Lynch syndrome, stand to benefit considerably by knowing their genetic status. Any woman with a personal diagnosis of ovarian cancer should be referred for genetic cancer risk assessment and tested for deleterious mutations in the BRCA1 and BRCA2 genes and genetic variance in mismatch-repair genes. Multiple studies have demonstrated that black women are less likely to know about genetic testing and to undergo genetic testing [82–85]. With the FDA approval of olaparib, a poly (ADP-ribose) polymerase inhibitor, for women with recurrent ovarian cancer and a deleterious BRCA mutation carrier, comprehensive testing of all women should be prioritized, especially for minority women currently least likely to get tested.

Through genomic studies, ovarian carcinogenesis appears to be characterized by tumor heterogeneity stemming from copy number alterations and genetic instability. Polymorphisms specific to certain racial groups are being discovered and may uncover the mechanism, at least in part, of why black women have different incidence and outcomes compared to whites. For example, short CAG repeat length in the androgen receptor (AR) gene increases ovarian cancer risk by twofold in black women but not white women [86]. A SNP close to tumor suppressor gene *TP53* has been associated with a modest increased risk of ovarian cancer among white women but not black women [87]. Currently, no such studies exist looking at genetic polymorphisms in Hispanic women with ovarian cancer.

### Treatment and Survival

Important determinants of the quality of ovarian cancer care include the completeness of the initial surgical effort for staging and cytoreduction,

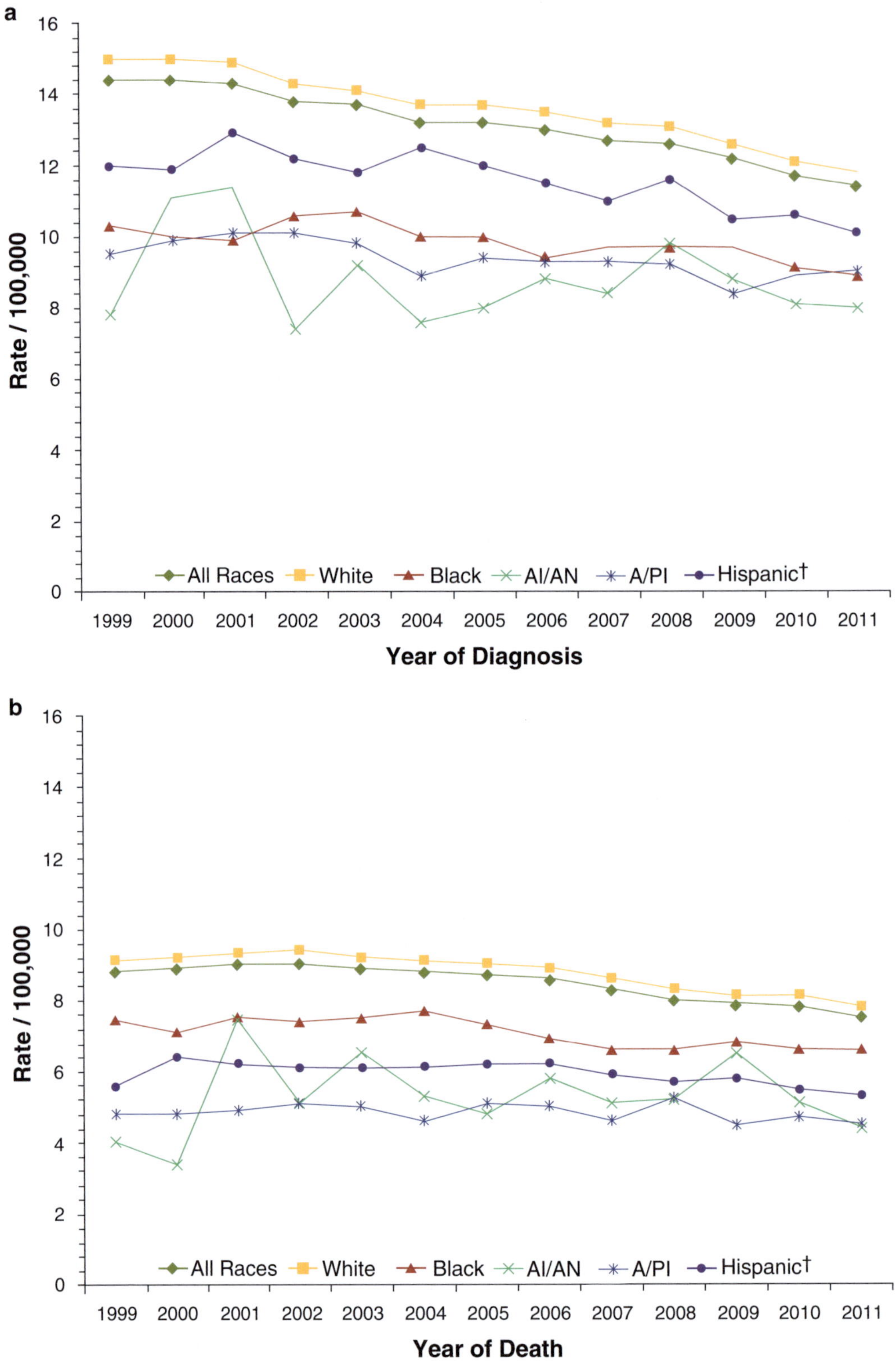


**Fig. 8.2** Ovarian cancer incidence (**a**) and mortality (**b**) rates by race and ethnicity in the USA, 1999–2011. Rates are per 100,000 persons and are age-adjusted to the 2000 US standard population (19 age groups—Census P25-1130). Incidence rates cover approximately 90 % of the US population. (*Dagger*) Hispanic origin is not mutually exclusive from race categories (white, black, A/PI = Asian/Pacific Islander, AI/AN = American Indian/Alaska Native). (National Cancer Institute and the Centers for Disease Control and Prevention, 2015)

receipt of recommended chemotherapy, and the specialty and surgical volume of the treating clinician and hospital [88]. Several studies have demonstrated a surgical treatment disparity among black and Hispanic women diagnosed with ovarian cancer [75, 80, 89–92]. In a study of 13,186 ovarian cancer cases from the California Cancer Registry, black and Hispanic women were less likely to be operated on by high volume surgeons [89]. In a study of 7933 ovarian cancer cases in California, both black and Hispanic women were less likely to receive ovarian cancer-specific surgical procedures compared to white women [93]. In a cohort of 47,390 advanced ovarian cancer cases, blacks and Hispanics were less likely to receive standard of care, surgery followed by chemotherapy [75].

Disparities in treatment administration or allocation are reflected by concurrent inequalities in overall survival. Unfortunately, in a recent study of racial disparities in mortality rates after diagnosis of ovarian cancer, Terplan et al. found that adjusted hazard ratios for all-cause and ovarian cancer specific mortality have worsened over the last three decades [94]. Data from the National Center for Health Statistics and the National Cancer Institute confirm that from 1975 to 2004, the 5-year survival rate for black women actually decreased from 43 to 38 % during the same time interval [95].

For ovarian cancer in particular, population-based studies have documented worse survival outcomes for black women [40, 96]. A comprehensive literature review published in 2013 highlighted that black women suffer discrepancies in care from diagnosis to treatment that detrimentally affects survival for all stages of disease [74]. This was confirmed in multiple large population based analyses [73, 97]. In an analysis of 47,160 women, including 3165 black women, that found that black race, Medicaid insurance status and not insured payer status each independently increased risk of death by 30 %, after adjusting for clinicopathologic, sociodemographic, and treatment characteristics [73]. Treatment at low-volume centers with low-volume providers has also now been linked with worse survival for women with advanced stage disease, which is disproportionately borne by black and Hispanic women, and women with Medicaid insurance and low SES [73, 98].

With better quantification of socioeconomic factors and the ability to estimate previously ill-defined metrics like distance to a high-volume surgical center, recent studies have more clearly delineated the impact of poverty and geography on the receipt of ovarian cancer NCCN guideline-adherent care. Bristow et al. found that black race, low-SES, and geographic location ≥80 km/50 mi from a high-volume hospital were independently associated with an increased risk of non-adherent care, with white patients more likely to travel ≥32 km/20 mi to receive care compared to all non-white counterparts [99]. Low SES was associated with location ≥80 km/50 mi from a high-volume hospital (6.3 % highest SES vs. 33.0 % lowest SES). On a smaller scale, investigators explored the impact of neighborhood disadvantage and ovarian cancer-specific survival for women with ovarian cancer in Cook County, Illinois [100]. Neighborhood disadvantage was negatively associated with ovarian cancer-specific survival, and after adjusting for tumor characteristics, age, and treatment, was able to diminish the risk of death for black women compared to whites ($HR = 1.59$, $p = 0.003$ to $HR = 1.32$, $p = 0.10$). Importantly, guideline adherent care appears to impact equally survival for women with advanced ovarian cancer across socioeconomic strata and racial categorization, supporting the delivery of standard of care to improve survival for all women with ovarian cancer [101].

The delivery of guideline-adherent care will help reduce disparities in survival; however, even in equal access environments, results are conflicting. In studies from two high-volume medical centers, the Surveillance, Epidemiology and End Results-Medicare database, and Gynecologic Oncology Group clinical trials have found that under equal access and treatment environments, the survival disparity of black women largely disappears [90, 102–104]. Conversely, in patients with advanced ovarian cancer enrolled in phase III clinical trials in the Southwest Oncology Group, black women saw a persistently higher risk of mortality despite adjustments for prognostics factors and SES characteristics [105].

## Conclusions

The issue of health disparities in ovarian cancer is complex and requires the provision of adequate health care coverage, improving access to care through education of patients and providers, and better understanding of the biologic mechanisms of carcinogenesis. The centralization of care at high-volume medical centers is one way to help ensure guideline-adherent care; however, methods to overcome geographic barriers are less concrete and also involve widespread community-based disparities through the segregation of neighborhood by race. More research is needed to help equalize care among all women with ovarian cancer to help ensure a comprehensive approach to treatment and maximizing survival.

## Vulvar and Vaginal Cancer

Vulvar and vaginal cancers are rare, and thus there is a paucity of data on patterns of care by race/ethnicity. According to a study using SEER data, vulvar cancer is far more common in non-Hispanic white women (83.8 % of cases) compared to black (8.9 %) and Hispanic (5.0 %) women [106]. There was no significant difference in stage at diagnosis between white, black, and Hispanic women in this study. However, in another study that compared white and black women only and did not include Hispanic women, black women with vulvar cancer tend to have a higher rate of distant metastasis compared to white women [107]. Similar to patterns of care seen with cervical cancer, after adjustment for stage, black women were half as likely (OR = 0.48, 95 % CI 0.31–0.74) to undergo surgery and 1.7 times more likely (OR = 1.67, 95 % CI 1.18–2.36) to receive radiation than white women [106]. In a multivariable analysis, there was no significant difference in risk of death by race/ethnicity group [106].

In a similar study of vaginal cancer using SEER data from 1988 to 2007, vaginal cancer is also far more common in white women compared to black women (85.8 % vs 14.2 %, respectively) [108]. Black women presented with more advanced disease compared to white women (30.4 % vs 23.1 %). In contrast to vulvar and cervical cancer, radiation therapy was utilized equally in both racial groups. However, white women underwent surgical treatment alone or in combination with radiation therapy more frequently compared to black women (27.7 % vs. 17.5 %). The 5-year survival was significantly better for white women (45 %) compared to black women (38.6 %). In multivariable analysis, compared with white women, black women had significantly worse survival after controlling for age, histology, stage, grade, and treatment modality (HR 1.2, 95 % CI 1.1–1.4, $p = 0.007$).

## Conclusions and Recommendations

National and governmental organizations have focused on eliminating racial inequities in health outcomes. From incidence differences in high-risk uterine cancer to screening variations in cervical cancer and treatment inequalities in ovarian cancer, there are several areas where intervention may help alleviate the disproportionate number of minority women with gynecologic cancer who are affected by health disparities. The issue of health disparities is complex and requires improving access to care through education of patients and providers, the provision of adequate health care coverage, and better understanding of biologic and genetic polymorphisms. In each of these areas, more research is needed to help equalize care among all women with gynecologic cancers. Addressing inequalities in access will help ensure that all women with gynecologic cancers have a comprehensive approach to prevention, treatment, and maximizing survival.

## References

1. NAACCR Race and Ethnicity Work Group. NAACCR guideline for enhancing Hispanic/Latino Identification: Revised NAACCR Hispanic/Latino identification algorithm [NHIA v2.2.1] Springfield, IL; September 2011 http://www.naaccr org/Research/DataAnalysisTools aspx.
2. American Cancer Society. Cancer facts & figures 2015. Atlanta 2015.

3. Surveillance EaERSP. SEER*Stat Database: NAACCR incidence – CiNA analytic file, 1995–2009, North American Association of Central Cancer Registries.
4. Jemal A, Simard EP, Dorell C, Noone AM, Markowitz LE, Kohler B, et al. Annual report to the nation on the status of cancer, 1975–2009, featuring the burden and trends in human papillomavirus (HPV)-associated cancers and HPV vaccination coverage levels. J Natl Cancer Inst. 2013;105(3):175–201.
5. Simard EP, Naishadham D, Saslow D, Jemal A. Age-specific trends in black-white disparities in cervical cancer incidence in the United States: 1975–2009. Gynecol Oncol. 2012;127(3):611–5.
6. American Cancer Society. Cancer facts & figures for Hispanics/Latinos 2012–2014. Atlanta 2012.
7. Watson M, Saraiya M, Benard V, Coughlin SS, Flowers L, Cokkinides V, et al. Burden of cervical cancer in the United States, 1998–2003. Cancer. 2008;113(10 Suppl):2855–64.
8. American Cancer Society. Cancer facts & figures for African Americans 2013–2014. Atlanta 2013.
9. Smith RA, Cokkinides V, Brooks D, Saslow D, Shah M, Brawley OW. Cancer screening in the United States, 2011: a review of current American Cancer Society guidelines and issues in cancer screening. CA Cancer J Clin. 2011;61(1):8–30.
10. Centers for Disease Control and Prevention. Chartbook on trends in the health of Americans 2010. Hyattsville, MD: National Center for Health Statistics; 2010.
11. American Cancer Society. Cancer prevention and early detection facts and figures 2012. Atlanta, GA2012.
12. Benard VB, Lawson HW, Eheman CR, Anderson C, Helsel W. Adherence to guidelines for follow-up of low-grade cytologic abnormalities among medically underserved women. Obstet Gynecol. 2005;105(6):1323–8.
13. Satterwhite CL, Torrone E, Meites E, Dunne EF, Mahajan R, Ocfemia MC, et al. Sexually transmitted infections among US women and men: prevalence and incidence estimates, 2008. Sex Transm Dis. 2013;40(3):187–93.
14. Weinstock H, Berman S, Cates W. Sexually transmitted diseases among American youth: incidence and prevalence estimates, 2000. Perspect Sex Reprod Health. 2004;36(1):6–10.
15. Ho GY, Bierman R, Beardsley L, Chang CJ, Burk RD. Natural history of cervicovaginal papillomavirus infection in young women. N Engl J Med. 1998;338(7):423–8.
16. Hariri S, Unger ER, Sternberg M, Dunne EF, Swan D, Patel S, et al. Prevalence of genital human papillomavirus among females in the United States, the National Health And Nutrition Examination Survey, 2003–2006. J Infect Dis. 2011;204(4):566–73.
17. Dunne EF, Unger ER, Sternberg M, McQuillan G, Swan DC, Patel SS, et al. Prevalence of HPV infection among females in the United States. JAMA. 2007;297(8):813–9.
18. Giuliano AR, Papenfuss M, Schneider A, Nour M, Hatch K. Risk factors for high-risk type human papillomavirus infection among Mexican-American women. Cancer Epidemiol Biomarkers Prev. 1999;8(7):615–20.
19. Villa LL, Costa RL, Petta CA, Andrade RP, Ault KA, Giuliano AR, et al. Prophylactic quadrivalent human papillomavirus (types 6, 11, 16, and 18) L1 virus-like particle vaccine in young women: a randomised double-blind placebo-controlled multicentre phase II efficacy trial. Lancet Oncol. 2005; 6(5):271–8.
20. Garland SM, Hernandez-Avila M, Wheeler CM, Perez G, Harper DM, Leodolter S, et al. Quadrivalent vaccine against human papillomavirus to prevent anogenital diseases. N Engl J Med. 2007;356(19):1928–43.
21. Future II Study Group. Quadrivalent vaccine against human papillomavirus to prevent high-grade cervical lesions. N Engl J Med. 2007;356(19):1915–27.
22. Paavonen J, Naud P, Salmerón J, Wheeler CM, Chow SN, Apter D, et al. Efficacy of human papillomavirus (HPV)-16/18 AS04-adjuvanted vaccine against cervical infection and precancer caused by oncogenic HPV types (PATRICIA): final analysis of a double-blind, randomised study in young women. Lancet. 2009;374(9686):301–14.
23. Paavonen J, Jenkins D, Bosch FX, Naud P, Salmerón J, Wheeler CM, et al. Efficacy of a prophylactic adjuvanted bivalent L1 virus-like-particle vaccine against infection with human papillomavirus types 16 and 18 in young women: an interim analysis of a phase III double-blind, randomised controlled trial. Lancet. 2007;369(9580):2161–70.
24. Markowitz LE, Dunne EF, Saraiya M, Chesson HW, Curtis CR, Gee J, et al. Human papillomavirus vaccination: recommendations of the Advisory Committee on Immunization Practices (ACIP). MMWR Recomm Rep. 2014;63(RR-05):1–30.
25. NIS-Teen. Vaccination coverage among adolescents aged 13–17 years—United States, 2012. 2012. http://www.cdc.gov/vaccines/stats-surv/nisteen/data/tables_2012.htm.
26. Jeudin P, Liveright E, Del Carmen MG, Perkins RB. Race, ethnicity, and income factors impacting human papillomavirus vaccination rates. Clin Ther. 2014;36(1):24–37.
27. Williams WW, Lu PJ, O'Halloran A, Bridges CB, Pilishvili T, Hales CM, et al. Noninfluenza vaccination coverage among adults – United States, 2012. MMWR Morb Mortal Wkly Rep. 2014;63(5):95–102.
28. Hamlish T, Clarke L, Alexander KA. Barriers to HPV immunization for African American adolescent females. Vaccine. 2012;30(45):6472–6.
29. WingroveFreeman HP, Wingrove WB. Excess cervical cancer mortality: a marker for low access to health care in poor communities. NIH Pub. No. 05-5282. ed. Rockville, MD: National Cancer Institute, Center to Reduce Cancer Health Disparities; 2005.

30. Brookfield KF, Cheung MC, Lucci J, Fleming LE, Koniaris LG. Disparities in survival among women with invasive cervical cancer: a problem of access to care. Cancer. 2009;115(1):166–78.
31. Rauh-Hain JA, Clemmer JT, Bradford LS, Clark RM, Growdon WB, Goodman A, et al. Racial disparities in cervical cancer survival over time. Cancer. 2013;119(20):3644–52.
32. Fleming S, Schluterman NH, Tracy JK, Temkin SM. Black and white women in Maryland receive different treatment for cervical cancer. PLoS One. 2014;9(8), e104344.
33. Farley JH, Hines JF, Taylor RR, Carlson JW, Parker MF, Kost ER, et al. Equal care ensures equal survival for African-American women with cervical carcinoma. Cancer. 2001;91(4):869–73.
34. Benard VB, Howe W, Royalty J, Helsel W, Kammerer W, Richardson LC. Timeliness of cervical cancer diagnosis and initiation of treatment in the National Breast and Cervical Cancer Early Detection Program. J Womens Health (Larchmt). 2012;21(7):776–82.
35. Horner MJ, Altekruse SF, Zou Z, Wideroff L, Katki HA, Stinchcomb DG. U.S. geographic distribution of prevaccine era cervical cancer screening, incidence, stage, and mortality. Cancer Epidemiol Biomarkers Prev. 2011;20(4):591–9.
36. Jemal A, Siegel R, Xu J, Ward E. Cancer statistics, 2010. CA Cancer J Clin. 2010;60(5):277–300.
37. Centers for Disease Control and Prevention. Uterine cancer rates by race and ethnicity. 27 Aug 2014. http://www.cdc.gov/cancer/uterine/statistics/race.htm.
38. Sherman ME, Devesa SS. Analysis of racial differences in incidence, survival, and mortality for malignant tumors of the uterine corpus. Cancer. 2003;98(1):176–86.
39. Setiawan VW, Pike MC, Kolonel LN, Nomura AM, Goodman MT, Henderson BE. Racial/ethnic differences in endometrial cancer risk: the multiethnic cohort study. Am J Epidemiol. 2007;165(3):262–70.
40. Jemal A, Siegel R, Ward E, Hao Y, Xu J, Murray T, et al. Cancer statistics, 2008. CA Cancer J Clin. 2008;58(2):71–96.
41. Hicks ML, Phillips JL, Parham G, Andrews N, Jones WB, Shingleton HM, et al. The National Cancer Data Base report on endometrial carcinoma in African-American women. Cancer. 1998;83(12):2629–37.
42. Wright JD, Fiorelli J, Schiff PB, Burke WM, Kansler AL, Cohen CJ, et al. Racial disparities for uterine corpus tumors: changes in clinical characteristics and treatment over time. Cancer. 2009;115(6):1276–85.
43. Smotkin D, Nevadunsky NS, Harris K, Einstein MH, Yu Y, Goldberg GL. Histopathologic differences account for racial disparity in uterine cancer survival. Gynecol Oncol. 2012;127(3):616–9.
44. Oliver KE, Enewold LR, Zhu K, Conrads TP, Rose GS, Maxwell GL, et al. Racial disparities in histopathologic characteristics of uterine cancer are present in older, not younger blacks in an equal-access environment. Gynecol Oncol. 2011; 123(1):76–81.
45. Cook LS, Nelson HE, Cockburn M, Olson SH, Muller CY, Wiggins CL. Comorbidities and endometrial cancer survival in Hispanics and non-Hispanic whites. Cancer Causes Control. 2013;24(1):61–9.
46. Rodriguez AM, Schmeler KM, Kuo YF. Disparities in endometrial cancer outcomes between non-Hispanic white and Hispanic women. Gynecol Oncol. 2014;135(3):525–33.
47. Díaz-Montes TP, Alberg A, Zahurak ML, Trimble EL, Bristow RE. Cancer of the uterine corpus among Hispanic women living in the United States: patterns of staging, diagnosis, and primary treatment. Gynecol Oncol. 2005;96(3):753–9.
48. Mahdi H, Hou H, Kowk LL, Moslemi-Kebria M, Michener C. Type II endometrial cancer in Hispanic women: tumor characteristics, treatment and survival compared to non-Hispanic white women. Gynecol Oncol. 2014;133(3):512–7.
49. Risinger JI, Hayes K, Maxwell GL, Carney ME, Dodge RK, Barrett JC, et al. PTEN mutation in endometrial cancers is associated with favorable clinical and pathologic characteristics. Clin Cancer Res. 1998;4(12):3005–10.
50. Maxwell GL, Risinger JI, Gumbs C, Shaw H, Bentley RC, Barrett JC, et al. Mutation of the PTEN tumor suppressor gene in endometrial hyperplasias. Cancer Res. 1998;58(12):2500–3.
51. Maxwell GL, Risinger JI, Alvarez AA, Barrett JC, Berchuck A. Favorable survival associated with microsatellite instability in endometrioid endometrial cancers. Obstet Gynecol. 2001;97(3):417–22.
52. Maxwell GL, Risinger JI, Hayes KA, Alvarez AA, Dodge RK, Barrett JC, et al. Racial disparity in the frequency of PTEN mutations, but not microsatellite instability, in advanced endometrial cancers. Clin Cancer Res. 2000;6(8):2999–3005.
53. Kohler MF, Carney P, Dodge R, Soper JT, Clarke-Pearson DL, Marks JR, et al. p53 overexpression in advanced-stage endometrial adenocarcinoma. Am J Obstet Gynecol. 1996;175(5):1246–52.
54. Clifford SL, Kaminetsky CP, Cirisano FD, Dodge R, Soper JT, Clarke-Pearson DL, et al. Racial disparity in overexpression of the p53 tumor suppressor gene in stage I endometrial cancer. Am J Obstet Gynecol. 1997;176(6):S229–32.
55. Alkushi A, Lim P, Coldman A, Huntsman D, Miller D, Gilks CB. Interpretation of p53 immunoreactivity in endometrial carcinoma: establishing a clinically relevant cut-off level. Int J Gynecol Pathol. 2004;23(2):129–37.
56. Santin AD, Bellone S, Siegel ER, Palmieri M, Thomas M, Cannon MJ, et al. Racial differences in the overexpression of epidermal growth factor type II receptor (HER2/neu): a major prognostic indicator in uterine serous papillary cancer. Am J Obstet Gynecol. 2005;192(3):813–8.

57. Ferguson SE, Olshen AB, Levine DA, Viale A, Barakat RR, Boyd J. Molecular profiling of endometrial cancers from African-American and Caucasian women. Gynecol Oncol. 2006;101(2):209–13.
58. De Vivo I, Prescott J, Setiawan VW, Olson SH, Wentzensen N, Attia J, et al. Genome-wide association study of endometrial cancer in E2C2. Hum Genet. 2014;133(2):211–24.
59. Setiawan VW, Schumacher F, Prescott J, Haessler J, Malinowski J, Wentzensen N, et al. Cross-cancer pleiotropic analysis of endometrial cancer: PAGE and E2C2 consortia. Carcinogenesis. 2014;35(9):2068–73.
60. Farley J, Risinger JI, Rose GS, Maxwell GL. Racial disparities in blacks with gynecologic cancers. Cancer. 2007;110(2):234–43.
61. Madison T, Schottenfeld D, James SA, Schwartz AG, Gruber SB. Endometrial cancer: socioeconomic status and racial/ethnic differences in stage at diagnosis, treatment, and survival. Am J Public Health. 2004;94(12):2104–11.
62. Rauh-Hain JA, Buskwofie A, Clemmer J, Boruta DM, Schorge JO, Del-Carmen MG. Racial disparities in treatment of high-grade endometrial cancer in the medicare population. Obstet Gynecol. 2015;125(4):843–51.
63. Trimble EL, Harlan LC, Clegg LX, Stevens JL. Pre-operative imaging, surgery and adjuvant therapy for women diagnosed with cancer of the corpus uteri in community practice in the United States. Gynecol Oncol. 2005;96(3):741–8.
64. Fleury AC, Ibeanu OA, Bristow RE. Racial disparities in surgical care for uterine cancer. Gynecol Oncol. 2011;121(3):571–6.
65. Farley JH, Tian C, Rose GS, Brown CL, Birrer M, Risinger JI, et al. Chemotherapy intensity and toxicity among black and white women with advanced and recurrent endometrial cancer: a Gynecologic Oncology Group Study. Cancer. 2010;116(2):355–61.
66. Fedewa SA, Lerro C, Chase D, Ward EM. Insurance status and racial differences in uterine cancer survival: a study of patients in the National Cancer Database. Gynecol Oncol. 2011;122(1):63–8.
67. Ko EM, Walter P, Clark L, Jackson A, Franasiak J, Bolac C, et al. The complex triad of obesity, diabetes and race in type I and II endometrial cancers: prevalence and prognostic significance. Gynecol Oncol. 2014;133(1):28–32.
68. Olson SH, Atoria CL, Cote ML, Cook LS, Rastogi R, Soslow RA, et al. The impact of race and comorbidity on survival in endometrial cancer. Cancer Epidemiol Biomarkers Prev. 2012;21(5):753–60.
69. Bristow RE, Palis BE, Chi DS, Cliby WA. The National Cancer Database report on advanced-stage epithelial ovarian cancer: impact of hospital surgical case volume on overall survival and surgical treatment paradigm. Gynecol Oncol. 2010;118:262–7.
70. Mercado C, Zingmond D, Karlan BY, Sekaris E, Gross J, Maggard-Gibbons M, et al. Quality of care in advanced ovarian cancer: the importance of provider specialty. Gynecol Oncol. 2010;117:18–22.
71. Kumpulainen S, Sankila R, Leminen A, Kuoppala T, Komulainen M, Puistola U, et al. The effect of hospital operative volume, residual tumor and first-line chemotherapy on survival of ovarian cancer – a prospective nation-wide study in Finland. Gynecol Oncol. 2009;115:199–203.
72. Elit L, Bondy SJ, Paszat L, Przybysz R, Levine M. Outcomes in surgery for ovarian cancer. Gynecol Oncol. 2002;87:260–7.
73. Bristow RE, Powell MA, Al-Hammadi N, Chen L, Miller JP, Roland PY, et al. Disparities in ovarian cancer care quality and survival according to race and socioeconomic status. J Natl Cancer Inst. 2013;105(11):823–32.
74. Chornokur G, Amankwah EK, Schildkraut JM, Phelan CM. Global ovarian cancer health disparities. Gynecol Oncol. 2013;129(1):258–64.
75. Chase DM, Fedewa S, Chou TS, Chen A, Ward E, Brewster WR. Disparities in the allocation of treatment in advanced ovarian cancer: are there certain patient characteristics associated with nonstandard therapy? Obstet Gynecol. 2012;119:68–77.
76. Edwards BK, Noone AM, Mariotto AB, Simard EP, Boscoe FP, Henley SJ, et al. Annual report to the Nation on the status of cancer, 1975–2010, featuring prevalence of comorbidity and impact on survival among persons with lung, colorectal, breast, or prostate cancer. Cancer. 2014;120(9):1290–314.
77. Morris CR, Sands MT, Smith LH. Ovarian cancer: predictors of early-stage diagnosis. Cancer Causes Control. 2010;21(8):1203–11.
78. Moorman PG, Palmieri RT, Akushevich L, Berchuck A, Schildkraut JM. Ovarian cancer risk factors in African-American and white women. Am J Epidemiol. 2009;170(5):598–606.
79. Parham G, Phillips JL, Hicks ML, Andrews N, Jones WB, Shingleton HM, et al. The National Cancer Data Base report on malignant epithelial ovarian carcinoma in African-American women. Cancer. 1997;80(4):816–26.
80. Chan JK, Zhang M, Hu JM, Shin JY, Osann K, Kapp DS. Racial disparities in surgical treatment and survival of epithelial ovarian cancer in United States. J Surg Oncol. 2008;97(2):103–7.
81. Buys SS, Partridge E, Black A, Johnson CC, Lamerato L, Isaacs C, et al. Effect of screening on ovarian cancer mortality: the prostate, lung, colorectal and ovarian (PLCO) cancer screening randomized controlled trial. JAMA. 2011;305(22):2295–303.
82. Armstrong K, Micco E, Carney A, Stopfer J, Putt M. Racial differences in the use of BRCA1/2 testing among women with a family history of breast or ovarian cancer. JAMA. 2005;293(14):1729–36.
83. Pagán JA, Su D, Li L, Armstrong K, Asch DA. Racial and ethnic disparities in awareness of genetic testing for cancer risk. Am J Prev Med. 2009;37(6):524–30.

84. Olaya W, Esquivel P, Wong JH, Morgan JW, Freeberg A, Roy-Chowdhury S, et al. Disparities in BRCA testing: when insurance coverage is not a barrier. Am J Surg. 2009;198(4):562–5.
85. Levy DE, Byfield SD, Comstock CB, Garber JE, Syngal S, Crown WH, et al. Underutilization of BRCA1/2 testing to guide breast cancer treatment: black and Hispanic women particularly at risk. Genet Med. 2011;13(4):349–55.
86. Schildkraut JM, Murphy SK, Palmieri RT, Iversen E, Moorman PG, Huang Z, et al. Trinucleotide repeat polymorphisms in the androgen receptor gene and risk of ovarian cancer. Cancer Epidemiol Biomarkers Prev. 2007;16(3):473–80.
87. Schildkraut JM, Goode EL, Clyde MA, Iversen ES, Moorman PG, Berchuck A, et al. Single nucleotide polymorphisms in the TP53 region and susceptibility to invasive epithelial ovarian cancer. Cancer Res. 2009;69(6):2349–57.
88. Vernooij F, Heintz P, Witteveen E, van der Graaf Y. The outcomes of ovarian cancer treatment are better when provided by gynecologic oncologists and in specialized hospitals: a systematic review. Gynecol Oncol. 2007;105(3):801–12.
89. Aranda MA, McGory M, Sekeris E, Maggard M, Ko C, Zingmond DS. Do racial/ethnic disparities exist in the utilization of high-volume surgeons for women with ovarian cancer? Gynecol Oncol. 2008;111:166–72.
90. Bristow RE, Ueda S, Gerardi MA, Ajiboye OB, Ibeanu OA. Analysis of racial disparities in stage IIIC epithelial ovarian cancer care and outcomes in a tertiary gynecologic oncology referral center. Gynecol Oncol. 2011;122:319–23.
91. Bristow RE, Zahurak ML, Ibeanu OA. Racial disparities in ovarian cancer surgical care: a population-based analysis. Gynecol Oncol. 2011;121:364–8.
92. Terplan M, Smith EJ, Temkin SM. Race in ovarian cancer treatment and survival: a systematic review with meta-analysis. Cancer Causes Control. 2009;20(7):1139–50.
93. Liu FW, Randall LM, Tewari KS, Bristow RE. Racial disparities and patterns of ovarian cancer surgical care in California. Gynecol Oncol. 2014;132(1):221–6.
94. Terplan M, Schluterman N, McNamara EJ, Tracy JK, Temkin SM. Have racial disparities in ovarian cancer increased over time? An analysis of SEER data. Gynecol Oncol. 2012;125(1):19–24.
95. Siegel R, Naishadham D, Jemal A. Cancer statistics, 2013. CA Cancer J Clin. 2013;63(1):11–30.
96. Barnholtz-Sloan JS, Schwartz AG, Qureshi F, Jacques S, Malone J, Munkarah AR. Ovarian cancer: changes in patterns at diagnosis and relative survival over the last three decades. Am J Obstet Gynecol. 2003;189(4):1120–7.
97. Howell EA, Egorova N, Hayes MP, Wisnivesky J, Franco R, Bickell N. Racial disparities in the treatment of advanced epithelial ovarian cancer. Obstet Gynecol. 2013;122(5):1025–32.
98. Long B, Chang J, Ziogas A, Tewari KS, Anton-Culver H, Bristow RE. Impact of race, socioeconomic status, and the health care system on the treatment of advanced-stage ovarian cancer in California. Am J Obstet Gynecol. 2015;212(4):468.e1–9.
99. Bristow RE, Chang J, Ziogas A, Anton-Culver H, Vieira VM. Spatial analysis of adherence to treatment guidelines for advanced-stage ovarian cancer and the impact of race and socioeconomic status. Gynecol Oncol. 2014;134(1):60–7.
100. Peterson CE, Rauscher GH, Johnson TP, Kirschner CV, Freels S, Barrett RE, et al. The effect of neighborhood disadvantage on the racial disparity in ovarian cancer-specific survival in a large hospital-based study in cook county, Illinois. Front Publ Health. 2015;3:8.
101. Bristow RE, Chang J, Ziogas A, Campos B, Chavez LR, Anton-Culver H. Sociodemographic disparities in advanced ovarian cancer survival and adherence to treatment guidelines. Obstet Gynecol. 2015;125(4):833–42.
102. Terplan M, Temkin S, Tergas A, Lengyel E. Does equal treatment yield equal outcomes? The impact of race on survival in epithelial ovarian cancer. Gynecol Oncol. 2008;111(2):173–8.
103. Du XL, Sun CC, Milam MR, Bodurka DC, Fang S. Ethnic differences in socioeconomic status, diagnosis, treatment, and survival among older women with epithelial ovarian cancer. Int J Gynecol Cancer. 2008;18(4):660–9.
104. Farley JH, Tian C, Rose GS, Brown CL, Birrer M, Maxwell GL. Race does not impact outcome for advanced ovarian cancer patients treated with cisplatin/paclitaxel: an analysis of Gynecologic Oncology Group trials. Cancer. 2009;115(18):4210–7.
105. Albain KS, Unger JM, Crowley JJ, Coltman CA, Hershman DL. Racial disparities in cancer survival among randomized clinical trials patients of the Southwest Oncology Group. J Natl Cancer Inst. 2009;101(14):984–92.
106. Tergas AI, Tseng JH, Bristow RE. Impact of race and ethnicity on treatment and survival of women with vulvar cancer in the United States. Gynecol Oncol. 2013;129(1):154–8.
107. Rauh-Hain JA, Clemmer J, Clark RM, Bradford LS, Growdon WB, Goodman A, et al. Racial disparities and changes in clinical characteristics and survival for vulvar cancer over time. Am J Obstet Gynecol. 2013;209(5):468.e1–10.
108. Mahdi H, Kumar S, Hanna RK, Munkarah AR, Lockhart D, Morris RT, et al. Disparities in treatment and survival between African American and White women with vaginal cancer. Gynecol Oncol. 2011;122(1):38–41.

# Index




A. Giordano, M. Macaluso (eds.), *Gynecological Cancers*, Current Clinical Oncology,
DOI 10.1007/978-3-319-32907-9